The Pill

In 1992 John Guillebaud was appointed by University College London as Professor (now Emeritus) of Family Planning and Reproductive Health, the world's first practising gynaecologist to be given a personal chair in the specialty. He worked as a consultant at the United Elizabeth Garrett Anderson Hospital and Hospital for Women Soho, in Euston Road, London, and until 2003 was the Medical Director of the Margaret Pyke Family Planning Centre. Margaret Pyke was the first Chairman of the UK Family Planning Association and a pioneer of the family-planning movement, hence the Centre was opened as a memorial to her by the Duke of Edinburgh in 1969. It is within the National Health Service, and provides a comprehensive one-stop reproductive health service. Hundreds of medical students, doctors, and nurses are trained each year through the Centre, and new methods of birth control are investigated with the help of the Margaret Pyke Memorial Trust (of which Professor Guillebaud is now a Trustee). He continues to work in Oxford, as Honorary Community Consultant in Reproductive Health, and at the Churchill Hospital's Elliot-Smith Clinic where he has performed a significant proportion of the 36 000 vasectomies there since it opened in 1970.

Professor Guillebaud's family are Huguenots who came to England more than 300 years ago, and so he retains the French name as it has always been spelled: it is *pronounced* in two syllables quite simply as '*gil-boe*'. He was born in Burundi, Africa, brought up in Rwanda, and educated in Uganda, Kenya, and Britain. At Cambridge in 1959 he attended an undergraduate lecture on the population 'explosion' which he describes as changing his life. He caught the vision expressed (much later) by the United Nations Children's Fund (UNICEF): that 'Family Planning could bring more benefits to more people at less cost than any other single technology now available to the human race'. If this was close to being the most important and at the same time almost the most neglected specialty in the whole of medicine, it was the specialty for him.

Soon after qualifying he spent six months as Medical Officer on the Royal Society Expedition to Mato Grosso, Brazil (1967–8). He has travelled to every continent promoting planned parenthood and concern for the environment, and in 1993 received the prestigious Evian/Birthright Health Award 'for his tireless campaigning on overpopulation: human numbers, a crucial factor in meeting human needs on a finite planet'. He is Co-Chair of the Optimum Population Trust; author or co-author of seven books, available in 10 languages, and of more than 300 other publications; and acts as a consultant to the World Health Organization (WHO) and other national and international bodies in the reproductive health field. His wife Gwyneth is a nurse in the local children's hospice and they have two sons and one daughter.

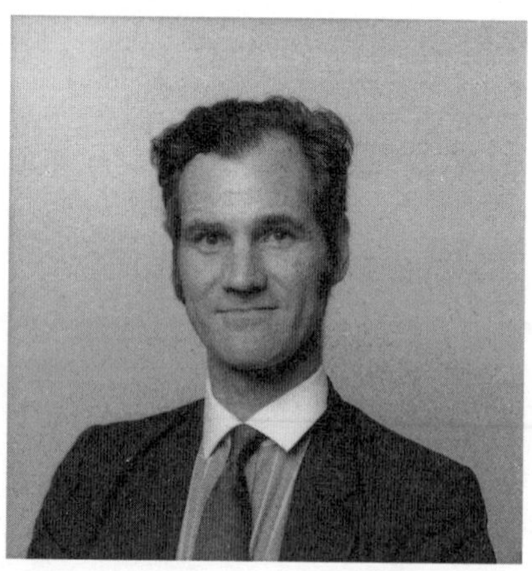

the pill and other hormonal contraceptives

the facts

sixth edition

Evidence-base and competing interests

This book represents the personal opinions of John Guillebaud, based wherever possible on published and sometimes unpublished evidence. When (as is not infrequent) no epidemiological or other direct evidence is available, clinical advice herein is always as practical and realistic as possible and based, pending more data, on the author's judgement of other sources. These may include the opinions of Expert Committees and any existing Guidelines. In some instances the advice appearing in this book may even so differ appreciably from the latter, for reasons usually given in the text and (since medical knowledge and practice are continually evolving) relates to the date of publication. Healthcare professionals must understand that they take ultimate responsibility for their patient and ensure that any clinical advice they use from this book is applicable to the specific circumstances that they encounter.

The author has received payments for research projects, lectures, short term consultancy work, and related expenses from the manufacturers of hormonal contraceptive products.

the pill and other hormonal contraceptives

sixth edition

---

the facts

JOHN GUILLEBAUD

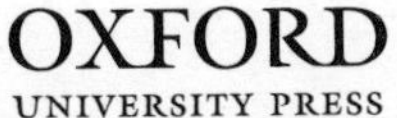

OXFORD
UNIVERSITY PRESS

Great Clarendon Street, Oxford OX2 6DP

Oxford University Press is a department of the University of Oxford. It furthers the University's objectives of excellence in research, scholarsip, and education by publishing worldwide in

Oxford New York

Auckland Bangkok Buenos Aires Cape Town Chennai
Dar es Salaam Delhi Hong Kong Istanbul Karachi Kolkata
Kuala Lumpur Madrid Melbourne Mexico City Mumbai Nairobi
São Paulo Shanghai Taiepei Tokyo Toronto

Oxford is a registered trade mark of Oxford University Press in the UK and in certain other countries

Published in the United States
by Oxford University Press Inc., New York

First published 1980
Second edition 1983
Third edition 1984; revised reprint 1987
Fourth edition 1991
Fifth edition 1997; reprinted 1998 (with corrections), 2001
Sixth edition 2005
Also published in German, Spanish and Japanese editions.

British Library Cataloguing in Publication Data

Data available

ISBN 0 19 856613 1

1

Typeset by Integra Software Services Pvt. Ltd., Pondicherry, India.
Printed on acid-free paper by Clays, Bungay, UK

foreword
by Gwyneth Guillebaud, RGN, ONC, FPA Cert.

Every day around 100 million women reach out for a pill packet and swallow a tiny tablet which alters the course of their lives. Well over 200 million have done so at some time. And millions more will do so.

What that means to you—whether you are taking the pill yourself, have at some time taken it, or are thinking of doing so, whether your lover is someone who is taking it, or you are in some other way involved or interested in oral contraceptives—what it means to all of us in fact is what this book is about.

The pill, very largely developed by men, produced by men, marketed by men, prescribed by men (written about by men!), and also undoubtedly of benefit to men, is taken by women. Should we as women be thankful? Forty years ago when the pill became available, first in America, then elsewhere, that question would have been very much easier to answer. It seemed that at last there was an answer to the prayer of so many couples through the ages—contraception without complication. Simple and safe. The publicity was enormous, expectations were high.

What now, after three decades? Should we be thankful? Many of us, feminists and non-feminists alike, who have come to see control of fertility as a necessity, a right, and a freedom, would now like to respond by asking further questions. Is the price for this freedom too high? Does taking the pill mean taking control or being controlled? Moreover, who has gained the freedom? Has the pill liberated men more than women? It is hard to deny that many men have come to assume that women will take it. Why won't they take their own share of responsibility? And anyway, shouldn't they use the condom *as well*, regardless of the pill, in all situations where sexually transmitted diseases could be transmitted?

The pill has not lived up to all expectations. There have been numerous press articles on the risks, and though many were wrongly scary, others were accurate. If so, why do so many women continue to reach regularly for the pill packet? There are several good reasons. Being an ostrich is not one of them. What is needed is a balance of healthy caution and practical common sense. The best reason for taking the pill is that it works. Whatever else experience has shown, it has proved that oral contraception is easy and effective. Secondly, stripped of sensationalism, the weight of informed opinion is that the risks relate to a very small number of women. Over the years it has become much easier to single out those who are at particular risk and the doses used in current pills are much reduced and believed to be correspondingly safer.

Society has to choose. One way to have no serious illnesses or deaths from the pill would be to ban it. Yet most women would then feel cheated, cheated from having the *choice*. Many see it as a necessity. At an everyday and practical level, it has relieved millions of women from the constant fear of unwanted pregnancy. For all those who do experience side-effects, there are many who take it without problems and with great relief that a major aspect of their lives is no longer a source of stress. Our grandmothers were less fortunate.

The introduction to the first edition of *The Pill* mentioned a British survey which revealed that, of 1000 women using the pill, one in three felt her health was being damaged and not properly monitored.

I can readily sympathize with those women—writing as a woman, with a woman's concerns about my body and the impact on it of the pill. I have tried practically all the recommended reversible methods with a record of success and occasional failure, of overall satisfaction, but also of having to live with some side-effects.

It is a startling fact that more than one woman in every three in England and Wales is expected to have at least one induced abortion in her reproductive lifetime. To reject all contraception or use very unsafe methods, as some couples do, simply because the ideal method does not exist, is to put the clock right back. That is not freedom. Almost nothing in life is completely safe and free of all health risks. Like every drug that has ever been devised, the pill can cause side-effects. And you are continually being reminded that it might do you harm by the tablet that you swallow each day. However, when I took it, I reminded myself that the betting odds were overwhelmingly in my favour, and for other routinely accepted risks (like using cars) are actually higher!

Since the first edition in 1980 we now have a number of new non-pill contraceptive methods, and more on the way. Although every one of them has one snag or another, I have proved like many others that it is possible to find an acceptable method for every stage of our life. Of course I am lucky, having a husband who is particularly well informed! But, even more important than the information, is a good relationship, the freedom to discuss one's feelings and fears. The eventual decision should ideally be a joint one.

Yet, if the method is one to be used by a woman, then the woman should make the final decision. The weight of medical opinion believes that for many women the known advantages of the pill and the new hormonal methods far outweigh any possible risks. But it is for the individual woman to decide whether she can be confident it is really right for her—whatever a doctor, or family planning nurse, or anyone else might say. She must weigh up many considerations: how big a risk of pregnancy might be accepted, how easy the method is, the likelihood and nature of side-effects, the acceptability of other alternatives, and personal preferences. We live our lives and base our decisions on what we know, and the best and right decisions are those for which we feel we have taken responsibility.

Knowledge is power. The introduction to the first edition described this book as 'a handbook for the owner/driver of a healthy pill-taking body'. The facts as far as they are known are here. They may confirm your doubts about the pill. They may equally give you new confidence in it. It is up to you now to make the decisions.

G.M.G.

preface
to the sixth edition

In 1959, while still a teenager, I attended a lecture. The biologist Dr Colin Bertram of St John's Cambridge discussed the daunting problems posed by ever-increasing human numbers meeting human needs. There were no visual aids, the audience was small, but the lecture changed my life. I decided then—and little has happened since to make me change my mind—that voluntary birth control was not only among the most important of all medical specialties but also the most neglected. I decided to make this my life's work. Indirectly, that explains how I came to write this book.

I wrote it chiefly to counter an accusation against doctors which can be summarized thus: that we knew a lot of worrying facts about the pill, but were not prepared to share them in case the knowledge interfered with women docilely taking their tablets! I decided to attempt to convey virtually everything I knew about the method, bad news and good, and then let people make up their own minds: 'here are the facts, now you decide.'

It remains, I believe, the most comprehensive handbook on hormonal contraception for non-specialists available anywhere. Updating changes have been necessary on the majority of pages. Sexually transmitted infections (STIs) including human immunodeficiency virus/acquired immune deficiency syndrome (HIV/AIDS) are very major problems connected with contraception, new progestogens have become established, and the pill's two hormones are increasingly being given by quite new routes: into or under the skin, and directly into the vagina or uterus. Indeed, there is one extremely significant arrival on the contraceptive method scene: the levonorgestrel-intrauterine system (LNG-IUS), otherwise known as 'Mirena' and described in Chapter 10. I see this as the most important new advance in contraception since the invention of the pill itself.

Reviewers of earlier editions made somewhat contradictory comments: some that the book would be too frightening, some that it displayed a 'pro-pill' bias. This perhaps means that the balance was roughly right.

I have tried always to follow two principles: accuracy about what is known, and honesty about what is still unknown—despite much more money being spent researching the safety of the pill than was ever spent developing it. I think any fair-minded reader of this, as of previous editions, will find that the facts still support the view that the pill *is* a reasonable option for fully informed women—but certainly not for all. It is important to insist on sufficient information to weigh up and choose between all the other options.

Though I would like to try everything myself, I still cannot write as a consumer: only as an understanding prescriber. There is still no marketed male pill or injection. A pity, because in a good relationship it would be nice to be able to be on the pill alternately, say for six months at a time, sharing the problems and benefits of contraception like everything else (see Chapter 9). Contrary to rumour, many men are interested in the whole subject of contraception: I have been pleased over the years to learn how many men have found this book helpful.

In addition to all those mentioned in the prefaces to the earlier editions, I should like to acknowledge particularly the help of Toni Belfield of the UK FPA, of my secretary Helen Prime and of all my colleagues at the Margaret Pyke Family Planning Centre and at the Alec Turnbull and Elliot-Smith Vasectomy Clinics in Oxford. The Margaret Pyke Memorial Trust has been and continues to be enormously supportive of all the work at the Centre, and even supplied the original word processor and printer which my son Jonathan and I used. Many thanks again to him, my other children, Lisa and Christopher (currently, as I write, both at medical school); and, last but not least, my uniquely considerate and supportive wife, Gwyneth.

John Guillebaud MA, FRCSE, FRCOG, Hon. FFFP
Professor Emeritus of Family Planning and Reproductive Health, University College, London April 2004

We have fought disease, we are eliminating malaria . . . the age of expectancy of life has gone up, and we have reduced child mortality. But believe me . . . all this is like writing in the sand. You write in the sand and the tide of population comes in and wipes out all that is written.
(M.C. Chagla, High Commissioner for India, 1963: speaking at an FPA symposium at Church House, Westminster)

We have not inherited the earth from our grandparents—we have borrowed it from our grandchildren.
(Attributed to the ancient Chinese)

Humanity is approaching a crisis point with respect to the interlocking issues of population, environment, and development.
(Statement of the World Scientific Academies' meeting at New Delhi, 1993)

Why Isn't Everyone as Scared as We Are?
(Chapter title from Paul and Anne Ehrlich, *The Population Explosion* [London: Arrow Books, 1990])

For more, see the Postscript!

contents

list of figures

list of tables

abbreviations

(See also Glossary, pp. 279–86)

AIDS	acquired immune deficiency syndrome
BBD	benign breast disease
BICH	benign intracranial hypertension
BMI	body mass index—see Glossary
BP	blood pressure
BTB	breakthrough bleeding
CASH	Cancer and Sex Hormones
COC	combined oral contraceptive
CPA	cyproterone acetate
CSM	Committee on the Safety of Medicines
DMPA	depot medroxyprogesterone acetate
DSG	desogestrel
DSP	drospirenone
EC	emergency contraception
ED	every day
EE	ethinylestradiol (estrogen of the pill)
FPA	Family Planning Association
FSH	follicle stimulating hormone
GnRH	gonadotrophin-releasing hormone
GSD	gestodene
GUM	genitourinary medicine
hCG	human chorionic gonadotrophin

HIV	human immunodeficiency virus
HPV	human papilloma virus
HRT	hormone replacement therapy
IUD	intrauterine device
IUS	intrauterine system
LAM	lactational amenorrhoea method
LH	luteinizing hormone
LNG	levonorgestrel
LNG-IUS	levonorgestrel intrauterine system
NET	norethisterone
NFP	natural family planning
NGM	norgestimate
PCOS	polycystic ovarian syndrome
PIL	patient information leaflet
POEC	progestogen-only emergency contraception
POP	progestogen-only pill
RCGP	Royal College of General Practitioners
SLE	systemic lupus erythematosus
SPC	summary of product characteristics (official instructions about a drug)
STI	sexually transmitted infection
TV	Trichomonas vaginitis
UNICEF	United Nations (International) Children's (Emergency) Fund
VTE	venous thrombo-embolism
WHO	World Health Organization
WTB	withdrawal bleeding

how to use this book

The Pill can be read straight through, or dipped into as a reference book. However you read it, be sure to include Chapter 6, which may help you to see 'the pill in perspective', and my Postscript.

Another possibility is to look first at the section '100 frequently asked questions about the pill' (p. 243). The brief answer there may be all you need; but, if you want a more detailed account, the pages to read are also given.

Unless otherwise stated, the word 'pill' on its own means the ordinary combined pill containing two hormones, an estrogen and a progestogen, as explained in Chapter 1.

The consultation: you, your doctor or nurse adviser, and the pill

Doctors and specialist nurses who still have a kind of 'God complex' and expect all their decisions to be taken on trust, with no discussion, will not like this book. I hope that they are a vanishing breed, or at least that any who are left refrain totally from forcing their religious or other views on people or ever telling them what method of contraception to use. If the pill is the method in question, in most countries doctors and nurses do the advising and the supplying, but that doesn't mean they should do the deciding: that is your right.

Nonetheless, even the most human and communicative providers are unlikely to appreciate being told that you read in this or any other book what they must do next in your case! You can be assertive, backed by published evidence, but you should still make allowances for the fact that your clinic or family doctor or nurse has much experience, and may have very good reasons for disagreeing with something suggested here. The golden rule is, if you are ever in doubt about any aspect of pill use, make sure that you talk things over with someone you trust, who knows the answers.

The ideal medical consultation is one between two specialists, two equally expert experts. Of course the health care professional is one of them. But the other is you! You are the specialist in absolutely all that pertains to you, your lifestyle, your ethics, what you retain out of your culture, and your sex life. I see this book as empowering your side of the deal: helping towards a 'contraceptive utopia' of patient-centred consultations where all the pros and cons of all the options are shared, and the outcome is the optimum for each couple for their stage of life.

One major block to that utopia, shared by all health-care professionals, is lack of time. So I think that, nowadays, most will be delighted if you are so well informed about the pill, through reading this book, that by the time you come to their surgery or clinic you only have one or two points left to clear up.

And if the pill is not for you . . .

If the pill does not suit you, or if for some reason you must avoid or give up the pill, remember the choice is not between it and 'crossing your fingers': other ways of getting effective reversible contraception include the *patch* or *ring*, an *injectable* or an *implant*, the *IUD or IUS* (intrauterine device or system), and *the male or female condom*. The last pair of methods has become especially relevant since the earliest editions of this book, with the increasing need for many to consider their risk of sexually transmitted infections (STIs) like Chlamydia and the human immunodeficiency virus (HIV) causing AIDS. Indeed in every family-planning waiting room there should be a notice reminding all present that *'we also supply condoms'—'these may need to be used as well, whatever your method of birth control.'* Because the Dutch have taken the lead in this, 'Double Dutch' has become the term for using an effective medical-type method for contraception but then a condom *as well* whenever there is need to protect against STIs.

It has been well said (Dr Elphis Christopher) that 'sex is hot, contraception is cold'. The wrong choice can lead to problems; not least an unwanted pregnancy, through using either an inefficient method, or a better method inefficiently. The main reason why contraception seems such an unavoidable bore, or rather why it often just isn't used, is that all our present reversible methods are tried and found wanting in some way. Either they have side effects, or they are a nuisance and interfere with love-making. If, as a result, nothing is used, don't forget the emergency pill (see pp. 54–8).

1 How does the pill work?

The idea and the name (Fig. 1.1) of an oral contraceptive have been around for at least 2000 years. But nothing very useful came out of centuries of magic, mumbo-jumbo, and a great deal of trial and error. It was only when the normal processes of male and female reproduction were better understood that scientists could begin to devise more effective methods for blocking them.

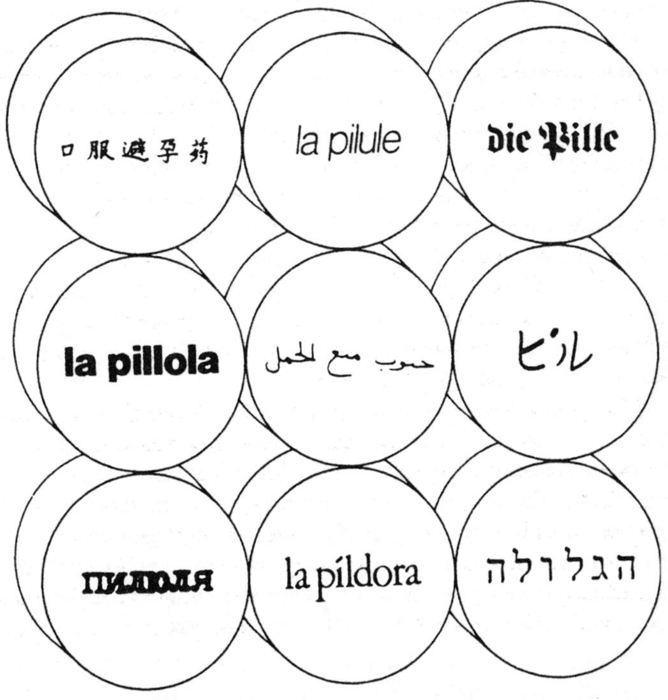

Fig. 1.1

The normal menstrual cycle

During their fertile years women are unique in having a more or less regular cycle of changes in their bodies. This cycle is caused by the ebb and flow in the bloodstream of various hormones or chemical messengers which are released into it by certain glands. The whole process is controlled by the brain, as is shown by the well-known fact that if a woman has a stressful emotional upset her periods can stop altogether for months at a time. Parts of the brain which are particularly involved have special names, including the pre-optic area and the hypothalamus.

As you can see in Fig. 1.2, just below the brain is the pituitary gland, sometimes called the 'leader of the hormone orchestra' because it is so important. Yet it is really quite small, just the size of a large pea. The ovaries and uterus are also 'in the orchestra' and blood flows through them all, connecting the whole system together. Any hormone released into the blood by one gland can therefore travel to all the others and can cause its own specific effects there or as appropriate anywhere in the whole body.

Egg release from the ovaries

The ovaries are about the same size as a peach-stone, though much less hard. Like the testicle of a man they have two functions: the production and the release of special sex cells (in this case eggs) and of hormones into the bloodstream. There are literally millions of potential egg cells in the ovaries of a baby girl before birth, but by the age of puberty the number has dropped to only 200 000. Yet there will be no shortage. Normally only one egg is released from one or other ovary during each menstrual cycle, which commonly lasts for 28 days. Thus only about 13 are required each year. As no woman can be fertile for more than a maximum of about 40 years, only something over 500 eggs will ever be required. Occasionally, of course, more than one egg is released, leading, if pregnancy follows, to twins or perhaps triplets. The egg is released from the largest one of several fluid-filled balloons or egg sacs called follicles and is picked up by the seaweed-like fronds (or fimbriae) of the outer end of one of the uterine (Fallopian) tubes (Fig. 1.3). It then starts its journey down the uterine tube, partly by the whole tube contracting and partly because there are microscopic paddles (cilia) within it which beat rhythmically in the direction of the uterus.

This happens about the middle of a cycle, if it is going to be four weeks in length. The time from egg release (often called ovulation) to the start of the next period is the only part of the cycle which is fixed in length and

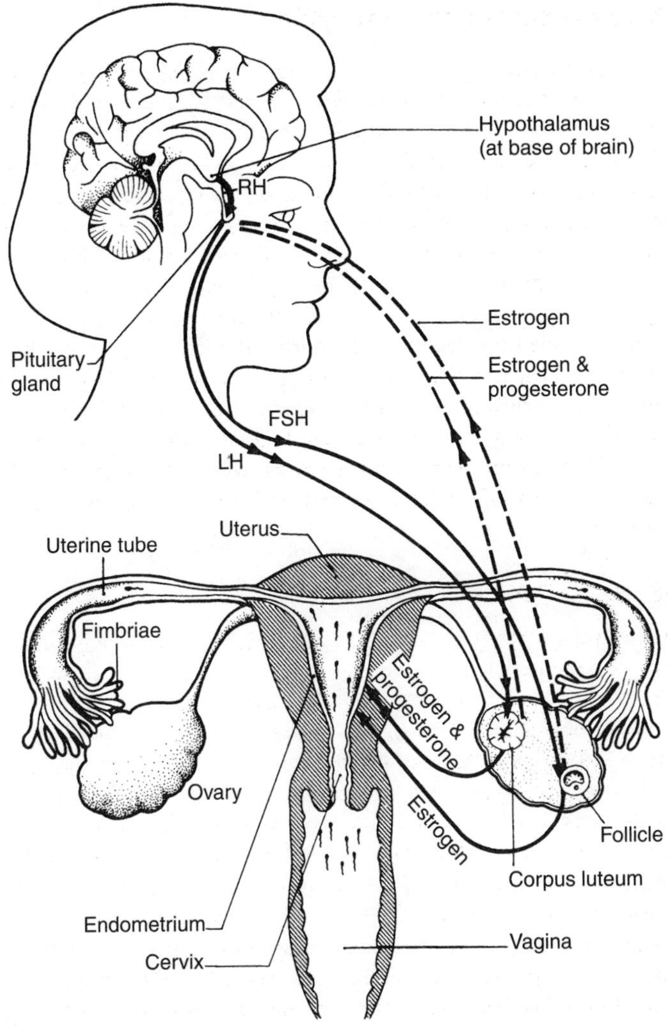

Fig. 1.2 The female reproductive system: control of the menstrual cycle

→	*events of the first half of the cycle (follicular phase)*
→→	*the second half of the cycle (luteal phase)*
– – –	*feedback effects (see pp. 8–9)*
RH	*releasing hormone*
FSH	*follicle stimulating hormone*
LH	*luteinizing hormone*

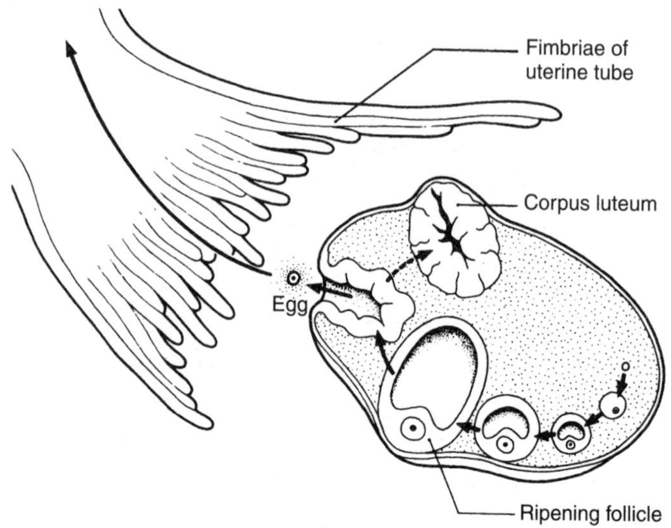

Fig. 1.3 Close-up of ovary to show growth of follicles and formation of corpus luteum after egg release

Note that this is a sequence over 28 days, not a snapshot at any one time.

lasts 14 (range 12–16) days. Many quite normal cycles last less or more than the usual 28 days. If so, the variability is almost all in the length of the first phase of the cycle from the start of the period up to egg release. The first day of menstrual bleeding is always called day 1. So if, for example, a woman has a 35-day cycle, egg release happens on day (35 − 14 = 21).

The cycle occurs because of a marvellously controlled interaction of hormones. The most important ones are two produced by the pituitary gland—follicle stimulating hormone (FSH) and luteinizing hormone (LH)—and two from the ovaries—estrogen and progesterone. Up to the time of egg release, the ovary produces only the one female hormone called estrogen. It is made in cells within the walls of the follicles, depicted in Fig. 1.3. These give their name to the first part of the menstrual cycle, the follicular phase. During the second part of the menstrual cycle, for almost exactly 14 days, the particular empty follicle from which the egg came that month now produces another hormone called progesterone as well as estrogen. It also turns yellow in colour, and so is given the name corpus luteum (which just means 'yellow body' in Latin), and this part of the cycle is called the luteal phase (Fig. 1.4*a*). The name luteinizing for the hormone which causes this change means no more than 'yellow-making'.

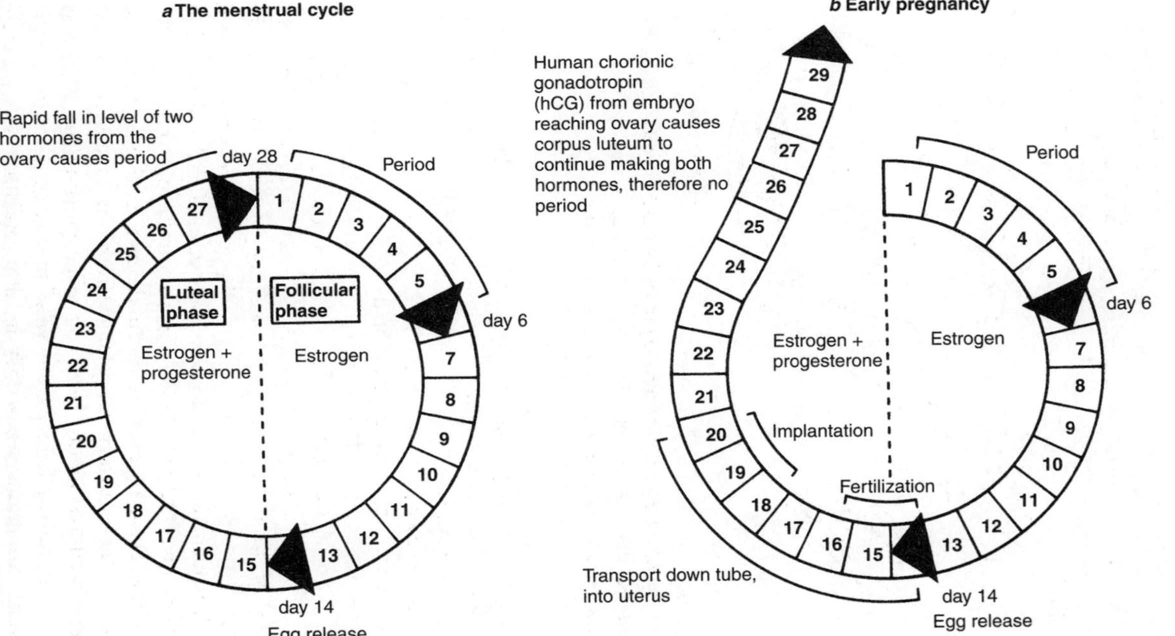

Fig. 1.4 (*a*) The menstrual cycle; (*b*) Early pregnancy

Note: Assumes standard 28-day cycle. Follicular phase is the part that varies, if the actual cycle is longer or shorter than 28 days.

The uterus

These hormones travel to the uterus during both phases of the cycle. Their main business there is to thicken its lining with extra glandular tissue and blood vessels so that it is ready just in case a pregnancy starts that month. If the woman has recently had unprotected sex, a sperm may reach the egg in the uterine tube and join up with it. This is fertilization. The fertilized egg starts just fourteen-hundredths of a millimetre in size. It begins to divide on its journey along the uterine tube towards the uterus, and embeds itself in the prepared lining around the 19th day of the cycle. This is called implantation (Fig. 1.4*b*).

The embryo, as it is called, now has just over a week to prevent the next period happening. This is vital, otherwise it will be washed out by the menstrual flow. It does this by itself producing a special hormone, whose name is human chorionic gonadotrophin (hCG). This sends an urgent message in the bloodstream to the corpus luteum to make sure it keeps on producing its hormones (estrogen and progesterone). These therefore keep coming in the blood to the uterus, and ensure that the lining of the uterus is not shed, so it can continue to provide nourishment for the developing embryo (Fig. 1.4*b*). Considering this intricate series of events, it is remarkable that a fully formed human being ever results.

Menstruation: the period

In fact, implantation very often fails—probably in up to 50 per cent of cases (see p. 209). Then the preparations for pregnancy come to nothing, just as if the egg had never been fertilized. The ovary stops producing estrogen and progesterone at about 14 days after egg release as regularly as if it had a timing mechanism programmed to switch it off. This rapid loss of the hormones which produce and maintain the lining of the uterus causes the lining to break down and leave the body through the cervix and vagina (Fig. 1.2). This causes the bleeding of the first day of the next period, which is day 1 of the *next* menstrual cycle (Fig. 1.4*a*).

The pituitary gland

Just as hormones from the ovary control what happens in the uterus, so the hormones from the pituitary gland tell the ovary to produce the correct hormones for each phase of the cycle. One of them, LH, is released in large amounts at mid-cycle, and this signal is what triggers off the bursting of the largest follicle to release an egg. This signal is never given in pregnancy because enough of the hormones estrogen and progesterone comes from the ovary to the pituitary gland to 'switch it off'. This prevents any further eggs being released and so explains why a woman who is already pregnant cannot go on getting pregnancies in the next nine months.

The pill

The combined oral contraceptive pill (COC) contains similar hormones to the estrogen and progesterone produced by the ovary. Hence the pituitary gland is, as you might say, 'fooled' into thinking the woman is already pregnant. From its point of view, there is no need to send out hormones to stimulate the ovaries if there are already high levels of ovarian-type hormones. So the pituitary cuts drastically its output of the hormones FSH and LH. In particular there are no more of those mid-cycle 'surges' of a large amount of LH which are essential for egg release. With so little of the hormones from the pituitary reaching them, the ovaries also go into a resting state, and produce minimal amounts of natural estrogen and progesterone. Both the pituitary and the ovaries are like factories where the main production line has stopped, perhaps for a works' holiday, but small-scale production and essential maintenance are continuing. Such a factory can start full-scale production at short notice as soon as the workforce returns. Similarly, when a woman discontinues the pill, the hormone factories in the pituitary and ovaries rapidly return to normal working.

While a woman is taking the pill, the normal menstrual cycle stops altogether. However, 'periods' of a sort are still produced, because the artificial hormones in the pill do have some effect on the lining of the uterus. When they are removed for one week out of every four this rather thinner lining comes away along with some bleeding. See p. 14–16 for more details about this.

So much for a brief summary of the menstrual cycle and how the pill works. Continue reading here if you would like a more detailed account, but otherwise you may like to skip to p. 10.

More about the menstrual cycle

The follicular phase

In order to start each new cycle, a special hormone called the gonadotrophin-releasing hormone (GnRH) travels from the hypothalamus, at the base of the brain, to cause the pituitary gland to release FSH. (See Fig. 1.2; you will find it helpful to keep referring to this and to Fig. 1.4 throughout this section.) FSH travels in the blood to the ovaries. Its main action, as its name implies, is to stimulate the growth of some of the many thousands of follicles which are contained in each ovary. Follicles are tiny, thick-walled, fluid-filled egg sacs, each lined by a layer of cells which are capable of producing hormones, and also containing an immature egg cell (oocyte). FSH usually stimulates about 20 of these follicles to grow, and also causes the lining cells to start to manufacture estrogen and release it into the blood. One particular follicle in one or other ovary is stimulated to grow and to 'ripen' more than all the others. Its egg cell is also maturing, ready to be released and, should it get the chance, to be fertilized.

Estrogens are the fundamentally female hormones which influence the whole body, producing rounded contours, breast development, and many other features of femininity. They also stimulate the uterus to grow its new lining to replace the one that was shed at the previous menstrual period. The lining is made of many little glands, set in several layers of cells which also contain arteries and veins. Estrogen makes the glands grow and the layers of intervening cells increase.

Meanwhile the rising levels of estrogen in the blood have been having a most important effect back on the hypothalamus and the pituitary gland. This is known as 'negative feedback' and it is important to understand this if you are to understand clearly how the pill works.

In general terms, negative feedback means that, if the level of a hormone in the blood goes *up*, the level of the stimulating hormone which caused it to go up is made to go *down*.

In the menstrual cycle, this means for example:

up ↑ estrogen in blood causes *down* ↓ FSH

The opposite is also true:

down ↓ estrogen in blood causes *up* ↑ FSH

Engineers call this a servo-mechanism.

So at the stage of the menstrual cycle we have now reached, the rise in the level of estrogen causes a fall in the pituitary gland's output of its FSH over several days.

By about the 13th day of a standard 28-day cycle, the stimulated follicles have produced a rise of estrogen in the blood to a peak level up to six times higher than it was on the first day. By negative feedback this has caused the level of the stimulating hormone FSH to drop. Now a most interesting and crucially different thing happens. Once the amount of estrogen reaching the pituitary gland gets to a critical level, it releases into the bloodstream a sudden surge of LH. In other words, the *rise* in estrogen is now causing a *rise* of a hormone from the pituitary. This is called 'positive feedback', to distinguish it from the negative type which operates all the rest of the time throughout the menstrual cycle.

This large amount of LH is conveyed by the blood to the active ovary. This is the one containing the largest follicle, now a balloon bulging the surface of the ovary and about 2 cm in diameter. The main job of this surge of LH is to cause the balloon to burst, resulting in ovulation and the release of a now mature and fertilizable egg. If all goes well, this is picked up by the fimbriae of the uterine tube and transported towards the uterus (Fig. 1.3). As this occurs, some women notice in their lower abdomen, on one or other side, a variable amount of pain which is given the German name Mittelschmerz.

Once the egg has been released, the follicle collapses and becomes that bright yellow body, the corpus luteum. Along with the change in colour of the cells lining its wall there is a change in what they do. As well as continuing to produce estrogen, for the first time these luteal cells start to manufacture and release into the blood a new hormone called progesterone.

The luteal phase

Progesterone, like estrogen, has effects all over the body; for instance, it is responsible for the slight rise in body temperature during the second half of the cycle which is used in the temperature method of family planning. But its main effect is on the lining of the uterus, to prepare it for a pregnancy. Indeed the word progesterone means 'pro-gestation': in favour of child-bearing. It thickens the lining of the uterus still further and causes its glands to release a nutritious fluid. Now if a sperm successfully fertilizes an egg, the resulting embryo (now called a 'blastocyst') travels down the tube and about five days after egg release begins to embed itself in that lining. This embedding process is called implantation. It is not complete until the 14th day (the same day as the next period would be due). The embryo produces hCG, a hormone which so exactly copies the action of LH from the pituitary that it prolongs the life of the corpus luteum in the ovary. This ensures that it continues to produce sufficient progesterone and estrogen. After about five weeks from ovulation the placenta (afterbirth) produces enough of these two vital hormones to maintain the pregnancy. As long as these hormones continue to be produced, from either source, there will be no menstrual flow and the embryo can remain secure within the lining of the uterus. A second effect of these two hormones, working in concert, is to lower the amounts of LH and FSH released from the pituitary by the more usual negative feedback process. This is important, as it prevents any more surges of LH.

If, however, a sperm fails to reach the egg on its way down the tube, the egg ceases to be fertilizable very quickly, about 12 hours after ovulation. For reasons which are still not clear, the corpus luteum abruptly ceases to function

12–16 days after it was first formed, unless hCG from a developing embryo dictates differently. There is therefore a rapid fall in the levels of both estrogen and progesterone. This has two results: first, by negative feedback, the amount of GnRH coming from the hypothalamus to the pituitary increases and therefore the amount of FSH released increases. When this extra FSH in the blood reaches the ovaries, another group of 20 or so follicles are stimulated to grow, one of them (or two if twins are to be a possibility) being destined to release its egg during the *next* normal menstrual cycle. Secondly, the sudden fall in the levels of both estrogen and progesterone in the bloodstream reaching the uterus causes local changes in its now thick lining which lead to it being shed during a normal menstrual period. How heavy and how long the bleeding is during the first few days of the next cycle varies considerably. Substances called prostaglandins are involved in this process: one of their effects is to ensure that the uterus contracts to expel the blood, but this can also cause menstrual cramping pain (dysmenorrhoea), which can be severe in some women.

The more detailed description I have just given is still simplified. 'Estrogen' is in fact a family of hormones, of which the most important member in the menstrual cycle is estradiol. The 'surge' of LH is accompanied by a smaller surge of FSH, and it is a myth that this is necessarily 'mid-cycle'. The duration of the pre-ovulatory phase of the 'normal' cycle can vary greatly, with successive waves of follicles growing until one to three truly dominant one(s) emerge(s). The releasing hormone (GnRH) normally reaches the pituitary in an intermittent, so-called pulsatile fashion, and this important mechanism is disturbed by progesterone (or any progestogen). Other hormones from the pituitary gland such as prolactin are involved; and the whole cycle can be affected by quite different hormones such as those from the thyroid gland, as well as by the nervous system.

How the pill was developed

To recap: so long as there are reasonably high levels of the two hormones estrogen and progesterone, the base part of the brain (the hypothalamus) and the pituitary gland are kept inactive (by negative feedback). This prevents:

- release of sufficient FSH to ripen any follicles in preparation for egg release
- any surges of LH, without which the actual process of release of an egg is impossible.

These results are regularly produced by the high levels of both the natural hormones during the second half of the normal menstrual cycle and throughout any pregnancy.

That the corpus luteum of pregnancy stops further egg release was first shown in the early 1900s. In 1921, the Austrian Dr Haberlandt was the first scientist on record to suggest that extracts from the ovaries of pregnant animals might be used as oral contraceptives. But in the subsequent years many pharmaceutical companies feared the controversy that might result and were reluctant to apply these hormones (now synthesized) for contraception, though they were happy for them to be used in the treatment of various gynaecological conditions. In the early 1950s Margaret Sanger, with her wealthy friend Catherine McCormack, provided the encouragement and resources to researchers that eventually led to the marketing of the pill. The leaders of this work were the chemists Russell Marker, George Rosenkranz, and Carl Djerassi, the biologists Gregory Pincus and H.C. Chang, and the obstetrician John Rock. They worked first with animals and then used a small group of human volunteers in Boston, Massachusetts. It soon became clear that the new hormones were very effective contraceptives, and produced no immediate or obvious harmful effects.

Trials with a larger number of women began in Puerto Rico in 1956, supervised by a young gynaecologist called Celso Ramón-Garcia and Edris Rice-Wray (the first female physician involved in testing the pill). The trials were highly successful—until, that is, the chemists got rid of an impurity in the pills. This impurity was the estrogen, mestranol. Immediately things began to go wrong. Irregular bleeding occurred and so did accidental pregnancies. So it was really by chance that the researchers learnt that a little estrogen was necessary for maximum effectiveness and control of the cycle. When they put it back in the amount previously present as an 'impurity', the combined pill was created. It took a few more years until June 1960 for the US Food and Drug Administration to release the first combination estrogen and progestogen birth control pill Enavid-10. This contained what we would now consider far higher doses of the hormones than are necessary or advisable. It is a fact that early pills gave as much estrogen in a day as is now taken in a week, and as much progestogen (norethisterone) as one current pill provides in a whole month!

The pill seemed to be safe but there was no certainty that it would prove to be so in the long term. So it was agreed from the start that these new and powerful medicines should be distributed only under close supervision and the initial recommendation was that they should not be used for more than two years continuously. That idea, of using it only for a very few years at a time, to make sure it was fully reversible, has persisted in many people's thinking—despite the latest evidence which shows that ex-pill-takers are *more* not less fertile than ex-users of alternative methods (see p. 100).

Figure 1.5 and Table 1.1 show the ways by which the usual combined pill and other combined hormone methods like the patch and the ring operate to prevent pregnancy. The main effect is to stop the normal hormone changes of the menstrual cycle and hence prevent both the maturing of

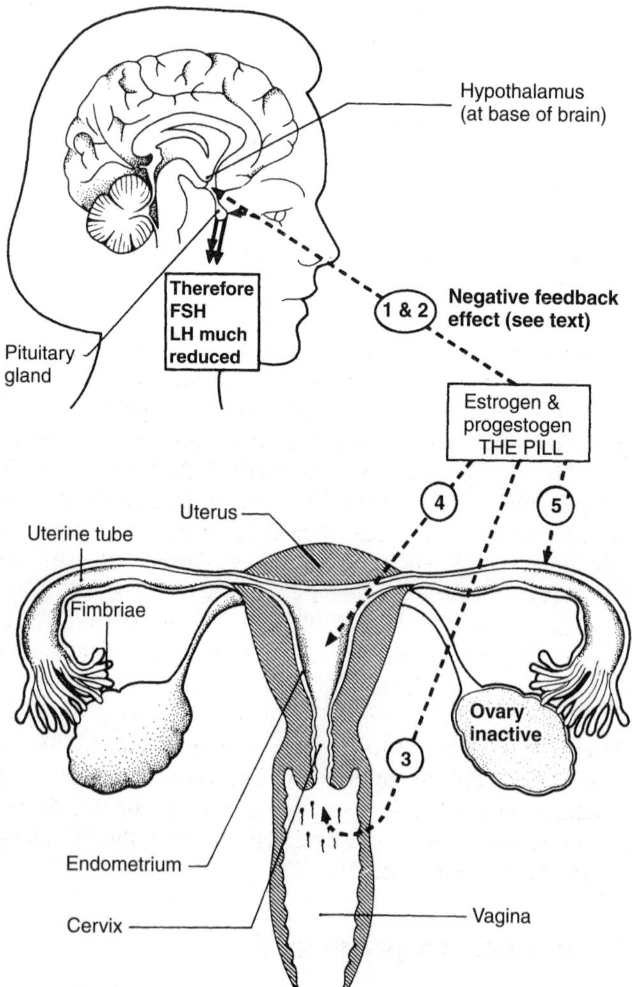

Fig. 1.5 How the combined pill prevents pregnancy

Note: Numbers 1–5 are the contraceptive effects of the combined pill as shown in Table 1.1.

Table 1.1 How combined pills prevent pregnancy

1. Reduced FSH therefore follicles stopped from ripening and egg from maturing	++++
2. LH surge stopped so no egg release	++++
3. Cervical mucus changed into a barrier to sperm	+++
4. Lining of uterus made less suitable for implantation of an embryo (uncertainty, whether this effect is sufficient alone to stop a conception)	+
5. Uterine tubes perhaps affected so that they do not transport egg so well (uncertainty about this also)	+
Expected pregnancy rate per 100 women using the pill method for one year (compare use of NO METHOD = 80–90)	<1 to 3

Notes:
1. The more +s the greater the effect.
2. The combined pill is very reliable, depending chiefly on effects 1 and 2 but with 3 as back-up. See Table 8.1 for the POP.

follicles and actual ovulation—rows 1 and 2 in the table. However, there is an important back-up mechanism to prevent conception even if egg release should occur. (The commonest reason for this 'breakthrough' egg release is forgetting to take tablets, especially after the pill-free time, p. 40.) The slippery mucus which normally flows from the cervix in the fertile part of the cycle and at that time is easily penetrated by sperm is transformed by the hormones—actually the progestogen—into a scanty, thick material which produces a quite effective barrier to sperm. This third way by which the pill may work is still clearly preventing fertilization.

There are also changes in the lining of the uterus which seem to make it less able to support and nourish a fertilized egg. But this fourth possible way is never needed by consistent pill-takers—fertilization gets blocked first by one of the first three methods. In other words, even though it might theoretically be able to do so (and this is uncertain and disputed by some), the pill never needs to block the implanting of a very early pregnancy: a mechanism some people would like to avoid (p. 207–10). Finally, it is unproven whether any hormones can be contraceptive through blocking egg transport (point 5 in Table 1.1).

Effectiveness against pregnancy

When it is properly used, apart from the levonorgestrel-releasing intrauterine system (IUS) and some injectables and implants (see pp. 215–16), there is no more effective reversible method of family planning than the combined pill and its 'clones' like patches and rings. This is explained because its back-up mucus method can work even if the prime effect of preventing release of an egg from the ovary were to fail. But failures do occur for two reasons: the method failing the user (which is rare) and the user failing the method (much commoner, e.g. by forgetting some tablets). If this second cause of failure is added to the first, the total failure rate rises from less than one per 100 woman-years in consistent users to three, or even more in very erratic pill-takers.

What does 'one per 100 woman-years' mean? The simple explanation is that, if 100 women used the pill for a year, one of them should expect to get pregnant. Put another way, if you the user were able to be fertile for 100 years, you would have an 'evens' chance of one pregnancy at the end of that time. Impossible, of course, but it gives the general idea. For healthy women who take their pills absolutely regularly at the same time every day, the failure rate is reduced about fivefold, even to as low as 0.3 per 100 woman-years with modern pills. This means just three pregnancies among 1000 users per year. You would have to be fertile for 333 years before you would have an evens chance of one pregnancy. However, that one true method-failure *could* of course happen in the very first year rather than the 333rd.

In practice, methods which depend on great care by the users, such as the condom and the diaphragm, may have overall (user) failure rates of about 10 per 100 woman-years. On average this means one unplanned pregnancy every 10 years. So a modern one to two-child family need hardly be 'planned', you could almost just wait for the failures! At the least, this statistic means that couples should always consider the likely failure rates of their chosen method(s) when planning their final family size.

What causes 'periods' on the combined pill?

When the pill is taken, the normal menstrual cycle is abolished. Just so long as sufficient amounts of the artificial estrogen and progestogen of the pill are in the bloodstream, there will be no bleeding from the uterus. It used to be believed that most women like to see some kind of period, as regular reassurance that the pill is working. We now know this is a myth—lots of women, if they knew it was not necessary for their health, would be delighted not to bleed at all. However, it may also be better to reduce the monthly intake of artificial hormones to a minimum, and there is a theory—not proved—that it might be preferable to give the pituitary and ovaries and one's body chemistry generally (see p. 122) a break from time to time during each year from the actions of the pill hormones. Solely for these reasons, most systems of pill-taking therefore include a pill-free time, usually one week in every four—but there is more of a choice now and it can sometimes be one week in every 10 or 13 (see Seasonale™, pp. 29–30).

The effect of thus cutting off the supply of pill hormones is to *imitate* the fall in the levels in the bloodstream of their natural equivalents at the end of a normal cycle. This causes shedding of the (rather thinner) lining of the uterus which the pill's hormones have produced during the previous 21 days (Fig. 1.6). Because the lining is different—caused in a different way, by the pill, and looking different under the microscope—its shedding usually leads to less bleeding, often darker in colour, than a normal menstrual period. It is also a lot less likely to be painful.

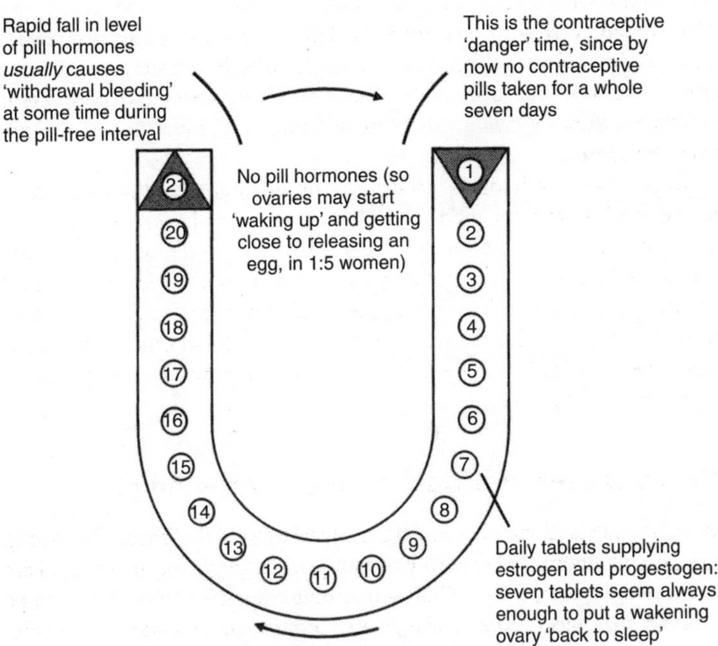

Fig. 1.6 The pill cycle (21-day system)

Note: Compare with Fig. 1.4a (see p. 5). The normal cycle shown there is taken right away and replaced by this simpler one. The bleeding from the uterus is caused just by withdrawal of the pill hormones.

2. Pill-taking is drawn in a horseshoe for the important reason that a horseshoe is a symmetrical object. Hence the pill-free interval can be lengthened, leading to the risk of conception, either side of the horseshoe: by forgetting (or vomiting) pills either at the beginning or at the end of the packet (see pp. 40–1).

So, if you are on the pill, your normal cycle is removed and replaced by something different. You are causing the 'periods' yourself by stopping the pills for one week out of every four. You could stop most of them altogether if you in fact made no break from pill-taking and this is a possible choice (p. 30). As they are in reality substitute periods, they are often (and more accurately) called *hormone withdrawal bleeds.*

An important conclusion from all this is that, if for some reason they fail to happen while you are on the pill, it probably only means that there was too little artificially produced lining of the uterus that month for the stopping of the pill's hormones to lead to bleeding. 'Bad blood' is not 'piling up inside'. There just is *no blood to come away.* If you have been taking your pills regularly, the explanation is very unlikely to be pregnancy. (If you are in doubt, this can be confirmed by a pregnancy test.) What is more, *absence of hormone withdrawal bleeds is totally irrelevant to any risk to your future chances of having a baby* (see p. 101–2).

Some pill-takers notice a quite different situation, in which they bleed too often: on the 'wrong' (tablet-taking) days. This usually settles with time, provided that the pills continue to be taken correctly, but if it does not, this needs to be discussed with whoever prescribed the pill (see pp. 164–7).

How unnatural is the pill?

People are often concerned that, even if it did not have unwanted side-effects (which I am going to discuss in some detail later), the pill's main contraceptive effect in suppressing the cyclical activities of the ovary and of the pituitary gland is 'unnatural'. But is it? It can be argued that having menstrual cycles and periods is actually not entirely 'natural'. Biologically, suppression of the menstrual cycle for years at a time may in fact be a much more natural state of affairs. It is a myth that periods are necessary to clean the bloodstream and 'flush out the flues', that they have a kind of excretory function.

In the past, before there was effective contraception, the normal thing was for a woman to be either pregnant or breastfeeding during all the childbearing years. A doctor working in Central Africa once told me that he had been visited some years ago by a woman in her early forties who was worried by bleeding. By excluding all the other possibilities, he eventually diagnosed this as a normal period. She had been anxious: she never remembered having such a thing before, since she had got married young and never used any contraception!

As support for this idea, that not releasing eggs and not having menstrual cycles is healthy, some cancers, notably cancer of the ovary and the endometrium (lining of the womb), are commoner in women who have had more rather than less natural menstrual cycles during their lives. Probably for this reason, the pill seems to protect against these very cancers (see pp. 116–17). Can we also be reassured by the fact that the pill's main action is to imitate the corpus luteum of pregnancy (p. 10–11 above)? Or that many of the changes in body chemistry caused by the pill (see p. 60), and not a few of the minor side-effects such as nausea, are so similar to those of pregnancy?

Although in many ways the effects of the pill are similar to those of pregnancy, they are by no means all the same: and pregnancy is anyway not free of risks. What is more, the hormones used are artificial rather than natural. (So far, experiments using natural hormones in the pill have not been very satisfactory, but they are continuing.) The dosage of the two hormones is not exactly tailored to each individual. It is roughly constant for three weeks out of four rather than continuously varying as in the menstrual cycle. (So-called phasic pills (see p. 160–3) imitate the menstrual cycle a little more closely, but not perfectly.)

So the most that should be said is that there are reasons to believe that the pill is *not nearly as 'unnatural'* as appears at first sight. And it has always puzzled me that some of the people who are worried by the so-called unnaturalness of the pill actually do something else which is even less 'natural', and certainly more dangerous—they smoke cigarettes! The pill contains two substances which are at least similar to hormones the body is used to handling. And pills are at least eaten—nothing in the animal kingdom takes food or alien chemicals on board deliberately through its lungs. The cigarette, however, is a chemical factory, manufacturing over 4000 unnatural compounds *which are absorbed via the lungs to travel in the blood all over the body.* Some are known cancer-causing agents.

Research continues, and we certainly know a lot more now about the use of hormones for oral contraception than we did at the time of those early tests in Puerto Rico. Indeed, more is known about the safety of the pill than the majority of drugs or food additives on the market (see pp. 133–4).

2 Should you take the pill?

Have you been hearing worrying things about the safety of the pill? If so, right at the outset, Fig. 2.1 and its caption may be reassuring. It is discussed more fully later (see pp. 132–4). But the main point is that the pill is significantly safer than many other risks in life, most of which we largely take for granted.

Getting advice

Before deciding whether the pill is right for you, you will need to know where to turn for advice. Everyone should have access to someone, usually a doctor but increasingly often a nurse trained in family planning, who can answer your questions about contraception and go over every aspect that applies to you personally.

Where to go? And what happens at the first family-planning visit?

The main choice is between general practice and a local community clinic. It is your right to choose where. Community clinics are often chosen by teenagers—and older women nearing the menopause. You may even go to a different general practitioner from the one who normally sees you for other medical matters. The arrangements vary: between different family doctors' surgeries, between different clinics, and in different countries. *As a minimum* you should always be asked some questions about your medical history and aspects of your family history in order to establish that you are suitable for the pill. Your age and smoking habits should be noted and you should be weighed and have your blood pressure checked.

In Britain and many other countries the addresses of family-planning clinics are to be found in the telephone directory (including the *Yellow Pages*) and through relevant websites (p. 267). Ring for an appointment, or they

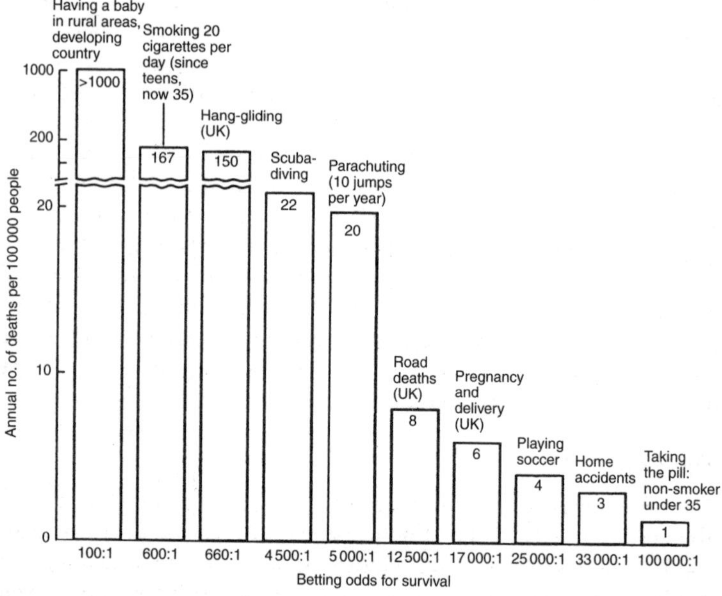

Fig. 2.1 Number of deaths per year for 100 000 people at risk

Notes:

1. The implications of this figure are discussed on pp. 132–4. The risks of pill-taking for non-smokers concern circulatory disease. Cancer is not in the reckoning, since, as explained on pp. 110–19, the benefits of the pill in cancer protection are believed more or less to cancel out the possible adverse effects.

2. The risks of pregnancy and delivery in all countries are much higher than pill-taking for non-smokers under 35. This statistic is not given to scare UK women about having a baby, since 17 000:1 in your favour represents pretty good odds. The point is the pill is even safer (and prevents pregnancy).

3. Note that road deaths in the UK have fallen since earlier editions—probably because of regular use of seat-belts.

Sources: various, listed in Guillebaud, J. (2004). Contraception Today, p. 27.

may have a 'walk-in' service. If you choose to go to one of them, you do not need to bring any doctor's letter with you. Your name is taken first at the reception desk—your partner is welcome too but there is no objection whatsoever if you are on your own—and your date of birth, address, and similar items are noted. A more confidential set of details is taken by a nurse in a separate side-room. She usually has a standard card to complete and all you have to do is answer her questions. She needs to know first about your general health, and then if you have had an abortion or miscarriage or ever had treatment for a sexually transmitted infection. The nurse plays a most important role in the modern family-planning clinic. It is she who usually checks your weight and blood pressure, and tests your urine if necessary.

Specially trained nurses often do much more, including examinations, and you may not need to see a doctor. If you do, again everything will be completely confidential. There will normally be no problem about your partner coming in with you, if you would both like that. The doctor describes and discusses the various methods of family planning, and answers your questions about the pill, if that is the method you are planning to use. Heart disease (see pp. 67–78) and cancer (see pp. 110–19) are important aspects usually discussed now, though if you have no special concerns they may be postponed until a later visit. If there are any special points—for instance, if you are a smoker over 35, or are uneasy and unsure about things, or are under age 16—then time should be made for a longer discussion on all the pros and cons.

The examination

Contrary to what is believed by many women and by some doctors, an examination is *not* a vital part of the first visit to start on the pill—apart, that is, from taking the blood pressure (which is indeed something you should insist on having done—see p. 77–8). However, if (and *only* if) you have noticed a change or abnormality, it would be right to have your breasts examined to ensure that there are no lumps. The first routine cervical smear test is now not advised until age 25 and then they should be done regularly, not just in pill-takers, but in all sexually active women aged 25–65. They are now recommended three-yearly till aged 50 and five-yearly up to 65 but stopping then (or by 60 in Scotland). However, especially if you have not yet started having intercourse, or are anxious about examination, there is absolutely no need for it just because of the pill.

If you have never had an internal examination, a brief description may be helpful. Women who were afraid of this beforehand often wonder afterwards what they were worrying about. In the *bimanual examination*—only done usually because of pain symptoms or as part of checking an intrauterine device (IUD) (p. 216–17)—the doctor or nurse uses both hands, the left hand on the abdomen and two gloved fingers of the right hand inside the vagina (usually, even if the person examining is left-handed). By applying gentle pressure between both hands, based on previous training and experience, they can then check the shape, size, and normality of the reproductive organs. The other part of the examination is with an instrument called a *speculum*, which enables the doctor or nurse to see inside. The speculum is designed to open out a little so that the walls of the vagina and the entrance to the uterus (the cervix) can be examined. Some women like to put the speculum in for themselves, so you have the choice to ask about that, if you wish. Using a flat wooden or plastic spatula the doctor then wipes some loose cells from the cervix on to a glass slide. A tiny 'bottle-brush' rather like a mascara wand, called a Cytobrush, is often rotated within the cervix as well. After being fixed with a special solution, all the smear material obtained is sent to the laboratory to check that the cells are normal. This examination, usually taking much less than five minutes, is all there is to the well-known cervical smear or 'Pap smear' test. (See also pp. 116 and especially p. 245, Questions 12 and 13.)

The speculum is also used if swabs need to be taken and sent to the laboratory, particularly to check for the absence of a sexually transmitted infection (STI) like Chlamydia. If you have recently been with a different sexual partner *or* are afraid your partner may have, because this infection usually causes no symptoms and other STIs might also be present, it is best to have a full check at a genitourinary medicine (GUM) clinic.

There is some good news on the way: a way of helping to avoid cancer of the cervix without having to have that uncomfortable metal speculum put in—indeed without even being examined. As I write (February 2004), research is going on at Cancer UK into a do-it-yourself kit, with which women will be able to take their own vaginal swabs of the human papilloma virus (HPV), especially the types 16 and 18 mentioned on p. 116 as being probably the main cause of that cancer. These will then be tested for in the lab, and the hope is that most women will then be able to be reassured and not need further investigation, perhaps for some years.

While we wait for that easier future, even now examinations should be few and far between, and never needed just because of the pill alone.

You should next be given a user-friendly explanatory leaflet—that produced by the Family Planning Association (FPA) still being the best—along with detailed advice about pill-taking, missed pills, and what symptoms need to be promptly reported (see pp. 37–43, 50, 53). Usually only three months' supply of the chosen pill is given at first, to see how it suits you.

You should return for a check-up as instructed, particularly of your blood pressure and any history of headaches (p. 83–8), and you will be given further supplies at that time. If you need special supervision because of slightly raised blood pressure or a similar medical reason, you may be asked to come back for the first follow-up sooner than three months.

What if I am under age?

If you are under a certain age (16 in Britain, with potentially more enforcement under 13), in many countries your partner will be breaking the law if you have intercourse. Plenty of couples do this, and the law will not lead to any prosecution if there is what it calls 'mutually agreed sexual activity within normal adolescent behaviour, where there is no evidence of exploitation'. But there is a lot more to consider (see pp. 232–42). If you are able to say 'let's wait', you will save yourself from a lot of worry, and some very real risks: emotional trauma as well as STIs and pregnancy. That is a factual, medical statement and not made in a judgemental way of those people who have decided not to wait.

If you are already having intercourse under age, know the problems and the risks involved, but feel that you will continue, you will find that most health-care providers are prepared to prescribe you the pill—without moralizing. The 2003 Sexual Offences Act still definitely permits them to do this, since they are acting to reduce the possible harm, like pregnancy at this age would cause. If you have not already done so, they will strongly encourage you to tell at least one of your parents, or some other trusted person like an aunt or older sister. The law recommends but does not enforce this—and actually you could be agreeably surprised by how helpful they turn out to be.

But you can certainly be prescribed the pill even without the definite consent of your mother or father, if it is the medical judgement of the doctor or nurse that this is in your best interests, and without it your physical or mental health might suffer through the even greater problem of an unwanted pregnancy. Above all they absolutely must keep your confidence: the law says you have the same right to confidentiality as any other (older) person. So they must not tell your parents or anyone else unless you want or allow this (as might be true in what the law calls abuse, where someone has been forced to do what they didn't want).

Many family doctor services are very welcoming, but if not you will find Brook clinics or the many equivalent young people's clinics in most areas particularly helpful, as they specialize in providing 100 per cent confidential help for teenagers in all sex and family-planning matters. They also provide excellent leaflets about sexual health, confidentiality, and talking to doctors. More details about your local clinics are available at www.fpa.org.uk or by telephoning the FPA's helpline: 0845 310 1334.

German measles (Rubella)

Rubella, although it is a mild illness in the mother, can very seriously damage a developing baby during pregnancy. If you plan to have a baby at any time and there is the least doubt about whether you were vaccinated against it as a child, it is sensible forward planning to have the simple blood test to show whether you have immunity to Rubella. Do not rely on a history of German measles in the past: this is often wrong, as other infections can imitate it. If you are not immune, the vaccination is not painful and it is well worth having. Like the blood test, it can easily be arranged by whoever supplies you with the pill.

Counselling and follow-up visits

Family-planning services are meant to provide total reproductive health care, meaning much more than just avoiding an unwanted pregnancy. For a start, they are also very ready to help those who are a bit late with a period and think they might already be pregnant. It is never too late to go to a clinic and talk things through. If the early morning specimen of urine (which you should take with you in a clean glass bottle) shows that you are in fact pregnant, clinics can arrange appropriate counselling about the pregnancy. Most family-planning nurses and doctors are easy to talk to, and are very helpful too if you have emotional problems or difficulties with any aspect of sex including becoming pregnant (infertility) or intercourse itself. Special counselling can be arranged for couples where sex has become a problem. At a major centre, such as the Margaret Pyke Centre in London or the Sandyford Initiative in Glasgow, there are also readily available services for screening, health education, testing for sexually transmitted diseases, male and female sterilization—in short a 'seamless' well-woman/well-man service.

Much of what I have described in the last few pages applies also if you go to your family doctor rather than to a clinic for your pills. The visits may tend to be briefer, partly because he or she probably knows most of the important medical facts about you already. It is entirely up to you whether you prefer to go to a clinic or to your doctor's—or any neighbouring doctor's—surgery. Better organized practices now run at least one special or 'dedicated' family-planning session each week. You should get more time there, for discussion and referral if necessary, perhaps for the fitting of an IUS or IUD, or maybe an implant.

For pill-users the first return visit is commonly after three months, sooner if special factors apply in your case, then the blood pressure check should be done as a routine every six months and then, if all remains well, perhaps just every 12 months (p. 152). An internal examination (often now done by the practice nurse) will be required *only* when you are due your next regular cervical smear. It is not necessary at any other routine interval, just because you are taking the pill.

Never hesitate to go back to whoever prescribed your pills, immediately if necessary, or certainly sooner than your next routine visit, if you ever have doubts or anxieties about using the pill, or about any effect it seems to be having on you.

Can anyone use the pill?

No, this method is not suitable for everyone. For a start, it is no good if:

- you think you might already be pregnant
- you have unexplained bleeding from your vagina (for example, between periods or after sex). This needs to be diagnosed and, if necessary, treated first.

Later in the book there is much more detailed information about risk factors, side-effects—whether nuisance-type or dangerous—and choosing pill brands. Chapter 6 is also very important, putting everything in perspective.

In brief, the doctor or nurse that you see at the first pill visit will need to ask you about your own and your family's medical history and any important illnesses or operations you have had. Some important conditions which need discussion, but may mean you should not use the *combined* pill, are:

- you smoke *and* are above age 35
- you are overweight (body mass index [BMI] being above 30, p. 146) *and* over 35 or have a BMI of 40 or above at any age
- you have, through some illness or genetically, a particular predisposition making you more likely to suffer—or you have ever had in the past—one of the following:
  - any *thrombosis* in any vein or artery
  - a *significant heart abnormality* you might have been born with, or a circulatory disease problem like *raised blood pressure* or *angina*
  - extremely bad *migraines* or any history of *migraine with aura* (which begins in the minutes *before* a migraine starts and mainly involves eye symptoms, pp. 84–6)
  - diabetes affecting the eyes, kidneys, arteries, or nerves
  - breast cancer
  - active disease of the liver.

Box 2.1 WHO classification of eligibility criteria for contraceptives, including the pill (*plus this author's supplementary comments*)

Group WHO 1. A condition for which there is no restriction for the use of the contraceptive method, indeed it may be beneficial.
'A' is for ALWAYS USABLE

Group WHO 2. A condition where the advantages of using the method generally outweigh the theoretical or proven risks.
'B' is for BROADLY USABLE

Group WHO 3. A condition where the theoretical or proven risks usually outweigh the advantages, so an alternative method is usually preferred. Yet—respecting the person's autonomy—if she accepts the risks and rejects or should not use relevant alternatives, given the risks of pregnancy the method can be used with caution and sometimes additional monitoring.
'C' is for CAUTION/COUNSELLING, if used at all

Group WHO 4. A condition which represents an unacceptable health risk.
'D' is for DO NOT USE, at all.

Source: www.who.int/reproductive-health

These usually mean the pill is *not* to be used in *any* circumstances—see Box 2.1 from the World Health Organization (WHO). This new WHO 1–4 scale is extremely useful. It will be my *basis* throughout the rest of this new edition. **It is important to note, though, that for numerous diseases (and for some new hormonal contraceptives) WHO has not yet stated its view. For those–and in some other situations where I say "in my opinion" in the text–the WHO Group given here can only be my own best judgement, from the data available to me.*

So the conditions listed above are in Group 4 or D ('do not use'), in the terminology of the WHO. But there are many other conditions, those in Groups 3 and 2, where there is more latitude: they mean the pill could be used if the woman is keen to do so, perhaps with special care and extra supervision (many examples are given on pp. 143–51).

Finally, and most importantly, there are situations where using the pill represents no problem at all, and could even be beneficial (Group 1 'ALWAYS USABLE', e.g. for someone who wants the best chance of having a baby in future, pp. 100–2). Box 2.2 gives an impressive list from within this Group 1 where the pill is especially 'usable', because there are likely to be real benefits.

Box 2.2 Contraceptive and non-contraceptive benefits of combined pills (for more details use index)

Contraceptive benefits of combined Pills

- Highly effective
- Convenient, nothing to be done during sex
- Reversible: indeed it may actually help to preserve fertility. In a study published in 2002, long-term use (more than five years) of the pill before planned conceptions meant it took less time to conceive, compared with ex-users of other methods (see p. 100).

Non-contraceptive benefits

- Reduction of most menstrual cycle problems: less heavy bleeding, therefore less anaemia, and less period pains (dysmenorrhoea); regular bleeding, and timing can be controlled (no pill-taker need have 'periods' at weekends; and upon request she may tricycle and so bleed only a few times a year, see pp. 29–32); fewer symptoms of premenstrual tension overall; no mid-cycle ovulation pain which some women are really troubled by
- Fewer pain-causing so-called functional cysts on the ovary
- Reduction in pelvic inflammatory disease (PID), caused by infections like Chlamydia, and therefore an expectation of less infertility from blocked tubes—but monogamy and condoms are more certain ways to protect the tubes
- Fewer pregnancies in a tube (ectopics)
- Reduced risk of cancers of the ovary, endometrium (lining of the womb), and possibly of the colon and rectum also
- Reduced risk of benign breast lumps and related disease
- Fewer fibroids in the womb causing symptoms
- Probably lower risk of the condition endometriosis (pp. 92)
- Probable reduction in thyroid disease (both overactivity and underactivity of the gland)
- Probable reduction in risk of rheumatoid arthritis
- Less acne (if certain pill brands are selected, pp. 107–8)
- Reduction in *Trichomonas vaginalis* infections
- Possible lower incidence of toxic shock syndrome
- Possibly fewer duodenal ulcers (not well established: the apparent link is perhaps due to anxious women who are more likely to get ulcers also tending to avoid using the pill)
- A positive effect on the bones in women who are at risk of osteoporosis (though, if the ovaries are working well, using the pill is no better for bones than the normal situation)
- No toxicity in overdose: you can't be poisoned by it (p. 59)
- Obvious beneficial social effects (such as making it possible for women to go to college without a baby to look after!).

3 How to take the pill?

This chapter is all about how to make sure the pill works and stays working in its main job of preventing pregnancy, and when to discuss a change of method with your provider. The progestogen-only pill (POP—formerly called the mini-pill) is considered in Chapter 8.

Systems of pill-taking

21-day system (with or without blank or dummy inactive tablets)

The most common system is the one in which you take one pill daily—morning, evening, or any other regular time that you find easy to remember—for 21 days, followed by a seven-day break taking nothing at all. There are also some every day (ED) brands available with 28 tablets in each packet, of which seven are dummies or 'blanks'. These are liked by many women. Care must be taken when starting these packets (p. 161) to avoid taking inactive pills at the wrong time, but the pills are then taken consecutively, one packet after another. There is no need to remember when to stop and start taking successive courses. (And I know if I were on a male pill, I would find it much easier to remember a pill every single day, rather than having to remember to restart after taking a week's break once a cycle!)

ED pills are particularly good for helping the user not to make the worst kind of pill-taking mistake: which is being *late in restarting* pill-taking after that regular seven-day break from the pill's contraceptive effects.

Tricycle system

There is also the *three-monthly* or *'tricycle' system* (see Fig. 3.1). In this, either four or three packets are taken in succession—therefore a pill every day for up to 84 days—followed by a break during which the 'period' normally

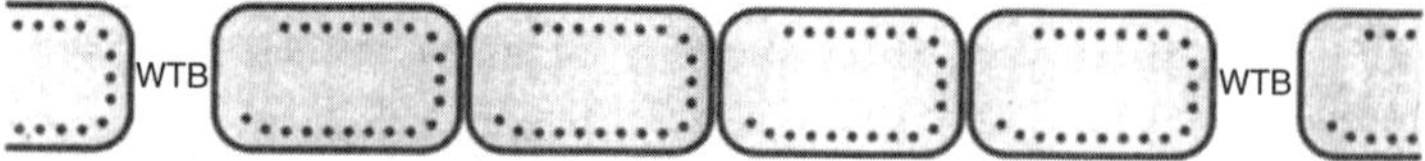

Fig. 3.1 Tricycling (using four packs)

Note that they must be monophasic packs. Duration of pill-free interval may also be shortened. WTB = withdrawal bleeds.

occurs. As explained in Chapter 1, pill 'periods' are in fact 'hormone withdrawal bleeds', created artificially by the taking of a seven-day break. So there is no particular reason why they should not happen every 13 weeks, with the four-packs-in-a-row system, instead of every four weeks. Once this has been explained, many find this four-per-year routine perfectly acceptable or even preferable. Indeed there is now a dedicated packaging in several countries called 'Seasonale', since the user only bleeds once a season—in the summer, autumn, winter, and spring!

Moreover, as shown in Box 3.1, there are some special reasons why the doctor may recommend this even without your particular preference.

A word of caution though: tricycle systems like Seasonale obviously mean you will need 16 packets of pills per year instead of the usual 13. Thus, unless the tablet dose is reduced, you take more hormone dose on board per year and this must imply at least the chance of increasing the risk of some side-effects (though this has not been found yet). Theoretically, also, the breaks themselves might be beneficial, in giving the body a regular 'rest' from the pill's effects (see p. 122).

Box 3.1 Reasons for tricycling of the pill

1. Own choice
2. If headaches are a problem and happen in the pill-free week. Tricycling really does help, meaning at most five bad headaches a year instead of 13 This can be the policy even for migraines, so long as they are not the type described on p. 84–6
3. If the 'periods' themselves are bad (unusual on the pill)
4. Sometimes when using the pill to treat premenstrual syndrome (PMS)
5. In managing epilepsy (see p. 88–9), and other conditions in which long-term use of an 'interfering' drug is needed (p. 44–8)
6. In treating endometriosis (see p. 97)
7. If there has been previous failure of the pill, leading to pregnancy. This important reason is discussed in detail on p. 150–1.

Secondly, annoying bleeding at the wrong times can occur, especially towards the end of the sequence of packs: you may then be advised to take a seven-day break from tablet-taking and restart. Thereafter fewer packs in a row—e.g. 'bi-cycling'—might work better for you.

But the important thing is that whether and how often to have bleeds on the pill is now a matter of choice. And watch this space: research is in progress to lead to absolutely continuous pill-taking systems, using exceptionally low doses. The studies suggest this produces fewer spotting and bleeding days per year but at the price of unpredictability, not knowing when those days will be.

I therefore recommend that this tricycle scheme is reserved for when there is one of the special reasons listed in Box 3.1, but definitely including the woman's choice after discussion of these pros and cons.

The tricycle system of pill-taking is of course completely different from triphasic pills, which are described on pp. 160–3. Indeed it does not work satisfactorily with any phasic pills: the more common single phase (monophasic) brands need to be used.

Postponing or improving the timing of 'periods'

Even if you regularly use the system of three weeks on, one week off, one advantage of the pill is that you always have the option of postponing your 'period'. When planning for your holidays, for example, this can be done either by taking extra pills from a spare packet, or more simply by just taking two or three packets in succession.

Also, if you happen to have pill 'periods' always at weekends, why not start one pack earlier (i.e. with a three- or four-day rather than seven-day break) one month? This will shift them to mid-week regularly in future. Note, starting one pack earlier will also work for phasic pills (see p. 160); and it is *not* so good to bring your 'period' on midweek by stopping pill-taking early.

Am I protected during the seven-day break?

Yes, whenever you take the seven-day break from pill-taking, your protection against pregnancy continues throughout it, provided three things are true:

1. you have been regular in your pill-taking during and through to the end of the preceding packet;
2. none of the other conditions which might reduce your protection, like vomiting back a tablet, has happened near the end of the previous pack (see pp. 40, 43);
3. above all, you do in fact start another packet on the eighth day, on time.

Never make the mistake of starting the next packet late or missing any of the first seven pills in the pack. Contrary to what many think, being late starting even by just one day is much more risky than missing, say, three or even four pills in the middle of the pack. This is because the seven-day break from pill-taking is a *contraceptive-free* time, during which your ovaries are not getting any effects from the pill. If you ever make this break longer than seven days, your ovaries might release an egg early in the following week. And then, of course, if you have already made love earlier, during the non-pill-taking days, the sperm might survive long enough to fertilize that egg. (If you do not want to conceive, there is still the emergency pill to think about taking—see pp. 54–8.)

But do not worry otherwise; if you *don't* lengthen the pill-free time beyond that critical seven days, then love-making is safe on any day of any month.

How to start taking the pill

If you are having normal periods up to the time of starting the pill, there are several different ways to start.

Starting on the fifth day of the period

This method is not often used now. You take the first pill on the fifth day of your period, whether your bleeding has stopped or not. Choose a pill from the section on the packet marked with that day of the week and press the plastic bubble so as to remove it from the foil on the reverse side. Then take a pill each day for 21 days. After a seven-day break you then start taking pills again on the eighth day: and from then on in each four weeks you follow the regular routine of 21 days of pill-taking followed by a seven-day break. (Avoid making a common mistake here, which is to start each new packet like the first on the fifth day of the period. This can cause a pregnancy, if the 'period' happens to come on late.)

The snag of this system is that some women frequently—and others 'out of the blue'—can have short menstrual cycles. There is then the small risk that there may already at this stage in the cycle be a follicle ripening. This could be producing so much natural estrogen that the pill may be unable to stop the surge of LH hormone from the pituitary which leads to release of an egg (see pp. 9, 10 and Figs 1.3 and 1.4). The WHO now reckons this risk is too low to worry about, but I continue to recommend that until the seventh pill of the first course has been taken you should use an effective alternative method of family planning as well, such as the condom.

Starting on the first day of the period (see also p. 161 for starting ED pills).

This is now the routine method in the UK. If, in the first cycle only of pill-taking, you start the tablets on the very first day of the period, egg release is effectively prevented even among women with short cycles. Thus no extra method of family planning need be used. The only problem is that in the first pill cycle this method does seem to cause a bit more breakthrough bleeding, which is bleeding on days when you are taking tablets; but this is common in the first month (Fig. 3.2), going away later. Also some of the days can't in fairness be called 'breakthrough' as they are only to be expected, during the first few days, when you are deliberately taking pills during the bleeding of the first period.

Another important point to realize is that your first hormone withdrawal bleed on the pill will come on sooner than usual. This is because you will be taking your twenty-first tablet only 21 days after the start of the previous period. As usual on the pill, your 'period'/hormone withdrawal bleeding follows only a day or two after that. Thus the very first pill cycle will tend to be only about 23 days long, but this matters not at all. The next packet is started as usual after seven days whether or not a 'period' happens and however long it lasts (Fig. 3.2).

Notice, by the way, in Fig. 3.2 that the woman had a bit of breakthrough bleeding and spotting, other than at 'period' times. But this minor problem cleared up by the time the third packet of pills was started. This is what usually happens. See pp. 164–7 for more about this.

Starting the pill without extra contraceptive precautions is absolutely fine up to day 2 of the cycle. If started on a day later than this, being a little more cautious than WHO or the FPA, I still advise that the pill should not be relied on for 7 days. (WHO says this only for starts after day 5).

'Sunday start'

Starting on the first Sunday after your period starts, with extra precautions just in the first cycle for the first seven days of *active* tablets, is usual in the USA and some countries. An advantage is that the twenty-first or last pill of that and of each subsequent pack—or the last *active* pill if ED packs are being used (pp. 29, 40)—will be on a Saturday. The withdrawal bleed will then begin on a weekday, probably the Monday, so no bleeding at weekends! (Although as we have seen (p. 31) there is an extremely easy way to shift the bleeding to mid-week, whichever of the starting routines is used.)

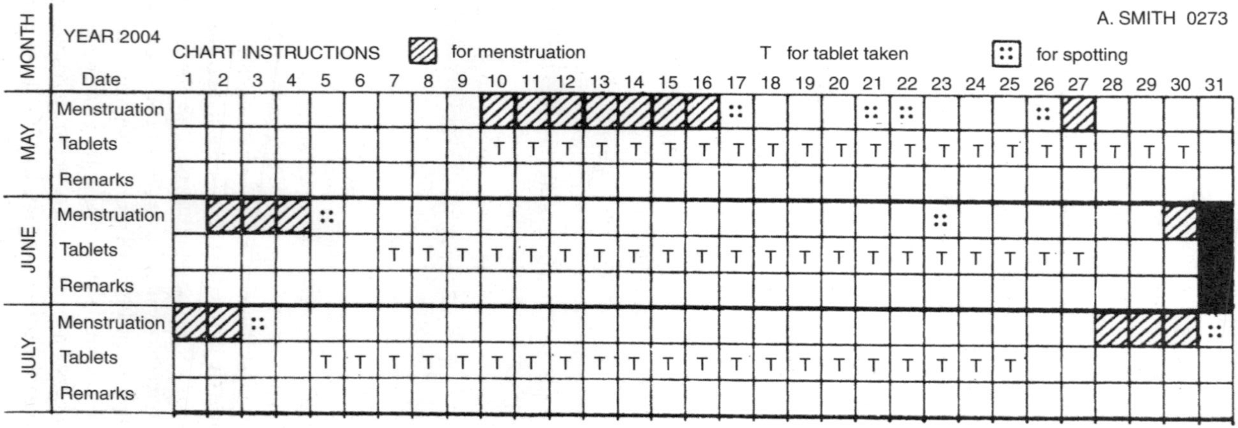

A. SMITH 0273

CHART INSTRUCTIONS — for menstruation; T for tablet taken; for spotting

MONTH	YEAR 2004 Date	1	2	3	4	5	6	7	8	9	10	11	12	13	14	15	16	17	18	19	20	21	22	23	24	25	26	27	28	29	30	31
MAY	Menstruation																															
	Tablets										T	T	T	T	T	T	T	T	T	T	T	T	T	T	T	T	T	T	T	T	T	
	Remarks																															
JUNE	Menstruation																															
	Tablets							T	T	T	T	T	T	T	T	T	T	T	T	T	T	T	T	T	T	T	T	T				
	Remarks																															
JULY	Menstruation																															
	Tablets					T	T	T	T	T	T	T	T	T	T	T	T	T	T	T	T	T	T	T	T	T						
	Remarks																															

Fig. 3.2 Diary card: first-day start of the pill

Note some expected extra days of spotting and bleeding in the first cycle, which is also short (c.24 days).

'Quick start'

If you have not had any sex at all since your last period began, or if you are 100 per cent confident that no sperm escaped when condoms were used, you could also start the pill on any day of your cycle, with condoms as well for at least the next seven days. If the risk of having conceived before the pill-start is acceptably low, the only other likely problem is irregular bleeding—which will nearly always settle in the first two to three cycles.

Quick start of the pill may also be acceptable sometimes after hormonal emergency contraception (p. 55), rather than as would be more usual (and officially licensed) waiting till the first or second day of the next period.

Starting after a recent pregnancy

There is no need to wait for your first period after a baby. Indeed to do so may well mean you conceive with the very first egg you release after the previous birth, and do not therefore see another period till the next baby arrives. Even if you do not breastfeed, egg release has never been proved to happen earlier than about four weeks after delivery. So, if you are *bottle-feeding*, the FPA recommends that you start taking the pill *from the 21st day* after the birth (no extra precautions needed). Twenty-one days later, when you finish the first packet, you should see the first withdrawal bleed.

It is better not to start earlier, as this might increase the small risk there is, after any birth, of thrombosis (clotting) in a vein of the legs. But starting later is a choice, so long as another method like condoms is used carefully up until starting the pill and until seven daily pills have been taken.

If you are *breastfeeding* and plan to continue, then the progestogen-only pill is preferable to the ordinary combined pill. This pill is also often started on about *the twenty-first day* following delivery. See Chapter 8 for all you need to know about this very different kind of pill.

After a *suction termination* of pregnancy, or a *spontaneous miscarriage* which has been treated in hospital by a dilatation and curettage (D & C; see Glossary), the pill can be started at once, on the very day of the procedure—or the next day if you are feeling a bit sick. Starting immediately like this protects you against pregnancy from the outset, and will mean that, as shown in Fig. 3.2, the first period will occur rather soon—after about 24 days.

If you get unexpected bleeding, as heavy as a period, and especially if it is painful, in the first weeks after any early pregnancy has ended, you should *not* call this breakthrough bleeding of the type shown in Fig. 3.2. It could mean that you need a second D & C as the uterus was not emptied out completely. So see your doctor or one of the doctors at the hospital *without delay*.

Starting *after another hormonal method*: generally you will be recommended to start the pill on the next day after the old method stops, without a break, or sometimes with an overlap with both methods working (e.g. with the injection depot medroxyprogesterone acetate, DMPA). Removal of IUDs, IUSs, and implants is also delayed until the pill has been safely started, meaning again a bit of 'overlap'.

If in doubt, e.g. if you have not been seeing any kind of bleeding or a proper cycle with your last method, bring a urine specimen with you and discuss how to start with your doctor or nurse.

Regular pill-taking

If the pill is the method for you, regularity is vital. It can be taken morning, noon, or night as long as it is at a roughly constant time, preferably within an hour or two. A very useful trick these days is to set a regular daily alarm on your mobile which is dedicated just for this. There is now estimated to be 24 hours' leeway in pill-taking for pregnancy prevention (at least twice the 12-hour margin allowed in previous editions), and maybe 48 hours according to WHO. This means that you can easily catch up if you forget overnight, for example: but it is decidedly unwise to make a habit of this. The reason for being consistent is that, after each pill is absorbed, your liver and kidneys, working in combination, are continually eliminating the hormones of the pill from your body. So a gap of more than the usual 24 hours between tablets certainly increases the chance of annoying breakthrough bleeding due to too little pill-support to the womb's lining. More importantly, if you are late in taking or miss out the first pill(s) of the *next* pack, you will risk breakthrough egg release and pregnancy—since this prolongs the time when your body has anyway just had a week's rest from the pill's effects (Fig. 3.3).

The risk of pregnancy if pills are forgotten is also greater:

1. if you are on one of the modern extra-low-dose (≤ 20 mcg) combined pills shown in Table 7.1 (p. 153); these are very reliable, but have a reduced margin for error;
2. if you are being treated with any drug which might interfere with the pill's actions (see pp. 44–8).

Fortunately, the extra contraceptive actions described in Table 1.1 (p. 13), especially the effect of progestogen making the mucus into a barrier, should still stop you conceiving if you do miss pill(s)—especially if you follow the rules which follow, in Fig. 3.4.

Missed pills

Do not panic if you forget to take a pill. This is one of the commonest worries that any pill-user ever has. It is unlikely that you will become pregnant. However, it is certainly not something to make a habit of, and most pill failures are caused this way. To be as safe as can be you need to follow some simple recommendations. *These have changed (more than once!) since early editions of this book.* The latest advice here (July 2004) is based on discussions at WHO in which I was involved—just using, for simplicity and safety, their recommendations for the very lowest dose ($\leq$ 20 mcg) pills.

What is the scientific justification for the modern advice shown in Fig. 3.4? The main point is that any contraceptive is most effective when it

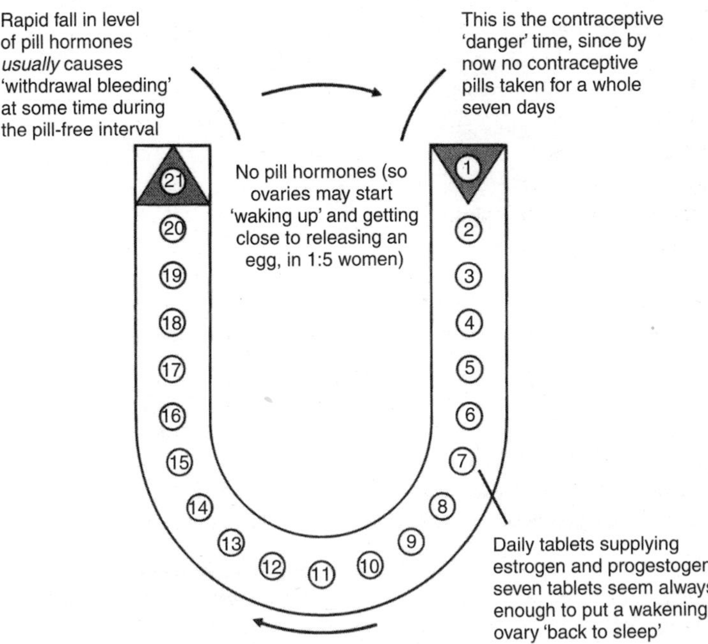

Fig. 3.3 The pill cycle (21-day system)

Notes:

1. Compare with Fig. 1.4a (see p. 5). The normal cycle shown there is taken right away and replaced by this simpler one. The bleeding from the uterus is caused just by withdrawal of the pill hormones.

2. Pill-taking is drawn in a horseshoe for the important reason that a horseshoe is a symmetrical object. Hence the pill-free interval can be lengthened, leading to the risk of conception, either side of the horseshoe: by forgetting (or vomiting) pills either at the beginning or at the end of the packet.

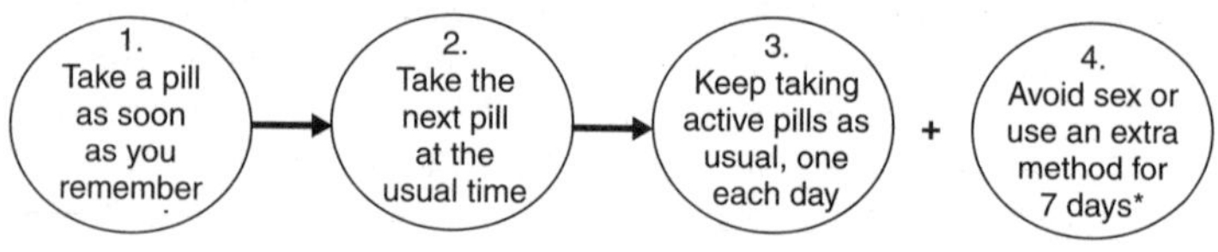

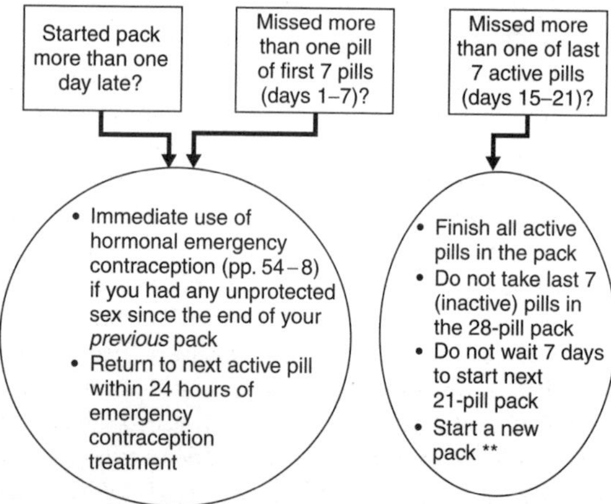

If you miss any of the 7 inactive pills (in a 28-pill pack only):
Throw away missed pills
Keep taking 1 pill each day
Start new pack as usual

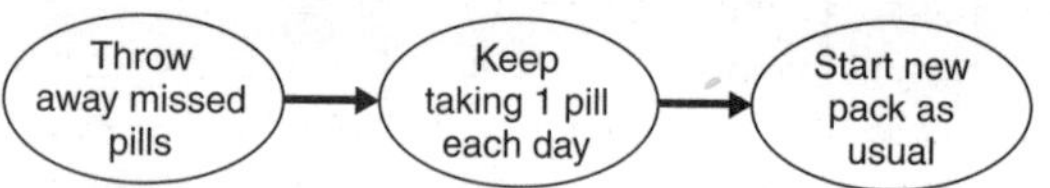

Fig. 3.4 Advice for missed pills – NB plural! **so that missing a single pill for up to 24 hours means only actions 1→3 at top of the figure**

**For what to do if more than 4 pills are missed in days 8–21, see pp. 41–2.*

***Even with triphasic pills, you should go straight to (the first phase of) the same brand. You may bleed a bit but you will still strengthen your contraception. This is quite different from postponing a 'period'. See pp. 162–3.*

****28-pill or ED packs such as Microgynon-ED can be very helpful, to minimize the risk of being a 'late restarter' of active pills, after the 7 day 'contraception-losing' time. See p. 40.*

is actually being taken, and bound to be least effective when it is not being taken. When you really think about it, the pill is a pretty strange contraceptive in that women are told not to take it, at all, for a whole week at a time. This contraception-free interval 'lets the body off the hook', so to speak. Though seven days is too short a time to allow egg release, in about one woman in every five anything more is too much. The advice has to cater for the most contraceptively risky tablets (whatever the brand) to miss, which are those which will lengthen the pill-free time—those at the start or finish of a packet, in fact.

*In all women the menstrual cycle is taken away during the 21 days of pill-taking (pp. 13–17). Indeed, research shows that once seven tablets have been taken the ovaries are inactive, or 'asleep' (see Fig. 3.3 and Box 3.2).

However, research at the Margaret Pyke Centre and elsewhere has shown a rise in the blood levels of FSH (from the pituitary gland) and estrogen (from a follicle growing in one of the ovaries, as can be observed with an ultrasound scanner) during the pill-free week. The rise is more marked in some women (about 20 per cent) than in others. If you refer to pp. 10–14, you will realize that this means that the pituitary and ovaries of these women are, if you like, close to escaping from the suppressing effect of the pill. Any lengthening of the pill-free time beyond seven days means a risk that the ovary 'wakes up'. If so, follicle growth and estrogen production in some women—and no one knows if they might be one of those 20 per cent at greatest risk—get high enough to cause a 'surge' of LH and hence egg release from the largest follicle. And with egg release comes the risk of pregnancy.

The modern advice for missed pills is therefore based on when, in each week of pill-taking, the pills were missed, and is summarized in Fig. 3.4. Notice that a single missed pill is defined as a whole day late now (previously 12 hours), and that *after the first week* the number of pills that are missable without having to even consider emergency contraception is four, perhaps surprisingly high.

Where an 'extra method' appears, in this Figure or (in later chapters) to do with other hormonal methods, the other method must *never* be the rhythm, temperature, or cervical mucus methods. The pill's hormones

Box 3.2 The seven-day slogan

- seven days of pill-taking puts the ovaries to sleep.
- seven days without pills is contraceptively safe.
- More than seven days since the last pill was taken risks the ovaries 'waking up' (egg release).

make these quite unusable. Contraceptive experts do not recommend spermicides for use alone either, and the IUD or IUS is unlikely to be useful for so short a time. So what is usually meant is either abstinence or a (male or female) condom.

The advice in Fig. 3.4 may be a bit different from what you read in the leaflet with your packet of pills: beware, sometimes in some countries and in the past the manufacturer's advice (see p. 42) has actually been contraceptively unsafe.

Missing pills at the beginning of a packet

The first obvious way a woman might accidentally lengthen the pill-free time could be by being late restarting after the pill-break, or forgetting one or more pills in the first week of a packet. Either will significantly lengthen the time without the pill's contraceptive actions. In fact, going away for a weekend or longer without one's pills, having sex while away, and then starting the next packet late (something a lot of people don't even reckon as 'missing pills') is a well-known cause of unplanned pregnancy. That is one reason why I strongly favour the more widespread use of 28 day ED (every day) pill packaging (as described on p. 29). Wouldn't someone who is used to taking pills all the time be more likely to have a packet with them wherever they went? I know I would, if there were a male pill.

The advice in Fig. 3.4 should protect you if you completely miss one or more pills early in a packet (see below re emergency contraception). You must also not rely solely on the pill method, for seven days from the moment you discover the problem. The first week of this time is the time of greatest pregnancy risk; there is no need to continue with precautions to the end of the packet (as used to be advised), if this means more than seven days.

Missing pills at the end of a packet

Another way a woman might lengthen the pill-free time would be by missing pills at the *end* of the previous packet, and then still taking the usual seven-day break.

In this case if you take no special action the dangerous time for conceiving would not be when the pills were forgotten, but *over a week later* when—once again—the pituitary and ovary have been 'let off the hook' for longer than usual. In fact, pregnancy could result from intercourse during or after the (falsely reassuring) 'period' which comes *after* the missed pills! (This is because that bleeding is not truly a period (see pp. 14–16), being caused only by the withdrawal of the artificial hormones. It has no connection with what is happening at the ovary.) The egg could be released around the end of the pill-free time *whenever it has been made longer than usual—unless you act.*

How should you act? The right-hand side of Fig. 3.4 for end-of-packet tablet omissions amounts to: 'Get back to pill-taking and miss out the next active-pill-free days.' It is really saying: 'You made your own pill-taking break early this month, through the pills you missed, so it would be crazy to add the routine seven-day break on top.' Moreover, unless you actually missed seven or more pills, having just the break you caused will make you even more secure against pregnancy this month than usual (see Box 3.2). Indeed, if you do run straight on to the next pack, the advice to use an extra method for 7 days is actually over-cautious . . .

This advice for pills missed in the third week means you may not have a period until the end of two packs in a row, but this does you no harm. (Nor does it matter, whenever pills have been missed, if for a while you see some breakthrough bleeding on subsequent tablet-taking days.)

Missing pills in the middle of a packet

Contrary to what most pill-takers—and some doctors—think, the middle of a packet is the least dangerous time to miss tablets (if you must!), even several in a row. If you follow the argument here, you will see that egg release and pregnancy are very unlikely, because the pills are missed after the pituitary and ovary have been 'put to sleep' by that 'magic minimum' of seven days of pill-taking (see Box 3.2). The advice to use condoms for 7 days (Fig. 3.4) is so ultra-cautious that if you fail to do so, you do *not* need emergency contraception unless (p. 42) you have missed more than 4 pills! It is still better not to be ever more than a day late even with one pill, though, because of the risk of causing the annoying symptom of breakthrough bleeding.

Triphasic pills? the rules are the same.

If you have missed pills at the end of a packet and therefore follow the advice and switch straight to the very low dose of the first phase (see pp. 160–3), you are a bit more liable to get a bleed than on a monophasic pill. But contraception will still be improved with either pill type. *If postponing bleeding more than restoring contraception is your main concern*, and a phasic pill is involved, see p. 163.

Missing/forgetting a succession of pills

What if you have been so disorganized that you forgot a large number(>4) of pills? Should you ask for emergency (post-coital) contraception?

To take a handful of missed pills all at once will simply make you sick!

Emergency contraception (EC described on pp. 54–8) is already advised in Fig. 3.4 for the worst situation, *where you were more than one day late in restarting after the break, or have missed more than one tablet out of the first seven*, and you also made love while not taking pills. It is also usually given, just to be on the safe side, if more than four pills in a row have been missed in the middle week; but however many pills were missed in the third week (tablets 15–21), running straight on to the next pack should always be enough. (*Not if you didn't run on, though: EC would be needed then, since the total pill-free time would be more than 7 days).*

Other rules

The 14-day rule which used to be recommended was a valid alternative and very simple to explain, but required more use of condoms or similar than is now considered necessary to restore contraception.

There is also one simple rule which is completely *wrong*, and that is the old-fashioned one: 'After any missed pills take precautions till the end of the current packet.' This is over-cautious in some situations—yet positively dodgy in others.

Breakthrough bleeding

Even if egg release does not occur as a result of missed pills, you are more likely to get the problem of breakthrough bleeding.

This is 'spotting' or sometimes a rather heavier blood loss, coming on at any time other than the pill-free week. It happens for the same reason as the normal pill 'period': too little at that time of the pill's hormones reaching the lining of the uterus. However, it will almost always stop if you simply disregard it and continue to take the pills regularly, using the usual routine of 21 days on, seven days off (see also pp. 165–8).

A missed 'period'

If your next 'period' does not come on, take advice from your doctor/nurse but continue using contraception. This is advisable because absence of this 'withdrawal bleeding' (see p. 16) is rarely due to pregnancy . It would be a pity to become pregnant unnecessarily just because you thought you already were. Taking the pill will not stop the pregnancy test becoming positive. If either you know you did miss pill(s), or you think they were taken regularly but new symptoms like nausea or having to pass urine very frequently occur, you should arrange for a pregnancy test.

Taking the pill in early pregnancy has not been proved to harm babies (see p. 102). All the same, if you do strongly suspect that you might be pregnant as a result of a pill-taking muddle, most doctors recommend that you transfer to using something like the condom method, carefully, until you know one way or another.

But if you have absolutely no reason to suspect reduced protection (including no vomiting or possible interaction with another medicine), then it is normally best to start the next packet even if there is no bleeding in a particular pill-free week. It would only be necessary to arrange a pregnancy test if you either went on to miss a second period, or began getting the symptoms of pregnancy.

Other causes of reduced protection

Stomach upsets

You can 'miss' pills by severe vomiting: it means the same for the body as forgetting to take pills. The risk of breakthrough egg release and of breakthrough bleeding are increased in just the same way. The advice to be followed is therefore not different to Fig. 3.4, based on when in the packet the vomiting occurred and the number of pills which were not kept down.

If any single episode of *vomiting* was more than *two* hours after pill-taking, according to the WHO no action is required at all, as by then the pill would have passed beyond your stomach. However, if you vomit back a correctly timed pill after less than two hours, you should take another as soon as you feel you will keep it down. If that one stays down and was taken within a day (less than 24 hours) of the vomited tablet then, again, you can continue to rely on the pill as your method. Should your stomach reject a second or even more pills, you should get back to taking tablets as soon as you are able to keep them down, and follow Fig. 3.4.

In summary, following Fig. 3.4 will mean:

- vomited up to four pills in the middle week, days 8–14: no special action
- vomited any pills from days 15–21: go straight on to your next pack
- unable to keep down 2 or more tablets after your pill-free time (for more than two hours), or vomited completely more than 1 pill during days 1–7:
  - take emergency contraception and
  - abstain or use condoms as well
  - while taking the next seven daily tablets.

If you have lost pills through vomiting, extra ones should ideally be taken from a separate packet or maybe from the end of the current packet, so that you can continue taking the right pill for each day of the week. (If you are using a phasic pill (see pp. 160–3), ensure that the replacement from the spare packet is the same colour.)

Diarrhoea alone (without vomiting) has to be 'as bad as cholera' to interfere with the absorption of the pill. If it is like that, which means like water and every few minutes, follow the advice just given for a bad attack of vomiting. Otherwise just keep taking your tablets.

The effect of other medicines on the pill

To be effective, the pill must be absorbed, be transported in the blood, perform its actions, and then be eliminated from the body. A number of other drugs can interfere with some of these complex processes. Such interference (interaction) can lower the blood levels of the pill hormones and so lead to the risk of egg release and therefore pregnancy (see Box 3.3).

*This weakening contraception effect can be caused in various ways. The most important is when *enzyme inducers* need to be prescribed. These

Box 3.3 Important drugs which are suspected of interfering with the pill, causing breakthrough bleeding and increased risk of pregnancy (see text)

Drugs to treat epilepsy

phenobarbitone (Luminal™) and other barbiturates
phenytoin (Epanutin™)
primidone (Mysoline™)
carbamazepine (Tegretol™) and *oxcarbazepine (Trileptal™)*
topiramate (Topamax™)
modafinil (Provigil™)—used to treat excessive sleepiness

Other drugs for epilepsy do not interfere at all, including sodium valproate (Epilim™), clonazepam (Rivotril™), and most newer ones such as lamotrigine (Lamictal™) and vigabatrin (Sabril™). But these may not suit every patient.

Drugs to treat infections

rifampicin (Rimactane™) and *rifabutin* (Mycobutin™) used in the treatment of tuberculosis and some other infections
griseofulvin (Grisovin™)—antifungal

Many other antibiotics, such as amoxicillin (Amoxil™) and tetracyclines, are also under suspicion of interfering minimally with the combined pill only, not the POP—see text, and important note below.

Miscellaneous drugs
Some anti-retroviral drugs used to treat HIV/AIDS (details at www.hiv-druginteractions.org).
St John's Wort ('Nature's Prozac')—its potency as sold is so variable that the CSM advises it is *not used* along with the pill.
Notes:
1. This is not a complete list. Other drug interactions remain to be clarified. Several here have been deliberately omitted because so far there is too little evidence that, in practice, they cause any problem for pill-users. Except for doxycycline which is a tetracycline (see above), anti-malarial drugs are OK.
2. Erythromycin (Erthrocin), co-trimoxazole (Septrin™), and metronidazole (Flagyl™) seem to actually enhance the pill's effects by inhibiting the liver's actions.
3. Italics in this box means the evidence of an interaction is stronger than in the other examples.
4. Common brand names are in brackets.

are medicines which, in addition to whatever may be their main effect, have a simulating action on special liver enzymes which normally inactivate pill hormones before they leave the body via the bowels and in the urine. So more inactivation means weaker contraception.

*Secondly, *broad spectrum antibiotics* are able, when they reach the large bowel, to kill certain 'friendly' bacteria which normally help to keep up the blood levels of the pill's estrogen, so allowing the bowel to reabsorb some of this (which is otherwise on its way out of the body). These antibiotics might therefore lower the estrogen levels. Though this weakens contraception in only a very small number of women (indeed the WHO considers this particular effect 'negligible'), no one knows which. So in UK practice it is still considered safest to assume all women taking these antibiotics might be affected. But fortunately, because of antibiotic resistance developing (explained below), this effect is anyway only short term. Also it does not affect progestogens at all, and therefore causes no problem whatever for users of the POP or injectables or implants.

In general, there are two golden rules:

1. tell the person who prescribes you the pill about all other medicines you are taking;
2. inform any other doctor about to prescribe you *any treatment* that you use the pill.

For safety, ask them specifically about any effect on the pill.

Short-term treatment: a treatment of less than two weeks

If you are put on a relevant medicine, especially one from Box 3.3, use another contraceptive method such as the condom throughout the treatment, and when it finishes continue extra precautions for seven more days; if you are now in the last week of a pack, run on to the next packet without a break.

Long-term treatment: a treatment for more than two weeks (could be much more)

1. *Relevant broad spectrum antibiotics* (*not rifampicin or griseofulvin*). The special system mentioned above, which in some women may help to keep estrogen blood levels up, depends on friendly bacteria in the bowel which are killed by the antibiotic. These become resistant to the antibiotic after about two weeks, and so they come back in large enough numbers to do their good work. This is why extra precautions are unnecessary if you are, say, already on long-term low-dose tetracycline for acne when starting the pill. The only time they are recommended (and not at all by the WHO!) is the other way around, if the antibiotic is started in a current pill-taker. This would be during all the treatment days and for one week thereafter, to a maximum of three weeks (i.e. two weeks plus one for contraceptive safety). If the last week of a pill pack is involved, as usual (Fig. 3.4) you should skip the next contraception-free interval.

2. *Enzyme inducers, used long term.* The drugs concerned are chiefly treatments for tuberculosis or epilepsy. If you are taking such drugs, you should first consider using another method of contraception altogether—perhaps an intrauterine method or injection (see Chapter 10).

After discussion, though, you may be able to continue to take the pill in a special way, which as it is not how the pill is licensed will have to be *authorised by a doctor* as a so-called 'named patient use':

- you should use two tablets totalling 50–60 mcg of the estrogen, making a higher-dose pill to compensate for the lowered blood levels caused by the enzyme inducer. This is still a low-dose pill for you, of course—it is a bit like climbing up a 'down' escalator to stay in the same place;
- you should also take fewer 'contraceptively dangerous' breaks than usual between pill packets, i.e. use the tricycling scheme (see pp. 29–32);
- for added effectiveness, the break after each run of three (or four) packets should be additionally shortened to four days.

Even if the other drug you are taking is not on the list in Box 3.3—but particularly if it is—watch out for bleeding on tablet-taking days (see pp. 165–8 for more details). This bleeding coming on for the first time after starting another drug can be the early warning sign of too low a blood level of the pill's hormones, so occasionally an even stronger pill combination may be required. But this would still be planned to avoid too much hormone *actually in your blood*, rather to be just enough for the pill to be effective in your particular case.

Sometimes breakthrough bleeding (BTB) is just a consequence of the tricycling itself, happening late in a sequence of packs (p. 31). Either way the BTB symptom should always be discussed promptly with whoever prescribes you the pill.

The effect of the pill on other drugs

The opposite kind of interference is also possible, in which the pill alters the action of another drug, usually raising its blood levels. Ciclosporin is an example, used after transplant surgery. Again, the main thing from your point of view is, *if in doubt*, ask if the other drug matters, either way. Very few make an important difference to treatment.

Fortunately, except for that herbal treatment, St John's Wort, none of the medicines available over the counter in the UK seems to weaken the pill's contraceptive effects. And so-called 'recreational' or illegal drugs have loads of other problems, but none of them are known to cause the pill to fail—though they may make the user so spaced-out she fails to take it!

Change of pills from a higher-to a lower- or ultra-low-dose variety

This matter of the different brands of pills will make more sense when you have read Chapter 7. However, the question of changing to a lower-dose pill needs to be considered here, as this is another time when there could be some loss of contraceptive protection. At the changeover time, the steady suppression by the pill of the woman's natural hormones from her pituitary and ovary is reduced, just enough perhaps to allow breakthrough egg release 'on the rebound'. However, once she is safely established on the new ultra-low-dose pill, she is effectively protected against pregnancy. The extra pregnancy risk is only at the time of the changeover and is believed to be small: indeed some experts question if it is real at all. It can be virtually eliminated by taking extra precautions during the first seven pills, if there is the usual gap between packets. More simply, the recommended method is to *start the new lower-dose variety the very next day after finishing the current higher-dose packet.*

If you follow this system, you may have bleeding like a pill 'period' during the first seven days of tablet-taking from your new low-dose packet. Or you may have no bleeding at all until after the end of that new packet. Either is quite normal, and your protection against pregnancy is maintained throughout.

Of course this problem never arises when moving to a definitely higher-dose pill, which can be done after the usual seven-day break. If you are ever left in doubt about what your new pill is, act as though it is lower dose.

Coming off a high-dose pill combination because of stopping an enzyme-inducer drug, e.g. because your epilepsy (pp. 88–9) is now better controlled

Take advice: you should normally stay on the higher dose you are on for one month at least, before going back to the planned single-tablet dose. The reason is that for a considerable time after the inducer drug is stopped, the liver goes on being more efficient than usual at getting rid of the pill's hormones.

For the rules about changing from a combined (ordinary) pill (COC) to a progestogen-only variety (POP) or back again, see Chapter 8.

Side-effects

Side-effects are all going to be considered fully later (Chapters 4 and 5), but a few general points need making in this practical chapter about pill-taking.

Side-effects of any drug are effects extra to the *main actions*, which in the case of the pill are those shown in Table 1.1 (p. 13). They can be good or bad, and the good ones which you can find in Box 2.2 (p. 27) are much too often forgotten. The effects which are unwanted fall into two main types: *common side-effects*, which are almost never serious but do cause enough nuisance or trouble to make some people change to a different pill or perhaps a different method; and *uncommon ones*, some of which can be serious.

Common side-effects

Common side-effects can be subdivided into two groups.

Side-effects related to the bleeding pattern

There are two likely variations to the bleeding pattern:

- breakthrough bleeding and spotting (bleeding or spotting on tablet-taking days—see pp. 164–7)
- absence of pill 'periods' (no bleeding on the tablet-free days—see pp. 14–16, 167–8).

Except on the advice of your doctor, neither problem should be allowed to affect your daily pill-taking routine. Let the pill packet rule your pill-taking, not the bleeding pattern—whatever that may be. Do not stop taking pills before the end of a packet because of bleeding, even if it seems like a period. Pregnancies have happened that way. Just keep taking successive packets and wait for the arrival of the normal bleeding pattern in due course. If in doubt, see your doctor—especially if reduced protection is a possibility.

More details about how these problems can be handled are given in Chapter 7 along with a helpful diagram (Fig. 7.3, pp. 164–8).

Other minor side-effects (so-called: they often do not seem so to the person affected)

These include nausea, headaches, breast tenderness or tingling, gain in weight, vaginal discharge, leg aches and cramps, mild depression, and loss of interest in sex. All these and more have been reported by pill-users. You should not, however, assume the worst. You may well have no side-effects at all and could even feel extra well while taking the pill. This is much more commonly so now that the dose given has been so much reduced. However, every woman reacts in her own way, and the first pill tried is not always the best for you. As there are more than 20 varieties of combined pill, if you do have problems, it is usually possible to find a different brand that suits you better. This is all fully discussed using the idea of 'pill ladders' in Chapter 7 (Figs 7.1, 7.3, 7.4, pp. 154–7, 164–9).

A very important point to remember is to give any particular brand a good try before giving up, and this usually means using it for at least three months. If either the bleeding or other-type minor side-effects occur, they usually do settle down after the first two or three courses of pills. If you look again at the list above, several of the symptoms, such as nausea, breast tenderness, and gain in weight, also happen in the first few months of pregnancy. This is partly because the pill imitates pregnancy in some ways, but it may be just a coincidence that, as in pregnancy, the symptoms usually improve after the third month!

More major or uncommon side-effects, and reasons to stop the pill at once

For completeness I am including here in Box 3.4 a list of those symptoms which, though most unlikely to occur, should lead you to contact a doctor at once and to inform him or her that you are taking the pill. They may or may not mean anything serious or even be anything to do with the pill.

Box 3.4 Important symptoms meaning 'stop the pill'

1. Severe pain in the calf of one leg, especially if linked with swelling (not the aching legs that so many people get, nor simple painless swelling of *both* ankles).
2. Severe central pain in the chest, or severe sharp pains in either side of the chest, aggravated by breathing.
3. Unexplained breathlessness, or cough with blood stained phlegm.
4. Severe pain in the abdomen.
5. Any unusually severe, prolonged headache, particularly if of migraine type, especially if it is the first-ever such attack, or is very different from previous ones, or gets worse with the passage of time, or keeps returning (see pp. 83–8).
6. Loss of part of the field of vision, right or left, either blackness or not; and if not black maybe with a bright zigzag line round it, usually but not necessarily *followed by* a one-sided headache (migraine with aura, see pp. 84–6).
7. *Marked* numbness and tingling coming on quickly to affect one side of the body (e.g. one arm, or the side of the tongue)—this is not to be confused with the carpal tunnel syndrome (see p. 108).
8. Sudden disturbance of the ability to speak normally.
9. A bad fainting attack, or vertigo, or first-ever epileptic fit.
10. A severe and generalized, perhaps painful, skin rash (see p. 107).
11. Jaundice (yellow eyes and skin).

Also, for completeness, three other situations where the pill should (nearly always) be stopped at once:

12. If and when found to have a very high blood pressure (see pp. 77–8);
13. Admission as an emergency to a hospital bed after an accident, or for a major operation;
14. *Any other kind of immobilization*, for any reason—especially for a *broken bone* or *badly torn ligaments in your leg*. These last two are discussed further below.

The symptoms in Box 3.4 mean that any pill user should:

- *stop the pill until further notice* (but transferring of course to another effective method of contraception);
- *come under medical care without delay*, so that the right diagnosis can be made and any necessary treatment started.

Importantly, the vast majority of pill-takers go for years and years without getting a single frightening symptom. Along with sudden immobilization of the whole person or of a limb as the result of an accident, or an emergency operation (p. 139), they are also practically the only reasons important enough for the pill to be stopped at once, in the middle of a packet. For any other symptoms, phone for advice or make a routine appointment to see your doctor and continue to the end of a packet. This reduces the chance of an unplanned pregnancy (and erratic bleeding). What's more, if the doctor is able to reassure you that a symptom from the list above is not due to anything serious and not due to the pill, you can restart pill-taking, following the rules of Fig. 3.4.

More about immobilization

Immobilization means being confined to bed, as might occur rather suddenly—for instance, after an accident. Should this happen, it is vital that you tell the hospital doctor you are on the pill and (almost always) stop the pill at once. Being kept in bed makes blood-clotting in the veins of the leg more probable, and the pill may increase that risk.

Having to live in a wheelchair is normally WHO 3 ('OK to use with caution', see p. 26), but can be WHO 4 ('do not use') if the thrombosis risk is considered to be above average, e.g. if the person is overweight as well.

IMPORTANT! Broken bone or badly torn ligaments in your leg. Immobilization might be of just part of the body, such as the leg after a fracture, not the whole person: but it is still essential to discuss stopping the pill. Thrombosis can occur in that immobile limb, so much so that the doctors who treat people with fractures or torn ligaments from the ski-slopes often put them on blood-thinning treatments anyway, like warfarin. If that is not done, at least the pill should be stopped. In a survey at the Margaret Pyke Centre, only one pill-taker in 10 knew they should stop the pill if they ever broke a leg.

Major operations, most leg operations, and varicose veins treatments

These important reasons for definitely stopping the pill, but in a more planned way, are discussed on p. 139.

Coming off the pill (routinely)

First, there is no need to make any routine breaks from the pill every few months or years in order to preserve your fertility or for any other reason (pp. 121–2). The pill is (truly) such a medically safe product, with such benefits on periods, etc., that it is not a bit illogical to stay on it even after the bust-up of a relationship, i.e. during the gap before you actually need it again for contraception.

If you do decide to stop it and use a non-hormonal method, it is very common for the first spontaneous or natural period to be a bit delayed. Two-thirds of women have their first period by six weeks after their last pill 'period', and by six months nearly all have got back their own periods. If this, or anything else, is a worry to you, do not hesitate to discuss it with your family doctor or with the clinic doctor who prescribes you the pill. Actually, many women find out the hard way that their fertility is in fine shape after stopping the pill—by getting pregnant so very easily that they cannot believe it! So if you are not ready for a baby, be warned and consider staying on the pill; or at least use another contraceptively safe method from the day you stop.

Even the first seven days off the pill are not OK, as you might think. The ability to have sex during the regular seven-day gap after each pack without conceiving depends a lot on starting the next one on time *afterwards*; as well as on correct use of the previous pack of course (see pp. 39–40).

Note that you cannot use the usual fertility awareness methods after stopping the pill. These are unreliable, generally, until after two normal periods have happened.

If after stopping the pill and getting the usual pill 'period' your next proper period is late, you may be worried that your new method of family planning has let you down. In that case wait until it is at least four weeks since your last pill 'period' started. Then arrange a pregnancy test on a small amount of your first urine of the day. Commonly it will be negative and remain so if repeated, until you see your first natural period in due course. But see your doctor or family-planning nurse if you have other symptoms, particularly pain which could (rarely) be from an ectopic (p. 96). This would happen because of a previously damaged tube, perhaps from a Chlamydia infection years earlier that you never knew you had (p. 22, 95)—and the pill would have been stopping you from getting the ectopic (perhaps for many years), just like it stops the more normal kind of pregnancy.

In about 1–2 per cent of women the first period is very much delayed, and if so it is sensible to take medical advice—but not until six months have gone by. Then a few tests are important, to check that your pituitary gland and ovaries are in good working order, though currently 'resting'. See pp. 100–2 for more about absence of periods.

Stopping the pill to have a baby

Women who stop the pill to have a planned baby are still usually advised to use another contraceptive method, such as the condom, until they have seen one natural period—which means one later than the bleeding which followed a few days after the last packet of pills. Box 3.5 gives a useful practical summary of this chapter so far.

Box 3.5 Take-home messages for a new pill-taker

After a doctor or nurse has assessed from your medical and family history that you are suitable to take the pill:

1. Your FPA information leaflet: this is not to be read and thrown away, it is something to keep safely in a drawer somewhere, for ongoing reference
2. It's worth asking for an ED pack (p. 40). The pill only works if you take it correctly: with any type of packaging, each new pack will always start on the same day of the week
3. Even if bleeding, like a 'period', occurs (BTB), carry on pill-taking. You can ring for advice if necessary. Nausea is another common early symptom. Both usually settle as your body gets used to the pill
4. Love-making during the seven days after any packet is only safe if you do go on to the next one: otherwise (if you are stopping the pill for any reason), start using a method like condoms after the last pill in the pack
5. Even if your 'period' (withdrawal bleed) has not stopped yet, never start your next packet late. This is because the pill-free interval (PFI) is obviously a time when your ovaries are not getting the contraceptive, so might anyway be beginning to escape from its actions
6. For what to do if any pill(s) are more than 24 hours late, see p. 38
7. Other things that may stop the pill from working include vomiting (within two hours) and some drugs (pp. 43, 44–8)
8. See a doctor *at once* if the things on p. 50 occur
9. To make sure all your future pill 'periods' (withdrawal bleeds) avoid weekends: as a one-off, you only need to shorten one PFI (p. 31)
10. You can usually avoid all bleeding on holidays, etc., by running packs together. Discuss this with whoever provides your pills if you want to continue missing out 'periods' long term, i.e. tricycling, pp. 29–31

Box 3.5 *(continued)*

11. Good though it is as a contraceptive, the pill does not give adequate protection against Chlamydia and the other STIs. Whenever in doubt, especially with a new partner, use a condom *as well*
12. Finally, always feel free to telephone or come back at any time (maybe to the practice nurse, or the local FP clinic in the *Yellow Pages*) for any reasons of your own, including any symptoms you would like dealt with. Thereafter there are really only three key things to be checked on during follow-up of the pill method (see also p. 152):
    - Blood pressure (pp. 77–8)
    - Headaches (pp. 83-8)
    - Whether you have any side-effects that bother you, or have been found to have a new disease or risk factor that affects your taking the pill.

Emergency contraception (post-coital contraception)

Available from nurses, doctors, and over-the-counter from pharmacists, the emergency pill—actually two pills swallowed at once, containing the single hormone levonorgestrel—is often called the 'morning-after pill'. This name is unhelpful because, although it works better the earlier it is taken, it can also be started *much later* than the next morning after unprotected sex—up to 72 hours later in fact. The other method, which is to have a copper IUD fitted, works up to five days after unprotected sex or five days after the earliest time you could have released an egg. Having that is obviously more uncomfortable and a bit of a hassle, but the IUD method is the more effective of the two and there can be other reasons to choose it (see below).

Either treatment could be necessary because of a contraceptive 'accident'—a condom rupturing or slipping off, for instance; or of course by being a 'late restarter' of the pill on top of the usual seven-day break (p. 40); or because no method of contraception has been used, perhaps because of alcohol, drugs, or in some cases rape. It acts mainly by stopping egg-release, but sometimes by preventing implantation (pp. 9, 13). Either way in my opinion it is not causing an abortion, though others may disagree (see pp. 207–10 for discussion of some ethical aspects).

How effective is hormonal emergency contraception (EC)?

In any group of women requesting EC, quite a few would not conceive anyway. If taken within 24 hours of the (earliest) unprotected sex it will prevent more than nine out of 10 (95 per cent) of the pregnancies that would have been conceived without EC. If taken later, between 48 and 72 hours, EC should prevent more than half (58 per cent) of the conceptions.

Can anyone use EC?

Almost, yes. Obviously you must be sure you are not already pregnant and a test may be done to confirm this. People with:

- a past history of serious allergy to any ingredients of the tablets (incredibly rare), or with
- a particular rare illness called acute porphyria

should avoid EC pills. And you should mention any treatments:

- medicines which are enzyme inducers (p. 44), including 'Nature's Prozac' (St John's Wort), mean the dose needs increasing. By how much is uncertain, since research is lacking: check with your doctor. Once the single tablet becomes available (p. 58) I believe doubling the dose will be advised.

What next? Does EC go on working afterwards, until my next period?

No. As the hormone method can sometimes work by just *delaying* egg release, not stopping it altogether, it is vital to use a method like the condom right through until the next period starts, sometimes longer when a new method takes some days to become effective.

You will need to think about a suitable future method (see Chapter 10): good choices might be the injection or implant, or maybe a pill or the POP. In all these cases you will normally need to be sure that the next bleeding is truly a period before starting the new method—and if this is before the third day, you can then rely on it right away.

What does 'quick start' mean?

Sometimes a doctor will be willing to advise immediate start of the pill or injection, without waiting for the next period. This is only in special cases where the chances of the EC failing are considered to be particularly low, and you yourself can be 100 per cent relied on to come back for follow-up.

What are the side effects?

Mainly nausea (15 per cent), with vomiting in about 1–2 per cent of women. If a dose is vomited back within two hours it should be replaced. Continuing vomiting may be a reason to use the IUD method instead.

What if hormonal EC fails?

The method can certainly fail, in about 1–3 per cent of cases treated overall, more if the risk was taken around ovulation or if other risks were taken earlier in the cycle. It is a sad fact that 2 per cent of all babies are not normal, so no one can ever be promised a normal baby; but if the method fails the EC pills have not been shown to harm a developing baby. After all, the treatment is given at such an early time, before the embryo even embeds and first starts to receive the mother's blood supply (implantation, see p. 9).

Additionally, if there is already a pregnancy, the hormone treatment has not been shown to cause an abortion. But as with any pregnancy there is a small chance it will be ectopic (p. 96).

Do I have to have an examination?

You will be glad to know that an examination is no longer routine. In individual cases examination might sometimes be necessary for special tests for infection or to check the size of the womb, especially if pregnancy is suspected—and also of course if the IUD method is used.

How will I know it has worked? What follow-up is needed?

If your next period seems normal in length and heaviness, it is unlikely that you will be pregnant. If you are worried, seek advice, but follow-up is usually only if you need it for your ongoing contraception (to see how the pill is suiting, and sometimes to remove a copper IUD [see below] if that was put in only to deal with the emergency situation). But you should always return three to four weeks later:

- if this is recommended in your case
- if your next period is more than seven days overdue or is exceptionally light (which can mean some doubt about whether the method has worked)
- after 'quick starts'
- if you get any abdominal pain. Always report this straight away: the method cannot cause an ectopic pregnancy (see p. 96), but it will not always prevent one in women who have got damaged tubes, something they can have without being aware of it (see pp. 22, 95).

Might I use the emergency pill as my regular method?

This is not a good idea, at least not until we have something much more effective. Even taking just the 1 per cent per month overall failure rate (which is an optimistic rate, anyway, because in the research it was based on only one unprotected sex act per month and a lot of the women treated would not have become pregnant), this rate must be expected each month it was used. This multiplies up to a 13 per cent pregnancy rate in a whole year, which is made up of 13 *lunar monthly cycles*. Irregular bleeding would also be a problem. So although it is not dangerous to use EC more than once, it should really be kept for use in emergency, not used repeatedly as a regular method. The need for it should be removed by arranging a recognized method for the future.

If I am on the regular combined pill or progestogen-only pill (POP) and have forgotten or vomited one or more of them, when would I need to take the emergency pill?

With the ordinary combined pill, many people think the most risky time is mid-packet, when actually that is the best time to miss pills if you must do so! Almost the only time you need to get this emergency after-sex treatment is if you have been more than 24 hours *late restarting a packet after your pill-free week, or have missed more than one pill in the first week of a pack*. See pp. 37–43 for more details; also pp. 181–2 for the advice which applies if you miss POP tablets.

You should take your next regular pill when it is due, and will also need to use an extra method like condoms or avoid sex until your combined pill or POP is effective again (7 days or 2 days, respectively).

Could getting the emergency pill be made less of a hassle? For example, could I have a supply in advance?

If you go to a pharmacy in the UK and some other countries, it already is easier than it used to be—though it will be quite expensive, unless there are special local arrangements. Moreover you can definitely ask for an advance supply if you have a special concern, e.g. because you are going abroad backpacking. Do not make this an excuse for not taking condoms as well, though, and using them in any situation (like a new relationship) where there is a risk of STIs.

Although the hormone EC method is much easier (and more usual), when might inserting a copper IUD be recommended instead?

The main reasons are:

- when you want the most effective method there is—and are prepared to handle the discomfort and potential risks (p. 217) of IUD insertion;

- when it is more than 72 hours but not yet five days after unprotected sex or;
- five days after the earliest time you could have released an egg, when this has been carefully and in good faith calculated by the doctor, working from information from you about your usual cycle lengths. This can make it possible to do something when other risks were also taken earlier in the cycle;
- when you are vomiting so much you wouldn't be able to keep down the tablets;
- because you actually want a copper IUD anyway as your long-term method. Putting one in will then solve both your immediate and your longer-term family-planning problem.

But if the IUD is not a good choice for the long term (as can be so for many, *not all*, who have not as yet had any children), it can also be removed after the next period, having dealt with the immediate crisis. You could wait until a new method, like an injection, implant or pill is fully effective first. Alternatively, if you have very heavy or painful periods your IUD could be exchanged for an IUS (p. 217)—but, unfortunately, the IUS should not itself be used directly in this emergency way.

Postscript: I understand that by the beginning of 2005 the dose for hormonal EC will be available as a single tablet—to be taken, like the current two tablets, as soon as possible after unprotected sex.

4 The effects of the pill, thrombosis, and the circulation

The pregnancy-preventing or contraceptive effects of the pill were described in Chapter 1. The next two chapters summarize what we know about its other effects, starting here with changes in the chemistry of the body, the very important effects the pill can have on the blood—then on the heart, arteries, and veins.

We all know that reading any medical book tends to be rather alarming because we immediately begin to feel that we are suffering from most of the diseases it describes. Do you tend to expect the worst all the time? If so, remind yourself how many millions of women take the pill (see Foreword) and that the majority stay entirely well. The list of side-effects which have ever been linked with the pill is a long one, and the next two chapters are bound to seem a bit threatening to some people. So be sure not to stop there but to carry on and read Chapter 6, to help you to see things in proportion. Provided you are not someone who should avoid the method altogether for medical reasons (see pp. 134–43), the chances of your getting any one of all the complications described here is very small.

Toxicity (poisoning)

One of the very good points about the pill is that, unlike so many drugs on the market, and that includes many such as aspirin and paracetamol which are considered safe enough to buy over the counter, it seems to be almost impossible to take a fatal or even dangerous overdose. Let us be clear what this means: it is certainly possible for particular individuals unexpectedly to be very seriously harmed even by the normal dose of the pill. What I am saying here is that the general 'average person'—whether woman or man, or even a young child—is unlikely to be harmed even by taking a large handful of pills. Toddlers have been known to swallow dozens of their mothers' pills and, apart from feeling or being rather sick at the time, have ended up none the worse for the experience.

If the patient should be a baby girl, after a few days she may well have a 'period'. This is because the hormones have stimulated the lining of her tiny uterus. It therefore grows just as it would do 15 years later in the menstrual cycle, or if she took the pill. Hence, as her body gets rid of the swallowed pill hormones, a harmless hormone withdrawal bleed follows in the usual way (see pp. 13–17).

Without emergency treatment, on the other hand, swallowing a large number of iron or paracetamol (Panadol™) tablets might be fatal. But obviously the pill, like all medicines, should be kept secure and out of the reach of children.

Body chemistry

All the effects to be described later must have their ultimate explanation in the chemistry of the body. So it seems logical to make this our starting-point. More than 100 different laboratory tests on blood, urine, and other bodily fluids have given abnormal results in women on the pill. See Table 4.1, which shows just a few of the more important changes which have been described.

Many of the alterations are similar to those that would be found in normal pregnancy. This is not surprising. It was explained in Chapter 1

Table 4.1 Some changes in body chemistry

	Blood level	Remarks
Liver		
Liver functioning generally	Altered in all users	These many changes cause no apparent harm to the liver itself, except in a tiny minority who develop jaundice. The liver is *involved*, however, in the production of most of the changes in blood level of substances shown in this table, including the important changes in blood sugar, fats, and clotting factors. These changes, hardly shown with the latest pills, may partly explain the increased risk of thrombosis in arteries.
Albumin (the main protein of blood)	↓	
Transaminases (special liver enzymes)	↑	
Amino acids ('building blocks' for body protein)	Altered	
Blood sugar (glucose) after a meal	↑	
Blood fats (lipids)	Altered (mostly ↑)	

Clotting factors generally	mostly ↑	Both the pill and smoking affect these interrelated systems, connected with the risk of thrombosis. Fibrinolysis is enhanced in the blood, but *reduced* in the vessel walls.
Anti-thrombin proteins (special anti-clotting factors)	↓	
Fibrinolysis (the system to get rid of blood clots once formed)	↑	
Tendency for platelets to stick to each other (platelet aggregation)	↑	
Hormones		
Insulin	↑	These hormone changes are thought to be connected with those affecting blood sugar and blood lipids (above).
Growth hormone	↑	
Steroid hormones from adrenal gland	↑	
Thyroid gland hormones	↑	
Luteinizing hormone (LH)	↓	Lowering the levels of these hormones is essential for the pill's contraceptive actions (see p. 12).
Follicle stimulating hormone (FSH)	↓	
Natural estrogen	↓	
Natural progesterone	↓	
Prolactin	↑	
Minerals and vitamins		
Iron	↑	This is a good effect
Copper	↑	Effects unknown, but not believed to cause any health risk in most pill-users. Pyridoxine is discussed on p. 81.
Zinc	↓	
Vitamins A, K	↑	
Riboflaine, folic acid	↓	
Vitamin B_6 (pyridoxine)	↓	
Vitamin B_{12} (cyanocobalamin)	↓	
Vitamin C (ascorbic acid)	↓	
Binding globulins	↑	These special substances carry hormones and minerals mostly in an inactive way in the blood. Because their levels increase in parallel with them, the effective blood levels of the hormones like from the thyroid or of minerals are not much altered.
Blood viscosity	↑	
Body water	↑	This retention of fluid explains some of the weight gain blamed on the pill (see p. 64).

Table 4.1 *(Continued)*

	Blood level	Remarks
Factors affecting blood pressure	Altered	
Renin substrate	↑	This is a very complicated story. Changes do not correlate as well as expected with the actual blood pressure levels.
Renin activity	↑	
Angiotensin II	↑	
Immunity/allergy system		
Number of white blood cells	↑	
Immunoglobulins (antibodies)	Altered	See p. 109.
Function of the lymphocytes	Altered	

Notes:

1. *In the table arrow up ↑ means the level usually goes up, arrow down ↓ means the level tends to go down. 'Altered' means that the changes are known to be more complex, with both increases and decreases occurring in different substances within the system concerned.*
2. *These changes make it extra important, if any blood tests are required, to tell any doctor you are on the pill.*

that, from the body's point of view, being on the pill in many ways mimics being pregnant. The fact that these changes are similar to those in pregnancy is somewhat reassuring. Pregnancy after all is a perfectly 'normal' condition, and many women have a whole succession of pregnancies and live long and healthy lives. On the other hand, pregnancy is linked with an increased risk of several conditions, including thrombosis, which I shall be considering shortly in connection with the pill.

In spite of much research, we have as yet no idea what some of the changes in body chemistry mean in practice. Quite a number, such as the changes in blood-clotting factors, connected with estrogen, have an obvious link with one of the known side-effects of the pill. Others which are so far unexplained may in due course be shown to lie behind a known or still unknown unwanted effect, or equally possibly some benefit of the pill. Others could turn out in the end to be entirely neutral changes.

As a general working rule (as proposed by Professor Victor Wynn, of London), to play safe means that '*if we can measure any substance in the pill-user's body, we would like it to be normal—or as near normal as possible*'. So a lot of research is in progress to produce new contraceptives with minimal effects on the system.

One consequence of the changes in the body chemistry is that whenever you visit a doctor it is most important to remind him if you are on the pill.

This is particularly necessary if some specimen, such as a blood test, is going to be sent to a laboratory. The laboratory may be unable to interpret the results of the test satisfactorily unless this information is given.

Effects on the blood levels of sugar and of fats

The earlier pill types altered glucose or insulin levels and caused changes to lipids (blood fats), similar to those which have been found in some women (and men) who have an above-average risk of heart attacks and strokes because of disease of their arteries. However, the newer pills in current use have less adverse effects on the lipids. And as we shall see later, in the child-bearing years the risk of heart attack and, with one exception (p. 84), of strokes is not increased by any pill on its own: you have to have an added risk factor like smoking.

If even before taking the pill you are known to have one of the rare disorders causing abnormal blood fats—sometimes called hyperlipidaemia—and you are informed that this already increases your risk of a heart attack, then the *combined* pill should be avoided (WHO 4 or sometimes 3). A family history of heart attacks or strokes occurring in young near relatives under the age of 45 is an important clue to this potential problem. If this applies to you, discuss the matter with your doctor even if you will not be taking the pill—you may be found to need a special diet or other treatment.

Effects on the body's own hormones

Some of the more important changes to the body's hormones which have been discovered are listed in Table 4.1. See the various comments in the Remarks column.

The thyroid gland

Although the total level of thyroid hormones rises in the blood, they are chiefly carried in an inactive way by the special thyroid hormone-binding globulin. So their effects on the body are generally not altered. In fact, there is now some reason to believe that the pill may actually protect the user against thyroid disease. This beneficial effect of the pill seems to apply to both over-activity and under-activity of the gland.

Effects on blood levels of minerals and vitamins

The vitamin and mineral changes shown in Table 4.1 have not been shown to cause any harm at all to most women. They have caused concern to some nutritionists that pill use might cause symptoms of deficiency diseases in poorly nourished women. However, studies among such women in developing countries have in general not confirmed this fear. And the WHO found that women who were already short of vitamins showed no further decrease in measured levels after one year's use of the pill.

Folic acid and vitamin B_{12} help to produce normal red blood cells. Anaemia due to the shortage of either of these substances has been described in pill-users, but very rarely and then only in women on poor diets. It might in fact have been a coincidence that they were pill-takers. The more frequent kind of anaemia due to shortage of iron is much less common. This is explained by the fact that pill-users tend to have lighter periods and therefore to lose less iron from the body each month in the menstrual blood.

The lowered levels of most vitamins may even be healthy and appropriate as the body adapts to being on the pill. *There is believed to be no true shortage. So pill-users should not feel pressurized to take extra vitamins,* whether by an expensive 'pill protection formula' or from any other source. The main thing is to rely on a normal diet, including plenty of fruit and vegetables.

In earlier editions of this book, research was reported that suggested that taking additional vitamin C could have the effect of turning a low-dose pill into a high-dose one, and result in more marked effects on the clotting factors. That research has now been disproved by the same experts in Liverpool doing more detailed work, and they no longer recommend taking each drug at a different time, four hours apart. *However,* it is now known that *grapefruit* juice, because of other ingredients it contains called flavonoids, should not be drunk in large amounts by pill-takers. It will raise the blood levels of ethinylestradiol. Ideally take your pill at a time which is four hours removed from when you drink your grapefruit juice!

See pp. 81 and 102 for more about *pyridoxine* and *folic acid.*

Retention of fluid and weight gain

Retention of fluid occurs more in some women than others, and is due to some complicated adjustments to body chemistry among pill-users. Except in certain types of heart and kidney disease (in which extra fluid can be dangerous and your doctor would not normally be recommending the pill), this seems to be quite harmless. It does, however, cause some of the weight gain for which the pill is often blamed, perhaps about a kilogram or so, just because of extra water being in the body. This is very temporary and the weight is lost if the pill is stopped. Some users notice in fact that they shed the extra weight regularly during the seven-day break from pill-taking each month. Yasmin™ (see below) can help a few women who get symptoms like breast swelling and bloatedness along with this kind of cyclical weight gain connected with fluid.

Fear of gaining weight is one of the things which most puts women off the pill. Yet in in a study of two modern ultra-low-dose pills (Femodette™ and Mercilon™), 70 per cent of the users of both brands stayed the same weight in the first year (plus or minus 2 kg). The remaining 30 per cent was split exactly, half (15 per cent) of the women actually lost more than 2 kg, with the rest (15 per cent) putting on more than 2 kg. That really adds up to the pill having had a zero effect with random or unconnected ups and downs over the year. But you can clearly see how the 15 per cent who put on the weight could so easily blame the pill unfairly.

Yasmin is discussed later (p. 157), its chief added advantage above some other pills being that it is good for acne. Its progestogen called drospirenone is a weak diuretic (meaning it helps get rid of fluid from the body) and since this fluid loss makes anyone slightly lighter, it got the unjustified reputation for being a good pill for not putting on weight. But as just mentioned we now know that other pills are equally 'weight neutral' for most people.

If, despite all that, weight gain after going on the pill seems to be a real problem in your case, make sure you discuss perhaps trying a different brand before you throw the method out of the window—pregnancy causes weight gain too!

Being actually overweight already will be coming up again below (pp. 71, 146), as it can be a reason to avoid the pill method altogether or maybe use it with caution; it is an important 'risk factor' for thrombosis in a vein or artery.

The prospective studies: how do we know about the pill's effects?

Much of the information in this book about the pill's effects, whether wanted or unwanted, came originally from the Oral Contraception Study organized by the Royal College of General Practitioners (RCGP). The study began in 1968 when about 23 000 pill-users from the practices of 1400 family doctors all over Britain were matched up with another 23 000 similar women who were not taking the pill. Ever since that time every episode of disease, treated at home or requiring hospital admission, and all pregnancies and of course deaths were recorded. Many women discontinued the pill for one reason or another, so that eventually there were three groups: pill-takers, ex-takers, and never-users. The ex-takers have been studied carefully for any possible harmful effects and also benefits of the pill which might carry on even after it was stopped.

Three similar prospective studies (forward-looking, following up pill-takers, and comparing with non-takers) supplement the information from the RCGP Study. One, referred to as the Oxford/FPA Study, was organized by the FPA working with Professor Vessey of Oxford University. Full details were obtained of all the hospital attendances of 17 032 women who were recruited between 1968 and 1974 from FPA clinics throughout Britain. A little over half the women were on the pill when first seen, the others used the cap or an IUD.

The Walnut Creek Study is named after a suburban township near San Francisco, California. Between 1968 and 1972, 16 638 women had a general health check-up provided by the Kaiser-Permanente Medical Care Program at Walnut Creek. They were subsequently followed up until 1977 and their health details were analysed. Those who had used or were currently using the pill were compared with the remainder, whose methods of contraception (if any) were not recorded. (This is a weakness of the Walnut Creek Study and applies to the RCGP Study as well.)

The American Nurses' Health Study is a big study started in 1976, in which over 121 700 nurses, all women aged 30–55 that year, returned a detailed questionnaire about their contraception, lifestyle, and health. The questionnaire has been repeated every two years since then, with the current and past users of the pill giving us much valuable and mostly reassuring information about their health as compared with those in the same study who have used other methods.

The findings of these four groups of researchers differ in some details but agree in most important respects. Most weight is given in this book, as it should be, to those findings which are *confirmed*:

1. by other studies;
2. by other types of research, in different populations.

The studies show that the overall death rate due to the diseases of the circulation that we are about to discuss is greater in pill-takers than in never-users. With regard to cancer, though, there are slight differences in which cancers pill-takers get and don't get—overall the cancer risk is not apparently increased (pp. 110–19). Among current users there is little evidence that increasing duration of use affects any risk, and there is good evidence that there are no persistent ex-use effects. The RCGP Study showed convincingly that the death rate from all causes is identical in ex-pill users after 10 years to that in never-takers.

There are very different risks for different subgroups of pill-users. *As the main serious problem is circulatory disease*, the women chiefly at risk are those with any of the risk factors listed on pp. 71–2, 74–5, 143–8.

Disorders of the circulatory system: bloodstream, heart, arteries, and veins

Most of this next section has to do with one basic problem known as thrombosis, which is the formation of blood clots in veins and (even more rarely) arteries. This causes most of the very rare major troubles blamed on the pill. But it should be remembered that thrombosis is also more likely in pregnancy, which is of course avoided by taking the pill.

The ability to clot is a most important function of the blood

Without the ability to clot, even a small injury to a blood vessel could lead to the injured person bleeding to death. But the estrogen of the pill tends to cause an increase in the blood levels of most of the important clotting factors and often reduces the amount of some important factors which tend to stop the clotting process.

These changes, among others, make clotting more likely to happen where it is *not* wanted—namely, in uninjured arteries and veins. Yet, if the changes occur to some extent in all pill-users, why do so few ever get any kind of thrombosis? An important reason for this seems to be that other systems are brought into play—particularly the one called fibrinolysis, whereby any blood clots which appear in the circulation are removed as fast as they are formed. Thus often, along with the increased tendency to clotting because of the raised clotting factors, there is at the same time a sufficient improvement of this process for getting rid of blood clots. Good health demands a balance between the two mechanisms. In pill-users it seems that this balance tends to be achieved by resetting them both at a higher level.

Very interestingly, it has been found that this balancing increase in fibrinolysis tends not to happen in smokers, especially heavy smokers. If smokers then take the pill, their increased clotting factors will no longer be counteracted by a better clot-removing system. Moreover, in the blood there are small particles which, among other things, have the ability to stick to each other at the start of clot formation. The tendency to platelet aggregation, as this process is called, is increased in heavy smokers. These effects partly explain why the most recent research cannot show an effect of the pill to increase the risk of thrombosis of the type occurring in *arteries*, unless the women also smoke (see below).

Clotting can occur either in veins or arteries. Because these are everywhere in the body and the effect of a clot is to block the flow of blood at that point, what exactly happens will depend on whereabouts the blockage has occurred. If an *artery* is involved, then the part of the body supplied by that artery may lose its blood supply altogether and it can be severely damaged. *Veins* take the blood at low pressure back from different parts of the body to the heart. If they are blocked by a blood clot, the effects locally are usually less severe. The trouble with venous clots, however, is that they themselves may move through the bloodstream, by a process known as *embolism*, and finish up somewhere else, where they can do more harm. This is most commonly somewhere in the lungs.

Clotting in veins (venous thrombosis)

Venous thrombosis was the first clotting problem to be linked with the pill, back in 1962. It was particularly highlighted in October 1995 by the UK Government's Committee on the Safety of Medicines (the CSM), causing a mega 'pill-scare'. It is uncommon, but when it happens it is most likely in the large veins of the leg—the so-called deep veins. Given a slightly increased level of clotting factors, which as we have seen the pill's estrogen does cause, the reason that clotting tends to occur in the legs is because the rate of flow is slowest there.

As a rule, thrombosis in a deep vein shows up by pain and tenderness in the calf of the affected leg, aggravated if the ankle joint is bent upwards. There may also be obvious swelling on that side. Whether or not there are these symptoms in the leg, rarely a piece of the blood clot may break off. After travelling in the great veins and right through the heart, it can finish up in the lung (*pulmonary embolism*). The combination of these events is called *venous thrombo-embolism* or VTE for short. If the clot is big enough, this can—in around 2 per cent of cases—even be fatal by stopping the blood flow through the lungs altogether. Otherwise there is a sharp pain in the chest, usually on one side or the other, made worse by every breath, and sometimes a small amount of blood may be coughed up. Hence these symptoms are on the important list on pp. 50–1 of the reasons for promptly stopping the pill. Every pill-taker should have this list of symptoms readily available to her (it is on the FPA leaflet).

The treatment (apart from stopping the pill *immediately, and forever*) is usually by admission to hospital for treatment designed to 'thin' the blood. This is done by drugs called anti-coagulants, and by other treatments which can dissolve clots. Most exceptionally, in a severe case, an urgent operation on the chest to remove the clot may be required.

Like all the conditions in this chapter and the next, this chain of events is not just a pill problem—it can also happen in women who have never taken a pill in their lives, and in men.

The 1995 'pill-scare'

The dust has finally settled on that media 'hype', which followed a letter about this same problem of VTE from the UK's Committee on the Safety of Medicines to all doctors on 18 October 1995. Many women were misled by the scary headlines and TV sound-bites into thinking the pill had been found to be really dangerous. They stopped their pills, didn't always use another method very well, and sadly during the next 12 months a real increase in unplanned conceptions often ending in abortions was the result.

It would have been far better if the same facts had been officially presented by the CSM as (roughly) a halving of the already very tiny risk of VTE with one lot of pills (previously called 'second generation'), rather than as a doubling with the others ('third generation'). The 'safer' progestogens were found to be levonorgestrel (LNG, which is found in Microgynon™) and norethisterone (NET, in TriNovum™).

What they should have said is something like:

- 'recent research has confirmed that all pills are very safe, but
- some pills have been found to be *even safer*, in regard to this one disease of VTE. On top of that, surprisingly
- the even safer ones are the ones that we have had for longest, not the new types.'

This would have come over to the public and all the media as 'the whisky bottle is half full, rather than half empty'. Same truthful statement exactly but it just seems a lot more positive!

Putting it that way round would also have been more accurate scientifically. Later research has confirmed that the 'different' progestogens really are LNG and (to a lesser extent) NET. Given along with the estrogen, which all combined pills contain, they seem to be able to oppose the estrogen's effects on the body. LNG-containing pills are, it seems, able to make the changes in some important blood-clotting factors known as Protein S and 'APC Resistance' less than expected, given the estrogen they contain. This action of LNG matches up with the reduced risk of VTE which was reported in 1995, since if estrogen makes thrombosis more likely, a progestogen which is 'anti' it in a relevant way in the blood would be expected to lessen the risk.

Hence it is no longer implausible, as was thought at first by many, that LNG would reduce the risk of thrombosis below what it would be with a given dose of the estrogen alone. All the other progestogens—the 'third generation' ones called desogestrel (DSG) and gestodene (GSD) and the related ones called norgestimate (NGM), drospirenone (DSP), and cyproterone acetate (CPA)—in this book seem (whatever else they do) not to have that opposing action. In short, when combined with estrogen these progestogens let the estrogen 'do its own thing', and so I call them 'estrogen-dominant' pills. Which is what we want for some conditions like acne that estrogen is good for, but not so welcome if we want the least possible effect on VTE-type thrombosis.

So what does this all mean in practice?

- First, it remains likely that the difference between the two types of pills is even less than the 1995 studies suggested. This is because prescribing practice at the time meant that LNG-containing pills were tending to be used by women who were less likely to get VTE anyway: obviously the LNG would get the credit wrongly in those cases. But, even more importantly:
- All the risks are very small, and the difference between the two kinds of pill especially so.

Let's consider some numbers, based on a worst case scenario (meaning accepting as real the whole difference shown in 1995, although it's probably less):

- Among one million women, each year between 50 and 100 will get a VTE-type thrombosis anyway, without the pill.
- This goes up to 150 for users of LNG- or NET-containing pills and about 250 for the other estrogen-dominant pills.
- So the difference between using (say) Microgynon with LNG—the commonest brand in the UK—and (say) using Marvelon™ without LNG is 100 cases per year.
- Using the top estimate of 2 per cent for the risk of dying from VTE, this means the calculated extra risk of dying from VTE caused by the non-LNG non-NET pills is two per million per year. Now take a look at Fig. 4.1. This risk difference is the same as you would get from just two hours of driving or two minutes on a motorbike.

Hence if a woman chooses, as is entirely her choice after counselling, to get rid of a side-effect (maybe acne spots or a mood problem) by switching from the Microgynon to the Marvelon in our example, all she needs to do *in a whole year* is to avoid two hours of being on the roads in a car and it is as though she was still on the Microgynon, as regards the risk of this one disease!

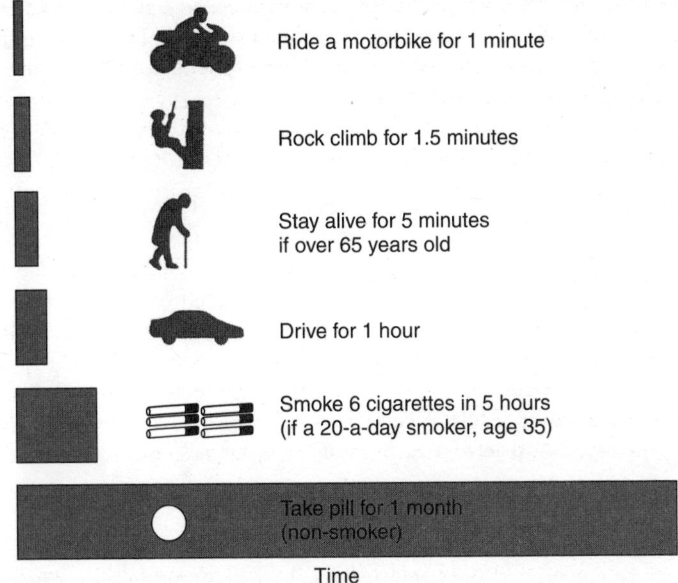

Fig. 4.1 Time required to have a one-in-a-million risk of dying

Adapted from Minerva, British Medical Journal (1988) and from Pharmacoepidemiology (1994).

What a 'storm in a teacup' that pill-scare of 1995 really was! Yet it is still worth not having even a two in a million extra risk if you don't need to, and this is why since 1995 there has been a massive shift in prescribing back towards the pills containing LNG or NET. Indeed in 2004 over 60 per cent of all women in the UK take the formulation in Microgynon. Which is fine as I see it, so long as they know that, if they get side effects, they can shift to one of the less estrogen-dominant non-LNG/NET brands and the extra risk would be so tiny. For more details about what this all means in practice, see 'Which pill?' in Chapter 7.

Other factors affecting venous thrombosis risk

The most important background factors which make clotting in veins more likely (or, as I'd prefer to say, less unlikely) are:

- being overweight or even obese
- being immobile

- not having blood group O (thrombosis in the veins is actually less common in people who have the blood group O. Fortunately, group O is the commonest one, possessed by about half the population)
- heredity, especially:
- having a particular family history.

Always tell the doctor or nurse if there is a history in your family of a close relative (parent, brother, or sister) who had a blood clot somewhere, especially in the leg or the lung, under the age of 45. Usually this means that detailed blood-clotting studies ought to be arranged: if they are not available or prove to be abnormal, you should use another method of family planning, not the pill.

These background factors will be discussed more later (pp. 143–8). In addition to them particular events and situations can increase clotting tendency or cause short-term reduced mobility, or both. These include:

- being unusually sedentary or confined to bed by illness, operation, or accident
- any recent surgical operation (especially bone or leg surgery, or even just having a broken leg in plaster, pp. 139, 147)
- recent pregnancy and delivery
- long-haul journeys, often but not only by aeroplane;
- following dehydration from excessive sweating, e.g. when flat out after a night of clubbing
- smoking. Though it certainly increases the risk of thrombosis in the arteries, it used not to be judged as particularly connected with this kind of thrombosis. However, new research suggests that it *may* affect this kind too.

What about the pill then? The added risk is much reduced in all the low-estrogen varieties, and as we have just seen probably even more so with LNG/NET brands. It is not worse with increasing duration of use, and it goes away quickly if the pill is stopped—within about four weeks.

Moreover, should you yourself, without any obvious explanation ever have suffered in any vein of the body from 'phlebitis' or thrombophlebitis, however minor, which the doctor says involved thrombosis, you should avoid or stop the pill. As a general rule, you also should *never take it in future in case you were to have a more significant thrombosis next time.*

A note on varicose veins

Many women and some doctors wrongly think that you should always avoid the pill if you have varicose veins, even if they have never caused any problems. This is just not so: the type of blood-clotting I am describing here which can be dangerous affects the *deep* veins, particularly of the calf.

Some women who would like to use the pill are frightened to take it because of really almost microscopic varicose veins. *Provided* the other risk factors which were listed above do not apply, and especially if you are not overweight, moderate varicose veins with no signs of any past thrombosis need not stop you going on the pill—one of the LNG/NET 'second generation' ones that have been recommended since October 1995. You may notice that the veins become a little more prominent and that you perhaps get some aching in your legs, particularly if you have to stand for a long time. Only if an actual *major* thrombosis in a varicose vein is ever diagnosed do you need to discuss whether you should avoid the combined pill in future (p. 137).

You should certainly stop the pill four weeks before *varicose-vein surgery*. The same caution is needed for anyone having *injection treatment* for veins, since this works by causing clotting, after which there is scarring inside them to seal them up. To prevent this intended localized clotting being overdone, you should stop the pill a month beforehand, stay off it during the period that you visit your doctor's surgery or the outpatient department for the treatment, and ideally for three months afterwards. During all this time you will, of course, need to use some other reliable method of contraception. As the clotting was caused deliberately, a history of this treatment should not stop you going on the pill once again, provided your doctor agrees.

Clotting in arteries (arterial thrombosis)

The main reason why clotting in arteries occurs is because of a disease of the walls of the arteries. This disease is often called arteriosclerosis ('hardening of the arteries') or atherosclerosis, and affects almost everyone in due course, men usually at a younger age than women. In the more developed countries of the world it has usually started even before the age of 20, and gets more marked as the individual gets older, especially if he or she is a smoker. It affects some much more than others, and one important factor seems to be high levels or an abnormal ratio of the levels of the various blood lipids mentioned earlier.

The changes in blood-clotting factors, especially those which affect the blood platelets, are also important. Once the walls of an artery have been damaged by atherosclerosis, clotting on the surface of the roughened bit of the wall can then occur and eventually this may block up the artery altogether. If it is an important one, such as an artery supplying the heart, the results can be very serious—i.e. a coronary thrombosis or heart attack. If the artery supplies part of the brain, then a cerebral thrombosis may result, leading to one type of stroke.

Once again, any of these events can happen, unfortunately, to women who have never taken a single pill in their lives and to *men*. There's some good news here about the pill in fact: all the recent studies have found the overall arterial disease risk to be essentially absent unless the woman is a smoker, or has one of the other recognized 'risk factors' discussed below.

Coronary thrombosis (heart attack)

A coronary thrombosis is caused by blockage of one of the arteries which supply the heart muscle, causing bad chest pain and—in severe cases—the risk of the heart stopping (cardiac arrest).

Risk factors. In the child-bearing years women almost never get heart attacks unless they are smokers (or have one of the illnesses [see below] which similarly speed up that atherosclerosis disease). You really have to be a smoker first and then yes, unfortunately, the pill is able to increase further your smoking-caused risk of heart attack.

- *Abnormal blood fats.* As discussed (p. 63), there is a group of people who have a 'high blood cholesterol' or other blood fat problem from birth and may be advised either not to take the pill at all, or that another method would be preferable. Many of them know about this, but a lot more do not: the appropriate blood tests need to be done if a near relative (especially mother, father, sister, or brother) suffered a first heart attack or other arterial thrombosis under the age of 45, especially if that relative was a non-smoker.
- *Diabetes whether type 1 or type 2 controlled by diet or tablets.*
- *High blood pressure (pp. 77–8).*
- *Cigarette smoking*, especially if heavy. Coronary thrombosis in otherwise healthy women before the menopause is almost exclusively an illness of smokers.
- *Increasing age*, especially beyond 35 in smokers.
- *Overweight, high BMI* (see Glossary). If the BMI is more than 30 this is WHO 3 (p. 26) for the pill; if it is 40 or more the pill should not be used at all (WHO 4).

- *Migraine.* This only figures as a risk factor for thrombosis in a brain artery leading to a stroke (see pp. 83–8).
- *A blood group other than group O.* (The other groups in this system are group A, B, and AB.) In other words, blood group O, though not routinely tested for, seems to give a bit of protection against clotting in *arteries* as well as in veins.

An important thing to understand about these factors is that, if more than one applies to a particular woman, there is a dramatic increase in the risk she runs. Let us take as an example a healthy 25-year-old woman who is not a diabetic, has normal blood fat levels and blood pressure, and does not smoke. If she starts to smoke cigarettes her chances of a coronary are something like three times greater than before, depending on how many she smokes. But if she swallows a daily pill and also smokes more than 15 cigarettes a day, her risk goes up by at most two for the pill *multiplied* by three (for the smoking), to six times the initial value. Double that if her daily consumption is 30 cigarettes. What would happen if she had a third risk factor, say a sufficiently raised blood pressure to add a further five-times risk? Multiplying again, she would then be five times 12 or up to 60 times less safe than a healthy non-smoker with normal blood pressure not taking the pill.

All these figures are very approximate. Research so far cannot give precise estimates of the risks, and they are only averages anyway whereas every pill-user is a unique individual.

The risk factors in the list above are also relevant to causing other forms of thrombosis in arteries, and to the concerns about some kinds of migraine. This is why they are so prominent in any discussion about who should avoid the pill, or perhaps use it with special supervision (see pp. 143–8).

If you look again at the list it will be clear that there is not a lot you can do about several of them. If you have that high blood cholesterol condition which runs in families, or you are unlucky enough to have diabetes, or have now developed high blood pressure—apart from taking your dietary advice and treatment, managing your stress levels, and increasing physical exercise—there is not much you can do about the situation. Nor, more's the pity, can you make yourself younger or change your blood group. However, if you are overweight you ought to be able to return to the ideal weight for your height (BMI less than 30 or better less than 25) by diet-plus-exercise—and this is well worth doing anyway. But what should be a wake-up call for some, is the number one risk factor that you can do something about, namely *smoking*.

Clotting in the arteries of the brain (cerebral thrombosis)

Cerebral thrombosis can cause one type of stroke: very suddenly the person notices weakness leading to loss of sensation or the ability to move the muscles on one side of the body; or loss of the power of normal speech. Other symptoms may be produced, depending on which part of the brain is damaged. Sometimes there can be almost complete recovery, but some people are left with permanent loss of power or feeling on one side and perhaps impairment of their speech. Stroke in general is very rare among women under the age of 40. However, we now know that the pill increases the risk of this type of stroke, though the risk can be minimized by careful attention to the nature of any migraine headaches (see below).

Strokes caused by bleeding

Among smokers, two varieties of strokes due to bleeding appear to be more likely. One is *intracerebral haemorrhage* (bleeding into the substance of the brain) causing damage and similar symptoms to those after thrombosis in the arteries supplying the same part of the brain. The other is known as *subarachnoid haemorrhage*, or bleeding into the cerebro-spinal fluid which surrounds the brain and spinal cord. This type leads to rapid and often prolonged loss of consciousness, from which the patient may or may not make a slow and not always complete recovery following medical or surgical treatment. Both these rare catastrophes are due to a localized weakness of the wall of an artery in the brain giving way.

There seems to be a very clear link between these strokes and smoking, and a weaker link with the pill if taken as well. *High blood pressure*, whether or not the pill has ever been used, is even more important. Some people are unlucky enough to be born with a weakness somewhere in a brain artery: raised pressure in that artery will make it more likely to give way. A British study concluded from all the known facts that subarachnoid haemorrhage 'should thus probably not be regarded as a serious cause for concern in healthy women using the pill, provided their blood pressure remains in the normal range'.

Prevention of strokes: beware rising blood pressure and severe or strange migraines

Sometimes a stroke may be avoidable by prompt action. This mainly entails stopping the pill if ever the blood pressure is found to be too high.

The pill should also be stopped if certain *unusual headache symptoms* appear. Among *migraine* sufferers, a few notice while taking the pill a marked change in the pattern of their migraine, so that it becomes either more severe or more *focal*, as it is called, with clear-cut asymmetry of their symptoms affecting one part or function of the body. The implications for pill-taking are discussed fully in pp. 83–8, 137, 146.

Thrombosis in other parts of the body

As there are arteries and veins everywhere, so thrombosis can affect other organs than those mentioned so far.

Mesenteric thrombosis

Mesenteric thrombosis is the name given to clotting in an artery or vein which supplies the bowel.

If a large mesenteric *artery* is affected, an emergency operation may be required to remove the affected bowel and stitch together the undamaged parts each side of it.

If one of the main *veins* leading from the bowel is affected, the results can vary between nothing, because the other veins take over, and serious, because of interference with the flow of blood taking absorbed food substances to the liver. There have also been isolated reports of blockage in the veins on the other side of the liver, on the way back to the heart.

The eyes

Exceptionally rarely, venous or arterial thrombosis (*or* bleeding) can cause damage to a part or all of the retina (the light-sensitive part at the back of the eye). This causes loss of vision in the affected eye, which is a disaster if it should be permanent: but it may be only temporary if the pill is stopped and expert treatment started at once.

Raised blood pressure

In most pill-users there is a measurable slight rise in blood pressure. However, in only about one woman out of every 100 who takes modern pills does this reach the level at which doctors term it hypertension. The reason why the rest are not more affected is still not clear. There are certainly changes in the circulation and in body chemistry (see Table 4.1) which may be involved, but those which have been measured often happen also in pill-users without a particularly high blood pressure. Some individuals are known to be more prone generally to raised blood pressure: those with a history of it in their family, those who have had kidney disease, and some black people. The pill may ‘bring out’ the blood-pressure problem in such women, particularly as they get older. One group of researchers has also shown that women with hypertension on the pill have higher levels of the hormone ethinylestradiol in their blood than other pill-users. So perhaps the few individuals who develop this problem are exceptional in the way their bodies absorb and handle the pill's hormones.

Whatever the reason, there are two main points about raised blood pressure. First, it usually does *not* make you feel at all unwell. Second, when large groups of both men and women with even very mild hypertension have been followed up, they have not remained as healthy over the years as comparison groups with entirely normal blood-pressure readings. Blood pressure seems to be linked with nearly all the diseases of the circulatory system and is often a feature of people who later suffer thrombosis in veins, heart attacks, and strokes. It also has the risk itself of becoming uncontrollable, even with drugs, leading to malignant hypertension, which is very rare but fatal.

As raised blood pressure is something that can be readily detected, it can be used as an early warning sign of other circulation problems with which it seems to be linked. *It is obviously vital, therefore, if you use the pill, that you have your blood pressure taken regularly.* Indeed in routine follow-up (see p. 152), apart from checking on headaches, almost nothing else matters. The pressure is measured in the main artery of the arm, the brachial artery. The highest (systolic) pressure reached in that artery during each pumping action of the heart is the first figure that doctors quote, and should not normally be above 140 mm of mercury. The lowest pressure reached before the next heartbeat is the other measurement, the diastolic pressure, and should not be above 90 mm. Several readings above these levels are needed before mild hypertension is diagnosed (WHO 3 for the pill).

Careful medical supervision is then required, with possibly the trial of a different combined pill (e.g. Yasmin, p. 157). If there are any other risk factors (like smoking in a woman above, say, 30), it would be safest to discontinue the pill at that time rather than persisting to age 35 when all smokers must stop. This then is an example of how *the blood pressure is used as an early warning sign.*

The pill has to be stopped anyway if the upper figure exceeds 160 mm or the lower 100 mm (these figures are those used by the WHO to define the "Do not use" levels, or WHO 4, for the pill method). Just stopping the pill generally brings the blood pressure back to normal within a month or two. Further treatment (with drugs) is rarely required for women during the child-bearing years. All brands of the combined pill tend to cause a recurrence of the problem, and so should be avoided, but the POP and DMPA (see Chapter 8) may be tried, often successfully.

Smoking, age, and the pill

All studies agree that the pill's hazards are heavily concentrated in cigarette smokers and older women. Smoking has been proved to do two things: not only does it increase the risk of getting an arterial disease, it also makes the attack more likely to be fatal. *The pill makes your smoking even more dangerous.*

The Walnut Creek and Nurses' Health Study researchers were even more emphatic. They could show the risk for pill-users who were also smokers, and for non-pill-users who smoked. In the absence of smoking, however, they could demonstrate no effect of the pill at all on arterial disease risk. The more recent reports about heart attacks by the RCGP and the Oxford/FPA studies say exactly the same thing. Of course this does not prove complete safety for non-smoking pill-takers, partly because the venous-thrombosis/pulmonary-embolism risk (see pp. 68–70) is still there, though less than with the older high-estrogen pills. Also this kind of research is not sensitive enough for us to say not finding a risk means no risk. But we can say that, if the risk is now undetectable, it must have become extremely small.

Why? Partly it seems because prescribers now know better who should avoid the pill, partly because we have available much safer brands than before, and partly because of better supervision and monitoring of pill-takers as the years go by.

These facts, plus a greater understanding of the *benefits* of the pill for older women (see pp. 105, 116–17), led the relevant Medical Advisory Committee of the American Food and Drugs Administration (FDA) to make an extremely important statement on 26 October 1989. This was a red-letter day for *choice* for pill-users. The Committee advised that *for women free of all risk factors, including excess weight and smoking, there need no longer be any upper age limit for the pill.* This instantly helped a large group of women who had previously been told that they must use another method from age 35 or perhaps 40 up to the menopause (in practice this is taken as age 51, p. 121). But there was *no change in the upper age limit for heavy smokers: this is still 35 years.* (The WHO would allow light or moderate smokers, <15 per day, to continue on a WHO 3 basis [p. 26], but this is not UK practice. And even WHO 3 means another method would definitely be preferable). *Fundamentally the combination of smoking with the inevitable steady increase of arterial risk with age produces an unacceptable combination.*

To avoid the pill but to continue puffing away, in response to the facts about the relative dangers of the pill and of smoking, is to 'strain out a mosquito and swallow a camel'; or a bit like a stunt motorcyclist refusing to play golf for fear of injury.

Smoking in effect ages your arteries and increases the risk of most diseases of the circulation for all women (and men), regardless of their method of family planning. On top of that, smokers are accepting some pretty frightening hazards, including bronchitis, cancer of the lung, larynx, bladder, and cervix, reduced fertility, and even gangrene of the legs. (The last four and others not listed are indirect through the effect of chemicals absorbed from the smoke into the bloodstream.) One in four smokers dies earlier than he or she would have done otherwise of a disease related to smoking: a bit like Russian roulette with only four rather than six chambers in the revolver!

Of course, you can get injured by a golf ball, and the pill certainly does have problems. But if you put together all of them mentioned in this chapter and the next, it still does not put the pill into the same league as the cigarette. And if you add the pill to your cigarettes, you make smoking even more dangerous than it would otherwise be.

The obvious if difficult answer is to get rid of the smoking—*research shows it is always worth giving up.* After a few years ex-smokers have no greater chance of dying than lifetime non-smokers. By stopping smoking they even benefit those around them. Breathing other people's cigarette smoke is dangerous for non-smokers, especially young children (not to mention the risks to unborn babies if their mothers smoke). Then there is the effect of example: 90 per cent of adult smokers began before they were aged 20.

Oddly enough, however, most surveys show that pill-users are *more* likely than users of most other methods to be smokers! This shows that the risk of the combination in young women is acceptably low; though not nearly as low as if the smoking was stopped.

5 Other side-effects of the pill

This chapter resembles a conducted tour of the systems of the body. Conditions which are primarily caused by a *disorder of the circulation* were dealt with in the previous chapter. This applies, for example, to strokes, which are disorders of the brain and central nervous system but are caused by arterial disease, and have therefore already been discussed. Within each system, the more common known unwanted effects are considered before those that are rare, followed by the known good effects.

The brain and central nervous system

Depression

The link between depression and the pill is a bit complicated. First, any depression which comes on regularly premenstrually in the normal menstrual cycle is, naturally, most commonly *improved* by the pill. Secondly, in the Oxford/FPA Study (see p. 66) there was shown to be no increase in the risk of severe depression—or indeed of any mental disorder so bad as to require a specialist opinion or admission to hospital.

However, most researchers do find that among women using the pill a few more than the expected number complain of mild or moderate depression. And there could sometimes be an explanation in body chemistry because, as shown in Table 4.1 (see pp. 60–2), pyridoxine (vitamin B_6) levels are lowered in the blood of some depressed pill-users. This vitamin is known to be involved in producing certain amines of the brain, substances which affect how it functions. Depressed pill-users with lowered levels of pyridoxine, but not those who were equally depressed with normal blood levels of the vitamin, did notice an improvement in one study in which they were given extra amounts of this vitamin every day. But most experts are against making it a routine that pill-users who complain of depression are given pyridoxine. The treatment would not benefit those who did not lack this vitamin. Those who lack it might be helped, so some doctors therefore prescribe it. A dose of 50 mg per day is plenty and should do no harm so far as we know. Foods that are rich in pyridoxine include wheatgerm, liver, meats, fish, milk, bananas, and peanuts.

As a matter of fact, it is very unlikely that most depression reported among pill-users is really due to the pill. The excess rate in the RCGP Study (see p. 65) was only about 30 per cent. Now depression is very common, and affects practically everyone—men as well as women—at some time or another. The pill is commonly used, so depression and use of the pill might well come together by coincidence. The pill may be blamed when really the depression is due to a combination of factors in the woman's whole life. But these may be so hard to tackle that it is very understandable to hope that stopping the pill will be the answer.

Another point is that the pill-users in the RCGP Study had to go to their doctor more often just to pick up their prescriptions, and so would be more likely than the non-users to mention the fact if they were depressed. This could lead to a bias against the pill. But if for the sake of argument we blame the pill for the whole 30 per cent excess noted among users, that still means that, out of every 130 depressed pill-users, 100 cannot really blame their depression on the method.

The pill has such a reputation for causing depression that this is one of the commonest reasons given by women who stop using it. Many could be giving it up unnecessarily. (Some of them may end up with a very depressing unplanned pregnancy.) Having said that, it is still true that there is a group of women who do find that their mood improves when they stop taking the pill and worsens whenever they start it again.

So, what should you do if you become depressed while taking the pill? The best advice is to discuss the whole matter with your doctor or nurse. Could there be other reasons for your mood change? Moving to a lower-dose pill may help, or to a different progestogen (see pp. 168–9, 171), and this is certainly worth a try if this is the only problem before transferring to another method altogether. Your doctor might suggest a trial of pyridoxine. If he or she suggests stronger treatment with an anti-depressant or tranquillizer, you may want to discuss whether another highly effective method of contraception such as the new IUS (see p. 217) might be preferable.

Loss of libido (interest in sex)

Loss of libido can happen as part of depression, but also for other reasons, such as relationship problems. Few people realize how common it is, especially after a recent pregnancy. Many women start taking the pill after having a baby, and blame the pill for the depression and loss of sex drive that follows, when they are really part of the postnatal 'blues'. Another possible explanation is that some women still feel that sex is primarily for making babies, and, as taking the pill makes pregnancy extremely unlikely, they lose their interest in love-making. However, these two explanations are not the whole story. Like depression, it is undeniable that some cases are indeed caused by the pill.

Just like normal men have a little estrogen in their blood, androgens are hormones produced in low amounts in women. Among other things they help to promote normal sex drive. There are a couple of pill brands known as Dianette™ and Yasmin containing progestogens that also have *anti*-androgen effects. This makes them good for conditions like acne, but if loss of libido came on after starting one of these it would certainly be worth trying a brand without the particular progestogens they contain (p. 170). Talk it all out with your partner, before and after seeing your doctor or nurse. Changing pills to one containing a different progestogen may help, even if you are not on one of the two brands just mentioned. Otherwise a simple solution can be that the vagina seems drier in some women because of loss of the natural lubrication. If this is the problem, it can be helped considerably by using something like a jelly lubricant (Sensilube™ or KY™) regularly, applied either to you or to him, just before love-making.

In a few cases the doctor may recommend some special sessions of counselling for you and your partner, to improve your general and sexual relationship. Only rarely should it be necessary for you to give up the pill solely because of loss of sex-drive.

Many women report an improvement in their sex lives once they go on the pill. Indeed most surveys have shown that, in general, pill-users have more intercourse than non-users each month. This may be because the pill avoids the 'turn-off' effect which some couples find with alternative methods. Or it may reduce the regular loss of libido due to premenstrual tension (PMT) which many women get in their (so-called) 'normal' menstrual cycles.

Migraine: a specially important matter for women using or about to use the pill

Migraines are unpleasant, variable, often severe headaches which definitely 'stop the person doing things'. They are usually one-sided and accompanied by sickness or actual vomiting. There are commonly other symptoms like extreme intolerance of bright lights (photophobia) or noise (phonophobia), and in the important type called 'migraine with aura' there are—*before* the headache starts—very specific short-lived disturbances of vision.

There is much disagreement as to what causes migraine. Changes in hormone levels can be an important trigger, which is why some women mainly or only get migraines when the hormone levels drop just before their periods when not on the pill, or while on it—see below—before or during their hormone-withdrawal bleeds (p. 30).

An important factor can be something in the diet: for instance, cheese, chocolate, sherry, and red wine are rich in an amine (tyramine), and can all precipitate migraine in some women. Whether or not they decide to take the pill, it can be helpful to avoid these foods.

Stress and allergy may also be factors in some people; smoking is highly relevant; and three out of every four migraine sufferers have a family history of some relative with the same problem.

How does migraine affect taking the pill?

Studies have shown a risk of the rare kind of *stroke due to thrombosis* in migraine sufferers and this is increased if they also take the pill.

There are certain features of the migraine which particularly go with this stroke risk—these are symptoms given the special name of aura, and always start before the headache. *It's very important to known about this, as having aura means the ordinary pill should not be used (WHO 4).*

So what is this 'aura'?

The word is used for strange symptoms, nearly always (99% of cases) affecting the eyes: typically the loss of part of the field of vision on the same side in both eyes. People tend to think at first that it's a problem in one of their eyes, but if they cover up each in turn they discover that the aura affects part of what each eye sees. Often there is a bright zig-zag line which gradually enlarges to form a big C-shape surrounding the bright (not black) area of lost vision.

Funny sensations may also happen, in about one-third of cases, but nearly always there is something affecting the eyes as well. There could be pins and needles spreading up one arm or one side of the face or the tongue. Some notice a particular disturbance of speech: they find it temporarily impossible to say the names of things, objects that they know perfectly well.

The timing is crucial: aura begins before the headache itself and typically lasts around 20–30 minutes. The headache may start as the aura goes away. Or there may be a gap of up to one hour. Occasionally the strange symptoms occur but no headache follows.

What things connected with a migraine are not 'aura'?

- Any symptoms along with the headache itself, like the photophobia or generalized eye blurring or other eye symptoms only occurring during the headache.
- Aura symptoms should also not be confused with *premonitions* that some people get a day or so beforehand: these can take the form of unusual tiredness or cravings for special tastes.
- Much more serious, though not aura, would be dark loss of vision (i.e. real blindness) in one eye, or loss of muscle power or sensation affecting the leg as well as arm on one side. These suggest a thrombosis has actually happened and would be reasons for going straight to the emergency department of a hospital: they still mean stopping the pill, but they are not 'migraine with aura'.

How can I be sure if what I get is or isn't really aura?

Dr Anne MacGregor of the City of London Migraine Clinic (www.colmc.org.uk) has a most useful tip, for use by doctors, nurses, or patients: people with true aura 'always' use a hand beside their head to describe their *pre*-headache eye symptoms.

They usually wave their hand beside their head and/or they draw a zig-zag line in the air on the same side as their partial loss of proper vision. Indeed if they don't bring up a hand beside their head at all in that way, they are unlikely to have true aura and so can usually take the pill if they want to.

As well as aura, what else increases the risk, rare though it is, of a stroke from thrombosis?

As usual, these are the risk factors on p. 74, especially smoking, raised blood pressure, diabetes, significantly overweight, and increasing age above 35 years.

What does this all add up to, in practice?

Only relatively few migraine-prone women must always avoid the (ordinary *combined*) pill (see Box 5.1).

If you are in one of these groups, even for you absolutely any of the methods which don't contain estrogen may be offered straight away—such as a POP or an injectable or implant or intrauterine method (see Chapter 10). You cannot be promised you will not get the bad headaches in future, but there will no longer be an *added* risk of getting a stroke.

Box 5.1 What kinds of migraine are WHO 4 ('do not use') for the COC?

- Any migraine with aura. It is the artificial estrogen that needs to be stopped and avoided in future. Aura with no headache following still means WHO 4.
- Other migraines even without aura if they are exceptionally severe, lasting more than 72 hours despite adjusting medication.
- Migraine which is being treated with ergotamine-containing products (check with your doctor or nurse).
- Migraines without aura but with two or more additional arterial risk factors (e.g. smoking plus being very overweight, BMI above 30).

Box 5.2 explains the case for others with migraine, where WHO 3 or even just 2 applies, and the diagram in Fig. 5.1 usefully puts it all together.

When they first go on the pill, a few women actually report some improvement in their migraines (without aura, of course). Rather more say that the pill makes their attacks more frequent, or has even brought this

Box 5.2 Migraine, but COC is usable at patient's choice after discussion

- WHO 3: migraine without aura with just one risk factor (see Fig. 5.1).
- A distant past history of migraine with aura. If this was five years earlier or only during pregnancy and there's been no recurrence, the pill may be started or restarted on a trial basis as WHO 3 ('cautiously usable'). But the woman must understand clearly what aura is (see description above) and what to do if it ever comes back:
  - stop the pill immediately
  - use alternative contraception (e.g. condoms in the short term)
  - seek medical advice as soon as possible.
- For the remaining migraine-prone women, the pill is 'Broadly usable' (WHO 2). This includes all with migraine *without aura* and not a single risk factor, and any drug treatment except ergotamine.
- If a woman is seen by a doctor during her first-ever attack of migraine without aura while taking the pill, it is usually recommended she stops the pill. But if there were no features of aura and no important risk factors, the pill can be restarted (WHO 2) with the usual teaching about what aura is (and what it would mean if she ever got it later on).

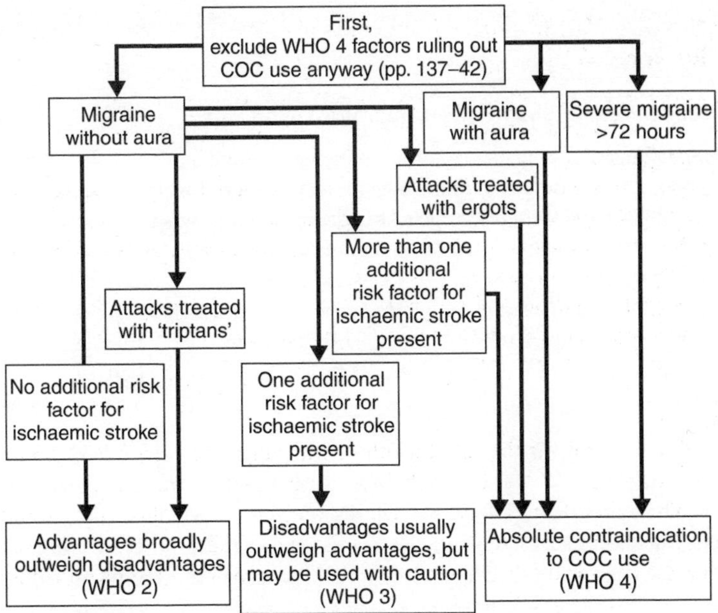

Fig. 5.1 Flow diagram for COC use and migraine

Reproduced from MacGregor, A., Guillebaud, J. (1998). British Journal of Family Planning, 24, 53–60.

problem on for the very first time. The headaches may only occur during the seven days while the woman is not taking tablets, probably because of the sudden drop in the hormone levels. A possible short-term solution is then, provided the headaches are never preceded by those aura symptoms, to take any ultra-low-dose monophasic combined pill on the tricycle basis described on pp. 29–31. For this purpose, a pill from as near as possible to the bottom of one of the 'ladders' in Chapter 7 (Fig. 7.1, p. 155) should be chosen. Transferring to a progestogen-only method like the POP (Chapter 8) can sometimes help, as this is taken steadily every day, with no hormone-free weeks. A third possible option which Dr MacGregor has studied is to stay taking your combined pill in the usual way, but use 100 mcg estrogen *patches* each day during the pill-free week. You could ask your doctor if you would like to try this.

Note that strokes, though serious, are very rare in young women with migraine, even with aura and even if they are rash enough to smoke. The reason for all the above cautionary words about the pill is to make them even more so.

When in doubt, discuss any strange symptoms promptly with your doctor.

Headaches: ordinary (non-migraine) type

Headaches are of course very common in women not taking the pill and also in men. Thus it is hard to know how much the pill can really be blamed for headaches that pill-users may get. After depression, this was the second commonest reason women cited for giving up the method in the RCGP Study. Apart from taking painkillers if necessary, the treatment is to use the very lowest-dose pill that suits you in other ways. If the headaches happen mostly during the pill-free week, your doctor may recommend the tricycle regime (see pp. 29–31), as for the tolerable non-focal migraines just discussed above. You could also try changing the progestogen in your pill—transferring to a different 'ladder' (see Fig. 7.1, pp. 154–5).

Epilepsy

The pill does not *cause* epilepsy. In fact many sufferers report fewer attacks when they go on the pill, especially if their attacks tend to come on either pre- or during periods in their normal cycles. However, a very few do get more frequent epileptic attacks, and may have to give up the method. There is also the distinct possibility that the tablets they take to control fits may interfere with the hormones of the pill once absorbed into the body, and reduce the protection it provides against pregnancy (see pp. 44–8). There are now a number of anti-epileptic drugs (sodium valproate, clonazepam, vigabatrin, lamotrigine) which do *not* do this, but they are not necessarily sufficient for all patients.

Those who are on the relevant treatments (the liver enzyme inducers shown in Box 3.3 on p. 44) should discuss the whole matter with their doctor. They may decide to use another method such as the injection, the IUD, or the IUS—the last (p. 217) has proved ideal for many women with epilepsy—but the pill can still be used (on a WHO 3 basis, p. 26) if that is what the woman strongly prefers. If so, it should definitely be a combination containing at least 50–60 mcg of estrogen to bring the pill method back up to strength despite the weakening effect of the enzyme-inducer medicine(s).

Tricycling. Since the pill-free break is the contraceptively risky time (pp. 37–43), I recommend that long-term users of these medicines which weaken the pill simply have fewer, shorter breaks. In other words, the woman *tricycles the pill* (pp. 29–31), taking three or even four packs of pills in a row, *without any breaks* at all. After that, a shortened gap between runs of packets is logical, usually four days. The woman should be more than usually careful to take her tablets regularly and will also have to report promptly back to the surgery or clinic should she develop breakthrough bleeding on tablet-taking days.

If that happens, she might be advised to run fewer packs in a row together (e.g. 'bicycling two packets in a row'). Or, it might rarely be judged appropriate to prescribe three pills a day. To her body this would still only be the same as taking one pill. The extra hormones are being got rid of faster by the anti-epileptic medication speeding up the liver's metabolism. This leaves only the same amount in the system as other pill-takers would get from one pill a day. It's a bit like climbing up a down escalator to stay in the same place.

Chorea

This rare condition causes the patient to make strange uncontrolled fidgety movements of the head, arms, and legs. It may have occurred in the past, during an attack of rheumatic fever or in pregnancy. With or without such a history, it has been found to happen in one or two pill-users. It generally seems to clear up if the pill is discontinued (and usually avoided in future).

Benign intracranial pressure, now known as benign intracranial hypertension (BICH) or 'pseudo-tumour cerebri'

This strange and rare condition of headache and loss of vision in many ways imitates a brain tumour. It nearly always occurs in young women who are distinctly overweight. Other drugs can cause it and cases occurring in pill-takers are not necessarily caused by the pill at all. However, it certainly might be to blame when, after investigation, the real problem is found to be thrombosis of certain important veins in the brain. In either type, urgent treatment to preserve the eyesight is needed.

If either BICH or the brain vein thrombosis problem is ever diagnosed: to be on the safe side, eye specialists recommend that all types of contraceptive hormone treatment should be discontinued and are WHO 4 thereafter (even the progestogen-only methods).

The eyes

Problems with contact lenses

Some contact-lens-users find that their eyes get sore for the first time when they start the pill. A possible reason seems to be that there is a slight corneal oedema, or increase in the amount of fluid in the cornea (the transparent covering in front of the iris). A possible reduction in tear production has also been reported.

If the eyes do become really uncomfortable, it is important that you do not persevere too long and that you take the lenses out to give the eyes a rest. (Otherwise it is possible to damage the surface of the sensitive cornea, or even cause a corneal ulcer.) You should then discuss the matter with your optician. This complaint is definitely less common with modern lenses, and with modern ultra-low-dose pills, indeed these days the FPA helpline "almost never" receives calls about this.

Other eye problems

Quite a range of eye problems have been reported in women who were taking the pill. In many of them pill-use may well have been coincidental. For example, no link has been proved between the pill and glaucoma (in which there is a rise in the pressure of the fluid within the eyeball).

See also p. 77 for *retinal thrombosis*, which can be a rare but very serious pill complication.

The respiratory system: air passages and lungs

Allergic rhinitis (hay fever)

Hay fever can sometimes become a problem for the first time when a woman starts taking the pill. The pill seems to be able to alter the immune systems of the body (see Table 4.1 and pp. 60,109), so this could be a genuine effect of the pill, though not yet proved to be so.

Asthma

Asthma does not appear to start for the first time more commonly in pill-users than other women, probably because it is a problem which tends to run in families and rarely starts for the first time in adults. Some women, especially those whose asthma is always worse premenstrually, notice that their symptoms are improved on the pill. In a few, they are worsened, maybe (again) because of the pill affecting an allergic factor in the asthma. In the majority there is no change. So the pill is an appropriate choice in asthma.

See also p. 68 for *pulmonary embolism*, which is really a condition of the big veins in the circulation although it finishes by affecting the lungs.

Disorders of the digestive system

Nausea (queasiness)

With modern pills nausea is quite uncommon, except in women who are underweight—including therefore many pill-users from the developing world. If you do get it, it can be bad—particularly during the first few days of pill-taking after the pill-free time, from each of the first two or three packets—and then usually disappears for ever. Perseverance, or taking the pills with a drink and a little food at bedtime so that you are asleep when the symptom appears, should be all you have to do. Otherwise see your doctor or clinic, perhaps for a lower dose of estrogen in the pill.

Do not forget the possibility that the nausea might be due to pregnancy, of course, particularly if it appears for the first time after several months of not getting it. Arrange a pregnancy test if in any doubt.

Duodenal ulcers

Here we have a possible (not certain) good effect of the pill. Both the RCGP Study and the Oxford/FPA Study are agreed that women on the pill were less likely than non-users to require treatment for severe indigestion due to this type of ulcer. However, it is hard to rule out the possibility that the anxious person who is prone to get such ulcers will also be particularly unlikely to use the pill.

Inflammatory bowel diseases (Crohn's disease and ulcerative colitis)

These uncommon but unpleasant bowel diseases cause pain and diarrhoea. In some research the diseases were more common in pill-takers. But in a big group of patients whose disease was well controlled with treatment, the women on the pill were no more likely to suffer flare-ups than the others. So that makes these conditions WHO 2 for the pill, generally.

A complication affecting the liver called sclerosing cholangitis means the pill should not be used (WHO 4). Also, if any patient gets a bad attack of bowel trouble itself, needing hospitalization, there is an increased risk of thrombosis. So the pill should be stopped and remain WHO 4 as long as the disease is severe. If all went well thereafter she could use it again (WHO 3).

Despite the diarrhoea the hormones are usually absorbed normally, so there is no need to take a stronger brand. Absorption could be affected in one of the conditions (Crohn's disease) if it badly affects the small bowel—meaning WHO 3 and a non-oral method (injection, implant, IUD, or IUS) would then be preferable.

See p. 77 for *mesenteric thrombosis*, which can go on to bowel trouble.

The liver and gall bladder

The liver has special receptors for sex hormones, and therefore its many functions are often influenced by the pill (see Table 4.1). The alterations—in clotting factors and blood fats, for example—mean that the liver is probably behind most of the unwanted effects of the pill which occur elsewhere.

Fortunately in most women the liver itself is not apparently harmed in any way. Exceptions are below, and see p. 118, *liver tumours.*

Jaundice

Jaundice is the sign of several liver diseases which make the skin and the eyeballs go a yellow colour. The reason for this is an increase in the amount of a yellow substance called bilirubin in the blood. Bilirubin is normally present in the bile, which is a fluid produced by the liver and carried in ducts to the small bowel. This fluid helps in the digestion of food.

If the liver is damaged from any other disease, usually causing at least some jaundice, the pill is stopped until after recovery (p. 140).

A very small number of pill-users may get jaundice of a special type, due to blockage within the substance of the liver to this flow of bile (cholestatic jaundice). There is then back-pressure, so that some of the bile spills over into the general bloodstream, so causing yellowness and also itching. If it is thought to have been caused by the pill, this means it should not be used again (WHO 4).

The same type of jaundice can occur sometimes in late pregnancy. In fact, if you had this jaundice in pregnancy, or if you had troublesome itching in late pregnancy which was produced by this liver disease, then you will be advised that it is usually best to avoid using the combined Pill (WHO 3) in future, in case it causes a recurrence.

Gallstones

The gall bladder is the reservoir for bile. Bile is a very saturated solution, and it has been shown that the hormones of the pill tend to make it even more saturated. In a few women this can lead to crystals separating out, followed by stone formation. The symptoms which may be caused by stones are a type of indigestion or heavy feeling in the upper part of the abdomen, particularly after meals containing a lot of fat. There may also be nausea and actual vomiting. More severe pain or jaundice may lead to hospital admission.

Apart from the obvious course of stopping the pill, treatment can be medical or surgical. Dissolving the stones with special drugs may be successful, otherwise they are removed, along with the gall bladder—nowadays often by keyhole techniques. Complete recovery of full health is the rule. And after definitive surgery the pill may once again be an option for you (WHO 2).

The urinary system

Cystitis and other urinary infections

Cystitis is the name for infection of the bladder. If the urine is cultured in the laboratory, a germ may be grown and the correct treatment is then usually an antibiotic. An increased tendency to cystitis has been found among pill-users in some studies. Even when there are no symptoms, bacteria are grown more commonly from the urine of pill-users than other women, and this would make actual infections more likely.

Women on the pill tend to have intercourse frequently, and frequent or vigorous love-making can cause cystitis—you may have heard of 'honeymoon cystitis'. Whether or not the pill is truly to blame for such infections, for some women they can be a real problem. If this is so for you, discuss the matter with your doctor. There are also some useful home treatments: for more on this ask for a leaflet about cystitis. It will probably help to empty your bladder both before and after intercourse and to use a lubricating jelly. You should take plenty of fluids—up to three litres in three hours—when you get an attack. Your doctor may sometimes advise taking a couple of antibiotic tablets shortly before intercourse as a regular preventive routine. Tests for vaginal infections such as thrush (p. 94) may also be necessary, as these infections can cause similar symptoms.

The reproductive system—gynaecology

Vaginal dryness and discharge

A few women on the pill complain of excessive dryness of the vagina. This can be quite a problem for some, and may be partly responsible for a loss of interest in sex. It can be due to thrush (see below). Or it can mean that a pill with relatively too high a dose of progestogen is being used (see p. 170). So you could ask for a change of pill. It may also help to 'slow down', with a bit more foreplay before penetrative intercourse; or occasionally to use a lubricating jelly such as KY or Sensilube. Be straight with yourself, though, and with your partner. Could the problem really be more to do with some aspect of your sexual relationship rather than the pill? Maybe some sex counselling would be more important than a change of pill brand or any lubricant.

Other pill-users complain of the opposite, an increase in their vaginal discharge. This might be due to the following.

Cervical erosion (preferred name 'cervical ectopy')

'Erosion' is a most misleading and unfortunate name for a common, quite harmless condition of the cervix. The normal covering of the outer surface of the cervix is what is known as squamous epithelium—that is, a covering of flattened cells a little like normal skin. The normal lining of the canal that leads up into the main part of the uterus itself is columnar epithelium (upright, box-shaped cells with a lot of mucus-producing glands). All that happens if there is an 'erosion' is that the normal glands lining the canal spread out over the outer part of the cervix. So it is not an 'ulcer', and nothing has been eroded or eaten away! It just looked like that to the doctors who gave it that name, before anyone had studied its structure under the microscope.

Ectopy (a much better name) is more common in pill-users than in non-users. The effect of having more of the type of surface which normally only lines the cervical canal is to have more mucus-producing glands: and hence an increase in the normal wetness of the vagina. Many women, pill-users or not, have this without noticing anything, but a few may call it a discharge.

All that is usually necessary is for the doctor to examine you and to take a cervical smear if you are due to have one. If, however, you are finding the amount of discharge a nuisance, perhaps requiring you to use a tampon or pad to control it, then there are very simple and painless out-patient treatments which can be arranged.

Thrush—otherwise known as candida or monilial infection

All three of these words apply to the same thing. It is due to a little yeast which is a very common inhabitant of the vagina, often in fact living there without causing any symptoms at all. However, it can cause an attack of intense itching of the vagina and vulva and sometimes burning on passing water, with or very *often without* a curdy, white vaginal discharge. It is more common in pregnancy, after a course of antibiotics, in women with even very mild diabetes, and seemingly in users of the older, high-estrogen pills.

Surprisingly to many, *the pill does not cause thrush.* Indeed those last six words were used as the title of a paper some years ago in the *British Journal of Obstetrics and Gynaecology.* If you get thrush, on the pill or off it, ask your pharmacist for some 'over-the-counter' treatment, usually with pessaries and cream.There is also an oral treatment, useful particularly in resistant cases.

In some women thrush is very troublesome, and keeps recurring. They, and also their partners, may then require extra help, perhaps from a genitourinary medicine (GUM) department.

Trichomonas vaginitis (TV)

There is some evidence from studies that this common STI, causing an itchy, fluid vaginal discharge, is *less* frequent than usual among pill-users. However, there is no proof as yet of this beneficial effect. If it occurs, as when Chlamydia is diagnosed, remember that checking for other infections, and getting your partner or partners properly treated as well as yourself, is vital—and that means visiting a GUM clinic.

Anaerobic vaginosis (AV) (or bacterial vaginosis)

This cause of a fishy-smelling discharge shares the same medicine as first choice for treatment as TV, but like thrush it has no known connection (either way) with the pill.

Pelvic infection

Pelvic infection is usually due to an STI, particularly Chlamydia but also gonorrhoea. It can seriously damage the uterine tubes, leading to infertility and/or the risk of ectopic pregnancy. Researchers in the USA and elsewhere have found that pill-users have half the rate of this kind of infection, compared with those using no contraception. This good effect is probably due mainly to the same mucus changes in the cervix which were described on p. 13, caused by progestogen. The altered mucus seems to obstruct bacteria as well as sperm (very probably they 'hitch-hike' because they are actually attached to the sperm!). This reduces, but does not of course remove, the risk of pelvic infections spreading up to the tubes. It is a useful benefit but not something to rely on—more effective choices to avoid these sexually transmitted infections are monogamy or condoms.

Toxic-shock syndrome

This is caused by a toxin (poison) getting into the bloodstream. The toxin, produced by a bacterium, the Staphylococcus, multiplying in the vagina, causes a high fever, bright red skin rash, vomiting, diarrhoea, and low blood pressure. The condition was given much publicity because of its link with menstrual tampons. It is extremely rare, the more so if women change their tampons frequently. But it is dangerous, and evidence is emerging that pill-users are even *less* likely to get it than other women. Another good effect!

Ectopic pregnancy

This is the name for a pregnancy in the wrong place—usually in a tube, instead of in the cavity of the uterus. It can lead to dangerous internal bleeding. While a woman takes the pill, she is (almost) completely protected from this, because she is not releasing eggs. Damaged tubes are the main cause of the problem, so if she has these she could still get an ectopic pregnancy later, after stopping the pill. But the pill makes even this less likely because, as we have just seen, it reduces the risk of pelvic infection while it is taken, and —worldwide— that is the main cause of tubal damage.

Fibroids

Here we find another *benefit* of the pill. Fibroids are lumps which can grow on the uterus. They are so common that most women get them eventually, though the size can vary from a pinhead to (rarely) something as large as a football. They consist of muscle and fibrous tissue. You will probably have heard of them as one of the causes of excessively heavy periods (menorrhagia) in some women in their late thirties or forties, who therefore require a hysterectomy (removal of the uterus). They are not cancerous. Indeed in most women no treatment at all is ever required.

How does the pill affect fibroids? First, by not causing them to appear in the first place. But in the days of the old-fashioned high-estrogen brands, in some individuals fibroids were noticed to grow very rapidly if they started on the pill. The same sudden increase in size is sometimes seen in pregnancy, and both in pregnancy and on the pill a fibroid can suffer what is known as 'red degeneration'. This is due to breakdown of tissue within it and causes pain.

However, the two main UK prospective studies (the RCGP Study and the Oxford/FPA Study) are now agreed that fibroids are *less* commonly diagnosed in users of low-estrogen pills than in non-users, and if they are present are *less* likely to require hospital referral. The heavy periods which lead to the diagnosis of fibroids if they are present simply do not happen on the pill, because the pill almost always diminishes bleeding from the uterus.

If fibroids are diagnosed, one of the more progestogen-dominant brands is best (see pp. 156, 170), or another method like an injectable or implant or the IUS. In most women the pill reduces the bleeding trouble that they may cause. But because in a few individuals the fibroids may enlarge, women found to have them should have regular annual examinations, with ultrasound scans as required.

Endometriosis

Endometriosis is an uncommon condition which is not entirely understood but causes misery to some women. Each month they suffer from a severe aching or bruising pain before and during the period, worsened by intercourse. This is described as being different in type from menstrual cramps, though it can be just as severe. They may also have to be seen by a gynaecologist for medical or perhaps surgical treatment before they can have a baby.

It is due to some of the same kind of tissue which normally lines the uterus being present in the wrong place—such as in the ovaries (where it is one cause of cysts) or elsewhere in the reproductive system, or even further afield. How this endometrium reached these sites is often unexplained. But, just as it bleeds in its correct place, in the uterus, so this wrongly situated endometrium bleeds regularly at period times; and bleeding into the tissues causes bruising pain. As in the uterus, the bleeding results from the fall in blood levels of estrogen and progestogen.

Continuous treatment or tricycling with a high-progestogen combined pill, or with similar hormones, to abolish egg release and therefore periods is logical and is often used as a way of preventing relapse if endometriosis has already needed treatment. A few studies have also suggested that this condition is also less likely to be diagnosed in the first place among women who take the pill in the ordinary way, and tricycling (as in Seasonale, p. 30) is expected to further increase the benefit.

Cysts on the ovary

Here we have another advantage of the pill: there are certain ovarian cysts (known as functional cysts) which are commoner in women who are not on the combined pill. These are not tumours: they are balloons containing fluid entirely surrounded by a tissue capsule, developing within the ovary. They are thought to arise because of minor imbalances in the normal menstrual cycle. They start life as a follicle, stimulated to grow by FSH during the first half of the cycle, as described in Chapter 1. However, instead of the follicle rupturing to release an egg, or simply losing its fluid and virtually disappearing like the other 19 or so stimulated follicles do, the mechanism can go a bit wrong. Instead, a particular follicle goes on accumulating fluid to produce a cyst. This can be just a few centimetres in size or grow to a fluid-filled bag up to 10 cm or more in size. (The egg it originally contained dies, of course, and is disposed of by the body in the normal way.)

Such cysts are usually painless but can sometimes cause quite bad pain, including pain on intercourse. They may cure themselves (by losing their contained fluid), or rarely lead to an emergency laparoscopy operation—especially if the cyst causes the whole ovary on either side to twist (torsion).

The good news for pill-takers is that the ovaries are made inactive and no follicles are stimulated to accumulate fluid ready for ovulation. Hence things are less likely to go wrong so as to produce this type of cyst. Here is a way that the combined pill may reduce the need for surgery.

There is a suspicion that the very lowest-dose pills may not suppress the activity of follicles so well and so may produce less of this benefit. And the progestogen-only pill described in Chapter 8 actually increases the risk of these functional cysts (see p. 186).

Polycystic ovarian syndrome (PCOS)

This is a different kind of cyst-producing condition in which little cysts appear all around the outside of the ovaries. It produces the wrong balance of hormones, including more androgen (male hormone) than would be normal in a woman (of course some is produced by all women). PCOS is not made either more or less likely through pill-taking, but the pill can be very beneficial in the treatment of its symptoms (chiefly acne and sometimes abnormal hair growth)—so long as the right kind of pill, an estrogen-dominant one, is chosen—see pp. 156, 171. When they stop the pill, some women can conceive a wanted baby without problems. But not infrequently PCOS does lead to the need for infertility treatment, especially in overweight women.

See also pp. 116–17 for two enormously important good gynaecological effects of the pill, considered separately: the reduction of the risk of *cancer of the ovary* and of *cancer of the endometrium.*

The menstrual cycle

For most women, almost everything about periods and the so-called 'normal' cycle is improved if they take the pill. I say so-called 'normal', because as a gynaecologist I know that many women suffer some extremely annoying symptoms from their normal cycles. These can be any or all of the following: short cycles (every three weeks or so); irregularity; ovulation pain (Mittelschmerz); premenstrual tension; painful periods (dysmenorrhoea); and heavy periods leading sometimes to anaemia. The 'normal' can be anything but 'nice'. (If men suffered similarly, how many would agree to such a catalogue of irritations being called normal, I wonder!)

However, since the pill abolishes the natural menstrual cycle altogether, and replaces it with an apparent cycle caused simply by the fact that the pill's hormone is withdrawn for seven days in each 28, most of these symptoms are dramatically improved. So much so that many women can be very reluctant to give up the pill, even if they should, perhaps, for reasons such as smoking, or being very overweight, and above age 35.

Periods

If you take the pill in the ordinary way, with regular breaks from pill-taking, you will notice that your 'periods' are very *regular* and can be accurately predicted and are usually also much *lighter.* As an extra bonus you are much *less likely to become anaemic.* This is because heavy periods can cause anaemia because more iron (in the blood) is lost from the body than you are able to take in your diet.

If you normally suffer with *painful periods*, then the chances are also very good that these will be improved if you go on the pill. Indeed many teenagers take it for this reason alone, even when they need no contraception. Period pains are caused by excessive contractions of the uterus, due mainly to substances called prostaglandins, released during the period. It seems that the thinner type of endometrium which develops in women on the pill causes less of these pain-producing substances to be released. Strangely, however, a few women, especially if underweight, actually complain of more menstrual cramping if they take the pill, especially some brands (the phasic ones). They may be helped by a single phase (monophasic) pill, and even more if it is 'tricycled' by running on the packets, as explained on pp. 29–31.

See pp. 164–8 for how to handle abnormalities in the bleeding pattern produced by the pill.

Ability to control the periods

This is another advantage of the pill. You have so much control that it is even possible, though not the normal routine, to take the combined pill continuously and then have no vaginal bleeding at all. This is perfectly acceptable short term, because of holidays and exams, and longer term when tricycling. You can also as a 'once-off' ploy start a new pack early, with a shorter pill-free week, to make sure you never have periods at weekends, for instance. This is all discussed on pp. 14, 29–31, and 162–3 (about phasic pills, which have special rules).

Mittelschmerz

This word means 'middle pain' and refers to the pain which signals ovulation or egg release. Quite a lot of women feel this slight ache in one or the other side of the groin, at around the middle of the cycle. In some months in a few women it can be very severe. The pain is due to the stretching of the rest of the ovary by the growing follicle at the middle of the cycle before it ruptures to release the egg: and when it does there may also be a small amount of painful internal bleeding. If the pain comes from the right ovary and is particularly severe, it can be very difficult to distinguish from appendicitis. Normal use of the pill prevents ovulation and so avoids both the regular monthly pain and this possibility of a mistaken diagnosis, which has been known even to lead to an unnecessary operation.

Premenstrual problems

In the days leading up to the next period, many women are troubled by depression, irritability, feelings of bloatedness, weight gain, tenderness of the breasts, backache, and headache. These and other symptoms are often lumped together as the so-called 'premenstrual syndrome', or 'premenstrual tension'. Just how awful this makes this time of the month varies enormously from woman to woman, and from cycle to cycle in the same woman. But the symptoms can be very bad. Statistics show that some women are more likely to have accidents, do less well than expected in exams, or even commit suicide at this time of the month than any other.

Probably because the pill gives a constant dose of both types of hormone, estrogen and progestogen, through the second half of the cycle, quite a lot of sufferers from premenstrual tension find it improved if they take the pill—especially if they tricycle it (pp. 29–31). However, some are not helped. And a few even complain of similar symptoms while taking the pill, particularly if it is a phasic pill (see p. 163).

The reproductive system—fertility and babies

Return of fertility after stopping the pill

From the beginning, doctors have been aware of the possibility that the pill, which acts by switching off the normal menstrual cycle, might delay its normal return. This might interfere with the ability of ex-pill-users to have babies when they wanted them. In fact every new year of research seems to reassure us more about this, culminating in a 2002 study of 8497 expectant mothers in the west of England. It was found that if they had used the pill for more than five years before they stopped to try for a baby, they had conceived faster than women who had never taken the pill! This and lots of other evidence shows that the pill probably improves fertility and certainly does not cause infertility.

But it can sometimes seem that way. There is a substantial minority of 10–15 per cent of all women who, whatever previous method of family planning they have used, do not become pregnant after trying for a baby for a year. This is the proportion of reduced fertility which is to be expected in any community, partly due in fact to fertility problems in male partners of the women. So, if a woman stops the pill and fails to get pregnant, although it is very natural to blame the pill, it is highly likely to be a coincidence.

Fertility also goes down with age. So sometimes the problem is partly connected with delaying too long before trying for a baby. This is a most important point. All methods of contraception share a common 'side-effect': they give modern women the freedom to delay starting their family, but this can sometimes mean they let their 'biological clock' tick for a bit too long. This is how some women suffer from infertility at 35, yet could have conceived easily at 20. Indeed a few proved that by an earlier unplanned pregnancy. If possible (having found the right father!—not always that easy, I realize), try to start your family in your twenties or early thirties.

Very few women, perhaps one in 200 who stop the pill, develop amenorrhoea—absence of ovulation and periods—for over six months. This is not normal and should be investigated. The pill gets blamed, but the rate is the same among women whose partners stop using the condom, yet no one blames the condom for absent periods! Experts believe that in only a few if any such cases was the pill truly responsible, and even then only by bringing out a natural tendency. Usually the previous pill use was a coincidence, and the regular substitute periods they were having on the pill were *masking* amenorrhoea which they would have had at that time if they were using another method. It has not been linked with any particular brand, has the same causes as when the pill has never been used, and can happen if the pill was used briefly or for a long time. Reassuringly, it is also now possible to treat this fertility problem when there are no periods with almost 100 per cent success.

What about taking a routine break from the pill every two years or so to improve your fertility chances? Everything is against that being necessary (see pp. 121–2). *The bottom line is that the pill is reversible, and on stopping it women get back the fertility that nature gave them—for the age they have now reached.*

Please note too that the problem of absent periods after stopping, or without ever having taken, the pill is a completely different one from absence of 'pill periods'. The latter has absolutely no connection with your chances of having a baby in the future. In fact, those few women discussed above who do have absent periods after stopping the pill very commonly had very regular 'periods'—hormone-withdrawal bleeds—all the time that they were taking it. See pp. 14–16 and 167–8 for further discussion of this matter, which many people find confusing.

Could the pill cause my next baby to be abnormal?

After stopping the pill

Providing the pill was discontinued well before conceiving, researchers have failed to detect any consistent increase—or decrease—in any type of abnormality. An expert scientific group of the WHO declared quite simply in 1981 that there was no evidence for any adverse effects on the fetus of pill use prior to conception—and this remains the considered view of the WHO based on more recent evidence.

What then should you do if you are on the pill and want to stop it for a baby? Those couples who are by nature extra cautious may, in addition, use a method like a condom to arrange that two natural periods or three months go by before their planned baby is conceived. This has not been proved to help, though it should certainly do no harm. You may find it reassuring to know that the vitamin and mineral changes shown in Table 4.1 (pp. 60–2) should all be back to normal by then, though most experts do not think this matters either way.

Should you take extra vitamins? Folic acid in the standard daily dose of 0.4 mg, bought over the counter at any chemist, is definitely advisable. But that is recommended prior to conception (and for the first 12 weeks of pregnancy) for everyone, and not just ex-pill-takers. Otherwise I would advise you only to take extra vitamins in tablet form, either at this time *or after conception*, if so advised by your doctor. A good diet throughout pregnancy plus avoiding, especially in the first third of pregnancy, all avoidable chemicals (certainly cigarettes and alcohol binges—but also ideally any drugs, where possible, and even food additives) is in fact the main thing.

Most importantly, any woman who conceives less than three months after stopping the pill should not be alarmed. Literally millions of mothers have done this without any harm befalling their babies. Any extra risk is unproven, and, if it does exist, it is clearly very, very small.

What about pill-taking actually during early pregnancy?

The RCGP Study researchers reported that 102 babies were born following pregnancies during which the pill continued to be taken for a while, usually by mistake. In the Oxford/FPA Study there were a further 66 such births. The rate of birth defects in these was no higher than would be expected in any group of women having a planned baby. But it seems that in these circumstances twinning may be more likely.

This is reassuring, especially when combined with the encouraging results of major surveillance studies in Scandinavia and elsewhere. Any bad effect on unborn babies of the hormones used in current pills—or if the higher dose in the emergency pill (p. 56) is inadvertently taken by a pregnant woman—must be very infrequent.

What does this mean in practice? Even though there is no proof that the pill could harm a baby, it is surely best to play safe. You should never *start* taking contraceptives or any other hormones (including the emergency pill) if you think you could already be pregnant. And if you think you might have become pregnant while taking the combined or progestogen-only pill, or (more commonly, see p. 242) had already conceived when you re-started either pill:- arrange a pregnancy test without delay.

If pregnancy is confirmed, and you did take contraceptive hormones of any kind of pills *after the conception*, the extra risk of an abnormality is described by the WHO and similar bodies as being 'negligible if not nil'. Not many people realize that 20 in 1000 of all babies have a serious defect at birth. That far higher risk is taken by all would-be parents.

The breasts

Breast enlargement

Most users of the pill notice some enlargement. The increase, not normally more than one bra cup size, is mainly fluid building up through the pill cycle, and it often lessens in the pill-free time. It tends to reach its maximum by the second packet of pills, and in the absence of weight increase your bra size is then likely to be stable until you come off the pill method again.

For some women and their partners, and in most cultures, a bit of non-surgical breast enhancement is seen as an advantage of the pill. Others may not see it this way, though, and if it's a problem to them a change of pill, perhaps to the new pill Yasmin, may help (p. 157).

The appearance of milky fluid from the nipples

Prolactin produced by the pituitary gland is a hormone whose levels in the blood tend to go up in pill-takers and in a few this leads to a milky fluid coming from the nipples. This can be a nuisance and should always be mentioned to your doctor. The level of the hormone ought to be measured, as, if it is particularly high, it could perhaps be coming from a pituitary adenoma, or micro-adenomas. These are 'lumps', tiny or even microscopic in size, formed in the pituitary gland. They can be treated very satisfactorily, either medically or, rarely, by an operation. The pill does not cause them but, like pregnancy, it could make them enlarge and cause dangerous pressure on surrounding structures if present. So, the pill is very much WHO 3 in this rare condition; it should be used only under expert supervision, along with the appropriate medical treatment to control the gland.

Tenderness of the breasts

Tenderness can be part of the whole range of symptoms of premenstrual tension, or it can occur alone. In some unfortunate women the tenderness can be so extreme that for a few days before each period they cannot bear their breasts being touched, even by clothing. If you have this problem (even if not quite as bad as that), you may find you are better off while on the pill. It is possible that you will not be helped; and, confusingly, a few women actually report the symptom for the first time on the pill, especially during the early months. (There is an enormous amount of variation in how people respond to drugs, and the pill is no exception to that rule.)

Breast tenderness and discomfort on one brand may often be helped by switching to a less estrogen-dominant pill (p. 170).

Benign breast disease (BBD)

BBD is the general term used to include a number of non-malignant problems of the breast which may be called fibromas, 'fibrocystic disease', and a variety of other names. They all refer to more or less generalized lumpiness of the breast which can be quite tender and vary from month to month and with the time of the month, usually worst just before a period. Here is a definite plus point for the pill, as the usual type of this breast trouble tends to be less common during pill use, especially long-term pill use. This therefore reduces the risk of special tests and procedures under local or general anaesthesia to make sure that changes or lumps due to this BBD are not due to an early cancer.

Once BBD is present it is a 'risk factor' for breast cancer. So there is a bit of a paradox here. On the one hand, the pill reduces the risk of getting BBD in the first place. But, on the other hand, doctors exercise extra caution if the breasts have the problem already, especially if a lump has had to be operated on. Established BBD is now seen as a so-called 'relative contraindication' (usually WHO 2) to using the pill. If you have ever had breast surgery for BBD, see p. 115(3).

Interference with breastfeeding

The combined pill can affect the volume and quality of milk flow in women who are breastfeeding after recently having had a baby. But it seems pointless to use the combined pill at this time anyway, when the POP is available which does not interfere at all with the flow of milk (see Chapter 8). In combination with full breastfeeding, the POP is close to 100 per cent effective.

See also pp. 110–15 for discussion of *breast cancer.*

Bones and joints

Premature closing of the epiphyses

There is a theoretical effect of estrogen in the pill that it might stop a young girl growing before she had achieved her full height. This idea arose because, in animal research, estrogen can affect the epiphyses (growing points) of the long bones, to cause them to close prematurely. This does not occur with the tiny dose of estrogen in modern pills, which after all contain progestogen as well. The pill should normally not be given until, at the earliest, menstrual cycles have become well and truly established, by which time a girl has almost reached her ultimate height. There are some relevant considerations about pill use in younger women (see pp. 22–3 and 238–42), but this is not one of them.

Arthritis

Women on the pill are less likely to suffer from the more severe forms of the fairly common and very troublesome kind of joint disease known as rheumatoid arthritis. Though some studies have not shown this good effect, most experts now think that use of the pill is definitely beneficial.

Osteoporosis

Osteoporosis means thinning of the bones, making them more likely to fracture even without much trauma. It is a problem chiefly of women past the menopause. But it often begins earlier, in the years leading up to the final menstrual period, as the ovaries work less well. Unless they are treated with estrogen, younger women who are short of estrogen from their own ovaries due to amenorrhoea—often connected with anorexia and weight loss, and sometimes in athletes—can also be affected.

If the ovaries are not fully functional, osteoporosis can be prevented by the pill, as by hormone replacement therapy (HRT), because of the estrogen it contains. As a result, pill-takers have been found to reach the menopause with better bone density than other women—another useful benefit apart from contraception.

So the pill can be of real value to older women free of risk factors who also want contraception (see p. 79). In women of any age at risk of osteoporosis, the pill is a valuable treatment, usually after special tests and under supervision from a hospital consultant.

The skin

Chloasma/melasma

These unusual words describe a fairly common brown discoloration which is mainly on the forehead and on each side of the face in front of the ears. It is obviously not a problem for black-skinned women, but can happen to other races in pregnancy (the 'pregnancy mask'), and, annoyingly, also to pill-users. It is usually first noticed when the weather is good. Some women also notice an increase of pigmentation in other parts of the body.

Chloasma usually fades a little when the pill is stopped, but can recur with progestogen-only methods. It may never entirely disappear, because of pigment having been actually laid down in the skin. Special sunscreen creams can be applied, especially during the summer, and careful use of make-up when required may help.

Photosensitivity (excessive sensitivity to sunlight)

Photosensitivity is reported in pill-takers, though it can affect women who have never been on the pill, and other medicines are more likely than the pill to cause it. If it develops, skin exposed to the sun's rays develops very itchy red weals (urticaria). Treatment for this is unsatisfactory and there may be only a slight improvement if the pill is stopped. It is fairly uncommon, but it may mean that the affected woman has to avoid sunbathing altogether. Very rarely it is the first indication of one of the porphyrias (see p. 140).

Increase in facial or body hair (hirsutism)

Hirsutism is fortunately very rare with the modern low-dose pills, and nearly always has another cause (i.e. being on the pill is a coincidence). Normally it's the other way around—an estrogen-dominant pill with one of the new progestogens such as Yasmin or Dianette may help in the treatment of this (see pp. 157–8). Extra hair may also have to be removed with the help of electrolysis or similar treatment from a skin specialist.

Loss of scalp hair

Loss of scalp hair can also occur in women who have never taken any sex hormones at all. There was no suggestion in the RCGP Study that this might be *caused* by the pill. However, hair growth is always in balance between the growth phase and the loss phase, with different waves of each phase happening all over the head, so that the loss which happens all the time is not normally noticeable. It is well known that pregnancy hormones can affect this, so that a greater proportion of the head hair than usual gets synchronized into the growth phase, which is fine while it produces the lush hair of pregnancy, but worrying after delivery when much more of it than usual is lost all at once. Things then return to the normal pattern.

Dermatologists consider that the pill in some women can do the same as the hormones of pregnancy, by bringing a greater proportion of the head hair than usual into the growth phase, but this all inevitably coming out when the time is up for the loss phase to begin. The good news is that this problem corrects itself spontaneously, though full recovery of decent-length head hair could take a year or more.

Other skin diseases

A range of other skin conditions has been described, occurring for the first time or apparently being worsened in pill-users. Yet others are improved. They tend to have rather complicated names. Out of a long list, those which are probably or possibly promoted by the pill include: telangiectasia, rosacea, eczema, neurodermatitis, erythema nodosum, and erythema multiforme. Some of these may be linked to the problem of allergy (see p. 109 for further discussion).

Pemphigoid gestationis is another one. It is interesting because, like the form of jaundice mentioned on p. 92, it can occur in pregnancy and is likely to recur or worsen if the same woman later goes on the pill (therefore 'do not use', WHO 4).

Even added together, these skin disorders are still uncommon. From the practical point of view, you should take advice from your doctor if you ever develop any skin problem which you think might be due to or made worse by the pill.

Skin troubles often made better by the pill

Acne

The RCGP Study showed that acne was particularly likely to be improved, but at the time all pills had 50 mcg or more of estrogen in them. The story is now a bit more complicated—any benefit depends on which pill you take.

Acne occurs chiefly because the tiny ducts or passages leading from the grease-producing glands of the skin, especially in the face and on the back, tend to get blocked. The estrogen in the pill may help to stop this happening. Some women are simply unlucky in the actual grease-producing glands they have been given by nature, and just going on the pill may not be enough to help the situation. However, if your own acne is not improved or seems to be getting worse on the pill, it is worth asking to change to a more estrogen-dominant brand using one of the new progestogens, such as Marvelon or Cilest™, or in the worse cases Yasmin or Dianette. Choosing such brands does mean accepting a possibly *less low* risk of venous thrombosis (pp. 69–71), compared with the more usual (less estrogen-dominant) types of pills like Microgynon.

There are also other treatments that a family doctor might use, including tetracycline antibiotics which have their own risk of causing photosensitivity (and BICH). Referral to a dermatologist may be necessary in the worse cases or those with hirsutism as well.

Hirsutism

Estrogen-dominant pills, including Yasmin and Dianette, can frequently also help this problem of unwanted hair growth (see p. 106).

NB. Both acne and unwanted hair growth are in reality very often features of PCOS, mentioned on p. 98. If those symptoms are present this can be diagnosed on an ultrasound scan. Fortunately the same type of pills (estrogen-dominant) are good for the treatment, whether or not that ovary problem lies behind the symptoms.

Less greasy hair and less wax in the ears

These are two more benefits of the pill–not hugely important perhaps, but benefits just the same! The wax-producing glands of the ears are affected in the same way by the hormones of the pill as the grease-producing glands of the skin and hair. As a result the RCGP Study also showed that women on pills (primarily the estrogen-dominant ones, again) were less likely to have their ears syringed for wax.

Other side-effects

As well as everything else mentioned in these two chapters, there is some weak evidence, weaker in some cases than others, for the following collection of possible side-effects: the carpal tunnel syndrome, in which there is a gradual onset of tingling and pain in one or both hands; cramps and pains in the legs; gingivitis (inflammation of the gums); dry socket after tooth extraction; voice changes in singers; Raynaud's syndrome (excessive whitening and 'deadness' of the fingers in cold weather); and chilblains.

There remain two very important but more controversial subjects, about which there are still as many questions as answers.

The body's immunity and allergy mechanism

The RCGP, Oxford/FPA, and Walnut Creek studies all showed that pill-users were more likely than non-users to have various infections, including chickenpox, gastric flu, respiratory, and urinary infections. Other inflammations, of soft tissues or of the bowel (tenosynovitis, bursitis, synovitis, and Crohn's disease), have also been reported more commonly in pill-users.

These facts suggest but don't prove that the pill can alter immunity. In addition, various skin troubles are often connected with allergy, and eczema, for instance, was twice as common in pill-users in the RCGP Study. Women can also develop an allergy, with specific antibodies (see Glossary for a further explanation of these), to either the progestogen or the estrogen of the pill itself. This occurs even more rarely than with other commonly used drugs like penicillins, but can show itself by troublesome rashes or by painful swollen joints (polyarthritis). These clear up completely only when the pill is stopped, and would recur if the same hormone were to be given again. So allergies to the pill itself certainly occur. Whether allergies to other substances happen more readily because the pill is being taken is not so clear, though the reported increased rate of hay fever is suggestive (see p. 90).

Another possibility is an allergy to a person's own tissues causing so-called auto-immune diseases. It does appear that the pill can sometimes aggravate the symptoms and signs of one of these, systemic lupus erythematosus (SLE), which affects connective tissues in the body. Thrombosis is more likely in SLE, so if it is diagnosed the pill is usually best avoided anyway (WHO 3, or 4 if the clotting tendency it can cause is established).

The immune/allergy system is involved in causing several types of thyroid disease and arthritis. As the pill seems to have possible protective effects (see pp. 63 and 105), perhaps some good effects too are due to an alteration in this system, caused by the pill's hormones.

What about cancer?

The pill does contain powerful hormones, and hormones have been shown to affect the growth of some cancers, in animals and in humans. So ever since the pill was first marketed there has always been a concern that it might be found to increase the risk of some type of cancer—balanced by a hope it would reduce the risk of another. Secondly, it is one of the best-known facts of cancer research that cancers may not develop until after many years—up to 30 years—of exposure to any cancer-producing agent. The pill has now been around for over 40 years, so we are beginning to obtain useful information about possible links between it and some forms of cancer.

In view of the widespread nature of the pill's effects, we should not be too surprised if it can in fact modify the risk either way: promoting some cancers but actually reducing the likelihood of other types.

So it's a bit like 'swings and roundabouts', or, as in the scales of Fig. 5.2, the good effects are tending to balance the bad. To sum up this section, among pill-takers the overall risk of cancer (anywhere in the body) currently appears about the same as that for the general population.

The breast

During the last four decades the pill has increasingly been used, and breast cancer rates have risen in many countries. In the United States, one in every 11 women will develop breast cancer at some time in her life (though many die, years later, of something quite different), and in the UK the

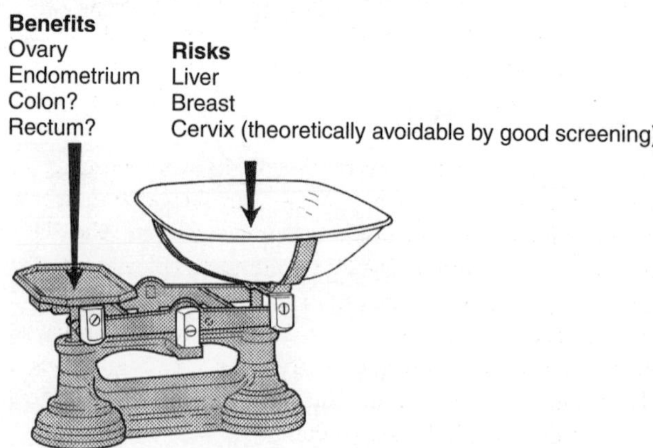

Fig. 5.2 Cancer and the pill: a balance

Box 5.3 Known risk factors for breast cancer

- Younger ages at the first menstrual period.
- Later ages at the menopause.
- More women delaying the birth of their first child to after age 30. (This is known to increase breast cancer rates, whichever method of family planning is used to do the delaying.)
- The family history of a close relative (mother or sister) with breast cancer, especially if it was diagnosed under age 40.
- More people being overweight.
- Possibly, the fact that more people are eating high-fat diets even at normal weights.
- Possibly, drugs like antibiotics; or other chemicals due to modern-day pollution of our air, water, or food. But surprisingly, smoking has not been shown to affect this cancer, unlike many other common cancers.
- The strongest risk factor of all, however, is *increasing age* (meaning more years of exposure of the breast to female hormones, whether from the ovaries or the pill). As a non-user of the pill the risk of breast cancer in young women is very small, being one in 500 in women up to age 35. But the cumulative (all added together) risk increases with age thereafter, to one in 100 at age 45.

figure is one in 12. It is obviously tempting to conclude that the pill is to blame. However, the statistics show a rise in breast cancer in all age groups, and the greatest rise among older women who never had a chance to take the pill. With such a high rate of this disease it must inevitably be expected to happen in women whether they took the pill or not. And many other things have changed in society during the same 40 years. Regardless of the pill, there have been increasing rates of several well-known breast cancer risk factors (see Box 5.3).

Unhelpfully, the research in this field is copious, complicated, confusing, and often contradictory! In the previous editions research indicated a pill-connected risk focused just on younger women who used the pill for long periods before age 35, with no sign of a continuing risk above that age.

Then a new publication came out in 1996, by the Collaborative Group on Hormonal Factors in Breast Cancer. They were able to reanalyse original data about over 53 000 women with breast cancer and over 100 000 controls without it, from 54 studies in 25 countries. This is 90 per cent of the world's epidemiological research data.

The new analysis has come up with a slightly different 'model' or framework for understanding how the pill affects breast cancer risk. This is now

Box 5.4

The increased risk of developing breast cancer while taking the pill and in the 10 years after stopping (Collaborative Group on Hormonal Factors in Breast cancer, 1996)

User status	Increased risk
Current user	24 per cent
1-4 years after stopping	16 per cent
5-years after stopping	7 per cent
10 plus years after stopping	No significant extra risk remains

accepted by the majority of experts in the field, though there is a minority who explain away the apparent pill risk as so-called 'surveillance bias'. The new research signals a very small risk in current pill-users at any age, but continues to show that it eventually completely disappears in ex-users. The most important thing now seems to be *recency of use* (i.e. whether a woman is still taking it now or stopped within the last 10 years)— see Box 5.4.

What does Box 5.4 really mean?

Pill-users can be reassured that:

- while the fact of a small increase in breast cancer risk for women on the pill noted in previous studies is confirmed, the increase of 24 per cent is *only while women are on it*, and becomes less over the next few years until:
- beyond 10 years after stopping there is no detectable increase in breast cancer risk for former pill-users. This lack of ex-use risk has now been confirmed in a big US study (2002). There is no 'time-bomb' of risk into the future, because of being a pill-user. If the extra risk had continued into much later ages when the ordinary background risk of breast cancer is so much higher, that would have meant many more actual cases.

The same 2002 US study also strengthens the evidence that the percentages of risk increase in Box 5.4 are not affected by many things we were previously worried about:

- if the woman was a teenager when she started the pill
- whether or not she used it before her first baby
- how many years she used it for (i.e. duration of use), or even
- the dose or type of hormone in the particular pill.

An important extra piece of good news

- The cancers diagnosed in women *who use or have ever used* pills are *less advanced* than those who have never used the pill; and are less likely to have spread beyond the breast.

An illustration using the Collaborative Group's own calculations may help you to put all the facts together. Think of a concert hall holding 1000 women (Fig. 5.3). Imagine it is filled with 1000 pill-takers, all now aged 45, but all having used the pill for varying durations of time then stopping when they reached age 35 (a common scenario). The (cumulative) number of cases of breast cancer would be 11 in that concert hall. However, imagine the same hall is filled with 1000 never-users of the pill also all currently aged 45: there would still be 10 cases. In other words, there is only one extra case linked with pill-taking, allowing for both the 'while-taking' and the 'ex-taking' risks in Box 5.4

Many experts believe that the one in 1000 extra case by age 45 shown in Fig 5.3 would have occurred later, anyway. The pill seems to be 'bringing out' a cancer already on board, whose *primary cause* is some other, unknown, cancer-causing factor acting in breast tissue, probably in the teenage years.

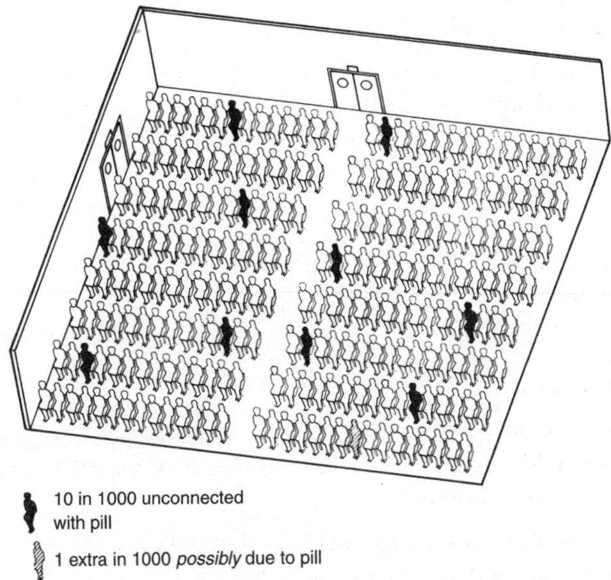

10 in 1000 unconnected with pill

1 extra in 1000 *possibly* due to pill

Fig. 5.3 Chance of being diagnosed with breast cancer by age 45 if pill is used until age 35

Note: The extra risk disappears completely 10 years after stopping (see p. 112)

This makes the pill what is known as a 'co-factor'. A co-factor is not the cause of a cancer but something that works along with the primary cause to make it finally happen, or happen earlier than it otherwise definitely would have.

Most importantly, the remaining 989 (past pill-using) women in the first audience will from this time on have only the same risk of breast cancer as never-users, meaning no ongoing extra pill-connected risk (above the one in 1000 risk which already touched someone else). Why? Because it is over 10 years since their last pill. This is reassuring to millions of women who took the pill in the past. Finally, the cancers diagnosed among the pill-takers, already and in future, will tend to be less advanced.

All this is still hardly good news. It would be preferable if the pill had been found to be neutral or even protective. But many women with whom I have discussed the illustration above have told me that the effectiveness and convenience of the pill and all its other benefits (which include protection against other cancers) do outweigh this problem, for them.

1. *What now, in practice?* First, the *whole* cancer story (not forgetting the balancing protective effects against at least two other cancers, see pp. 116–7) needs now to be discussed as part of routine pill counselling with all pill-takers—either before they start or at some more appropriate time in the first few years of use. The known contraceptive and non-contraceptive benefits of the pill may seem so great to many (but not to all), as to counterbalance a small lifetime excess risk of breast cancer.

2. *What if there is a close family history of breast cancer (occurring young, in sister or mother before age 40)?* Family history can rarely be WHO 4 ('do not use', p. 26) if the woman is then proved to have one of the known breast cancer genes (BRCA 1 or 2).

But in the great majority of women with this kind of family history, there is roughly double the risk of them getting breast cancer. Therefore the percentage increases shown in Box 5.4, which apply to them while they are users (or recent ex-users), do mean more additional cases compared to pill-takers with no extra risk factor. This is because a 24 per cent increase when you would have 100 cases anyway in never-takers of the pill is 24 extra cases; but if because of having the family history there were going to be 200 cases anyway, it means 48 extra. After explaining this, and thinking of all the advantages of the pill to them as a method, some women with a relevant family history will still be happy to take that extra possible risk. Others say they would rather not chance adding anything to the inborn risk they already have (and cannot change) and so would prefer to use another method. No one can decide for them, this must be their own decision after weighing up all the known facts.

In short, family history is mostly now seen as WHO 2 (p. 26). This means the pill *may* be used, probably starting with the lowest dose of estrogen available (20 mcg), with extra counselling about the pros and cons and then reassessment every five years or so.

3. *What if the woman has benign breast disease (p. 104)?* If you had a minor operation in the past for a lump or lumpiness in the breast, enquire whether it is advisable to continue with or start taking the pill. If the laboratory found any tissue with what is called epithelial atypia (abnormal cells), in that unusual case the pill really would be best avoided altogether (WHO 4). Otherwise this *personal* history is only WHO 2 (p. 26).

4. *What about pill use by older women?* A choice they have if they are completely healthy, risk-factor-free non-smokers of normal weight. There is no change in percentage extra risk, as in Box 5.4. But there is an increase in the number of cases, because of the crucial fact that the background chance of getting breast cancer goes up with age.

Looking again at Fig. 5.3, if we move things on 10 years so the 1000 ex-users of the pill who stopped 10 years ago at 45 are now aged 55, the numbers have to change. There would now be 26 cases in all: the pill-connected ones would be three, to be added to 23 cases that would happen anyway in 1000 non-users by the same age 55. So now the pill-connected risk is three times the one in 1000 risk when the pill is stopped at 35 not 45. This *might* be acceptable, with the balancing (see below) from the pill's protection against cancer of the ovary and endometrium. But many older women might now prefer instead to choose new options. See pp. 121, 224–6 and Table 10.2, p. 227.

5. *What if a woman has actually had breast cancer treated?* She is normally advised to stop or avoid the pill (WHO 4) and all similar sex hormones. A progestogen-only method such as the IUS may sometimes be allowed in selected women after five years free of any spread of the cancer, if their breast cancer specialist agrees.

6. *All women should ideally breastfeed any babies they have* as long as they can, especially those with a positive family history. There is some research which suggests that this is protective, over and above the known protection from having one's babies young.

We can be sure that the last word has not yet been said on this whole matter . . ..

The uterus: the cervix

Cancer of the cervix is really a sexually transmitted disease. It is caused most probably by a virus or a combination of viruses (chief among the suspects being known as HPV 16 and HPV 18) that are transmitted sexually. Hence barrier methods like the condom are protective. The risk for someone with many sexual partners can be many times that of a one-man woman whose partner is a one-woman man. The pre-cancer stages can be picked up from cervical smears (p. 22) and then eradicated, if found (p. 151).

A 2003 review of lots of studies—including those which checked and controlled for the presence of the relevant HPV viruses—leads to the conclusion that the pill is not the cause of this cancer but (like with breast cancer) may act as a co-factor (pp. 113–14). Cigarette smoking acts even more strongly as a co-factor. They seem to *promote the abnormal cell changes once they have been started* and so speed the transition through all the stages of pre-cancer of what is called cervical intra-epithelial neoplasia (CIN).

In practice, the main point is that pill-users (like all women) should be sure to have their regular cervical smears, which ought to catch the earliest *pre-cancer* abnormalities in plenty of time for preventive treatment. How often for pill-users, especially if they also smoke? Three-yearly from the age of 25 onwards is sufficient, routinely, with extra tests as advised by the laboratory if any abnormal cells have been found.

May you stay on the pill if you have, or have had, an abnormal smear? The short answer is 'yes'. Abnormal smears while awaiting or following treatment to the cervix are only WHO 2 (p. 26) for the pill. Condoms would be more protective for the future, but if, after full discussion of all the facts, you prefer the pill to any of the alternatives, your choice should be respected. It will of course be vital to have repeat smear tests, initially more often than usual, or colposcopy examinations as ordered by your gynaecologist—whether you take the pill or not.

The uterus: the endometrium

Good news! Researchers from an excellent American study, known as the CASH (Cancer and Sex Hormones) Study, showed a halving of the risk of cancer of the endometrium (the lining of the womb) if the pill is taken for at least one year, and a threefold reduction after five years. This *protective effect* has now been confirmed by many other studies, and encouragingly seems to persist in ex-users—for 15 years, possibly even longer.

The ovary

Even better news! More than 10 large studies consistently report a clear-cut protective effect which is again greater the longer the pill has been used. This is really important, since this cancer kills more than any other gynaecological malignancy. After five years the CASH Study reported a threefold reduction in the risk, and protection continues among ex-users for at least 15 years, maybe even for life.

It is probably not coincidental that both the last two cancers are beneficially affected by the pill: both are commoner in those (older) women who have had many menstrual cycles. This is an *unnatural* state of affairs (see pp. 16–17) which is avoided by pill-takers who do not have *true* periods at all. In other words they seem to share some of the health advantages of women who have many pregnancies.

Choriocarcinoma and trophoblastic disease

Sometimes there is complete failure of the normal development of a pregnancy, resulting in one of these strange disorders. Trophoblastic disease is the commoner, not itself a cancer, but with a very small risk of turning into one. No embryo or baby develops, and the afterbirth fills the uterus to make it seem like a bag full of very mushy grapes. These produce large amounts of the special pregnancy hormone hCG (see pp. 5, 9). Sooner or later, as this is never going to be a successful pregnancy, bleeding occurs. Eventually the uterus has to be emptied under anaesthetic in hospital, by a dilatation and curettage (D&C).

Subsequently, the patient has to be very carefully followed up. The main thing that has to be done during follow-up is a regular special blood or urine test to measure the hCG level. In the UK, these tests are mailed to specific regional centres. In nearly all patients, the level falls steadily to nil in a few months, and that is really the end of the story. In a tiny minority, however, the level of hCG stays up, and this means that powerful drugs must be given, as it is due to the very beginnings of a cancer called *choriocarcinoma*. If this is treated early, the outcome is almost always complete cure.

The pill does not make the original trophoblastic disease more likely to happen, but researchers in London showed that, if the pill is taken before the hCG level in the blood has declined to zero, the chances of needing the powerful drug treatment for the early cancer are about doubled. Other research workers in the USA have failed to confirm this and WHO currently classify it WHO 1 to use the pill even when the hCG level is high.

In the UK, until the uncertainty is resolved, both combined and progestogen-only pills and injectables are usually avoided (WHO 3) by a woman who has had this unusual trouble—but only until she is informed by the lab that her hCG test is back to normal. After discussion with her gynaecologist or other doctor, any form of hormonal contraception would then be fine (WHO 1).

Melanoma

Melanoma is a cancer which can develop from a mole, one of those black patches which people have on their skin. Almost everyone has a few of these. The change to cancer is more likely in skin exposed to a lot of sunlight. In areas like California and Australia where there is a lot of sun it seemed possible, in some studies, that the pill might slightly increase the chances of the transformation of an ordinary mole into this cancer. But the pill-users in the research populations may have sunbathed more than non-users, and other researchers found no link at all with the pill. Most experts now think the pill does *not* promote this cancer.

Hence anyone who is given this diagnosis while taking the pill may stay on it if she so wishes, or even start using the method for the first time (WHO 2).

Liver

The pill may promote primary liver cancer, an exceedingly rare disease, and also tumours of a non-cancerous kind. The latter can still be dangerous, through causing sudden internal (abdominal) bleeding. Most of the reports were in the days when much higher-dose pills were being used. If modern pills still have this risk, in the UK the background rate is fortunately so low (1–3 per 1 million women per year) that very few extra cases would be caused by the pill.

If any type of liver tumour is diagnosed the pill (and POP) would be WHO 4 in future.

Is there any other information about cancers?

One other possible link is with cancers of the large bowel (either the colon or the rectum), but it's good news—a 60 per cent reduction of risk was found in ever-users of the pill in one large study (1998). However, this benefit is not yet fully established, unlike the similar protection against cancer of the ovary and endometrium.

To conclude, if all the pros and cons about cancer overall and about the individual tumours are carefully weighed up, the evidence so far does not disprove the following statement (confirmed visually by Fig. 5.2 p. 110 above):

The average informed pill-user may continue to take modern ultra-low-dose pills without fearing any increase in her OVERALL cancer risk.

But, how long is it safe to continue? See pp. 121–3. And remember, the situation is constantly under review as new facts emerge.

How reliable are the research studies on the Pill?

Although they are the best we have, we do have to be a little cautious when applying the results of research like the RCGP, Walnut Creek, Oxford/FPA, and Nurses' Health studies. For a start, there are differences between the sort of women who help in research and other women; and within a study between those who use the pill and those who do not. These differences could lead to any trouble or apparent benefit which arises being put down to the pill when it was really connected with some other feature of the woman herself. In general, pill-users seem to be generally healthier than non-users, rather than the reverse.

Secondly, in all the studies except the Oxford/FPA one, the pill-users went more often to their doctors as a routine, to collect their prescriptions. While there, they could be more likely to mention a problem they had noticed than the non-pill-users with whom they were compared, who would have to have made a special visit. As the research workers are aware of this possible bias, attempts have been made to allow for it.

Thirdly, most studies so far omit teenagers, people with highly relevant chronic illnesses like diabetes, and use of the most recent pill formulations.

What about the risks of the pill in less developed countries?

Risks in less developed countries have been inadequately examined so far. The research has nearly all been done in 'over-developed' countries, where diseases of the circulation such as heart attacks and strokes in relatively young people are commoner than in developing countries. This is probably because there are so many things wrong with the diet, combined with the popularity of smoking and the unpopularity of exercise, among other things. This would suggest that use of the pill should be even more reasonable for women in less developed countries—particularly in comparison with the tragically high rate of death and serious complications of pregnancy and childbirth in the absence of good medical care (see Fig. 2.1, p. 20) which many of them have to face.

A special advantage of the pill is connected with anaemia of the type which is due to shortage of iron, which is more common because of malnutrition and conditions such as worms. The pill reduces both blood loss at 'periods' and loss of iron to the baby in repeated pregnancies.

More research is needed. But so far no reports have identified any definite extra risk for pill-users in developing countries compared with those in Europe and North America. Everything points instead to the benefits being even greater for them in comparison to the risks they run—especially those of pregnancy.

What are the long-term or long-delayed effects of taking the pill?

For an individual woman, this question needs to be broken down to three different but closely connected questions:

1. What is the upper age limit for continuing to take the pill?
2. Should one take breaks every two years or every ten years?
3. How long should one continue taking the pill?

From the point of view of preserving future fertility, the answer is clear to all these questions. The upper age limit for the best chance of success when it comes to trying for a baby is the same, whether discontinuing the pill or any other method: if circumstances permit, try to start your family in your twenties or early thirties. And there is no connection between fertility problems and how long the pill was previously used, with or without breaks. Routine breaks at any set time interval are therefore illogical (p. 101). The combined pill seems to be truly a reversible method of contraception, and may even enhance ex-use fertility (p. 100–1).

What about long-term use and unwanted effects?

The RCGP Study (p. 65) showed convincingly that the death rate from all causes is identical in ex-pill users after 10 years to that in never-users. Most of the non-death-causing risks (and benefits) also seem to apply only or mainly while the pill is actually being taken. If the pill is stopped, things seem to return to normal within a few weeks. These statements apply to the studies of body chemistry which were described earlier (see Table 4.1 and pp. 60–5); to the risk of many of the serious side-effects such as venous thrombosis, and of the less serious but annoying ones such as weight gain and headaches; and of course to the beneficial effects on the menstrual cycle. Any risk (or benefit) to do with cancers persists longer—see below—but still eventually disappears.

Long-term current use and diseases of the circulation

Most available research does not show any increase in the risk of arterial or venous disease with increasing duration of pill use in current users, over and above the risk which always goes up with increasing age and made worse of course if the person smokes or has raised blood pressure. But raised blood pressure is itself diagnosed increasingly often, the longer the pill has been used.

How then do we minimize the risk of diseases of the circulation?

Age

Smokers should consider stopping the pill at age 30 and must transfer to another method at the age of 35 (WHO 4: though WHO itself is a tad more permissive for light smokers, p. 79). For others the situation has changed due to that statement by the US FDA (see p. 79), which means that healthy non-smokers, without migraine or any other disease or risk factor, may continue to use the appropriate pill brands on their request (WHO 2) right up to the average age of the menopause (51 years). The reasons for this policy are: we now know that the risks of the pill, although greater in older women, are much less than used to be thought for those without risk factors, and can be minimized by careful monitoring; and we know more about the extra benefits as women get older, especially protection against gynaecological problems such as ultra-heavy periods leading to the risks of hysterectomy, and against cancer of the ovary.

But breast cancer risk argues the other way (p. 115) and now we have so many exciting new choices in contraception (see Chapters 8 and 10), many healthy pill-takers who have the choice to continue into their 40s decide instead to switch, often to an IUD or IUS.

Breaks

We can, I think, give a definite answer 'no' to the question about taking breaks every two or every 10 years as used to be advised. One way of looking at this is: because you take the pill for only three weeks in four, if you have been on it for 10 years you have really only taken it for seven and a half years. What is more, you have already taken 130 breaks: how many more do you want?

Various fascinating studies of body chemistry have now reported that abnormal measurements on pill treatment, including changed clotting factors, often return towards normal during the pill-free interval of (normally) seven days. Could these breaks be important as a time of 'rest' for the system, a time when the body adjusts before the next three weeks of pill-taking?

That is so far only hypothetical, but there is no research to suggest that taking additional breaks over and above those regular ones would reduce overall risks, unless the breaks were long enough to have a definite impact on the *total accumulated duration* of use. In other words, suppose a pill-user decides to take a six-month break every two years: after 12 years she will have accumulated 10 years of use, without, so far as we know, lessening her risk as compared with someone who took the pill continuously for 10 years.

In short, repeated breaks from pill-taking are a nuisance, are of no proven benefit for health, and also have been known to lead to unplanned pregnancies.

Duration

As far as the circulation is concerned, how long to go on might first be faced and discussed after, say, 15 years of accumulated use (with or without breaks). Smokers should consider 20 years as the absolute maximum, provided they are also under 35 and have normal blood pressure. Non-smokers who are free of risk factors using modern low-dose pills no longer need consider that there is any fixed upper limit for duration, just like for age (up to max. 51), on the grounds of circulatory disease. Yet, even though the choice is there, many do decide on a more 'forgettable' intrauterine method, especially when they are pretty sure their family is complete.

Cancer and duration of use/ex-use

Please read pp. 110–19 above, if you have not already done so. If the pill is finally proved to increase the risk of any cancer, the harmful effect is likely (not certain) to be greater the longer the pill is used, and might persist for a few years in ex-users. If the pill reduces a risk, as it does for cancer of the ovary and endometrium, the protective effect is definitely greater the longer the duration of use, and continues among ex-users.

Once again we have 'swings and roundabouts': good effects (here of long-term pill-use) tending to balance the bad. So the conclusion I am drawing here is that no-one ever need feel under pressure to take a break from the pill just because an arbitrary time like 10 years has gone by. Breaks should basically be because you either want a baby or want to try a new method, or maybe no longer have a partner (but even then women with a good likelihood of a new relationship may find it better to stay on rather than keep starting and stopping).

Nothing I have said overrides the importance of your own views and intuition. You may just feel like a short-term or longer break: you feel it will help your own peace of mind. In that case all I will say is: do be careful in your use of another method, without gambling—unless you really want a baby.

6 The pill in perspective

Table 6.1 is a summary of most of the effects for which there is at least some evidence of a link (either way, good or bad) with the pill. It is, of necessity, not entirely comprehensive. The emphasis to be given to any one effect depends on the answers to four important questions:

1. *How strong is the evidence?* Has it been consistently shown by more than one group of researchers? And/or is there a reason for expecting the effect, such as a known change in body chemistry?
2. *How important is the condition being caused, worsened, or improved?*
3. *How large is the effect of the pill?* (How many times more or less common is the condition in pill-users?)
4. *How common is the condition anyway?*

Questions 3 and 4 are linked in the way to be described on p. 130 (attributable risk), and they all apply to the good as well as the bad effects, of course. At the end of the day, the conclusion, based on the answer to all four, depends on the individual judgement of the informed person, whether doctor or pill-user. Try answering these questions: which is the more important in deciding about the pill today, some very preliminary and unconfirmed evidence that the pill might increase the chance of a severe allergy in a tiny number of women? Or the certainty that abnormal pigmentation (chloasma) will develop in a larger number? And how do you match either with the certainty that an even larger number of pill-users will not get the iron deficiency anaemia due to heavy periods which they would otherwise suffer?

Although the actual amount of the extra risk or benefit may be hotly debated, the evidence linking it with the pill to some extent is at least adequate for most of the conditions mentioned in the last two chapters. In Table 6.1 those side-effects about which the evidence is weakest, or where the net effect of the pill is uncertain, are in parentheses. There is no doubt

Table 6.1 Side-effects of the combined pill

Good effects

Common	Uncommon or rare
• (Acne—less with some pills) • Benign breast disease—less • Breast tenderness—usually less • Effective—nearly 100 per cent (hence relief of fear of pregnancy) • Intercourse—unaffected by the method • Menstrual cycle improved: – more regular bleeding – timing of 'periods' can be controlled – no ovulation pain – (less pre-menstrual tension) – less period pain – less heavy bleeding, therefore: – less anaemia • Pelvic infection—less • Poisoning—almost impossible • Reversible—nearly 100 per cent • (Trichomonas vaginitis—? less) • (Unwanted hair growth—less with some pills) • Wax in the ears—less, overall	• Bones—prevents osteoporosis • Cancer of ovary—less • Cancer of endometrium—less • (Cancer of rectum and of the colon—? less) • (Duodenal ulcers—? less) • Ectopic pregnancies—much less • Endometriosis—less • Fibroids—fewer troubles • Ovarian cysts—less • Rheumatoid arthritis—less • (Thyroid disease—? less) • (Toxic shock—? less)

Bad effects

Common	Uncommon or rare
• Absent bleeding in pill-free week • (Allergies) • Bleeding on pill-taking days • Breast enlargement* • Cramps and pains in legs, or in arms • Cystitis and other urinary infections • (Depression) • Ectopy of cervix with increased vaginal discharge • Fluid retention/bloatedness • Gum inflammation • Headaches • (Loss of libido) • Migraine • Nausea	• Breast pain • Cancer of breast—in current or recent users • Cancer of cervix—co-factor • Chloasma or other skin troubles • Crohn's disease • Contact-lens troubles • Delayed return of fertility • Eye troubles • Fibroids—rarely enlargement and pain • Gallstones • Heart attacks • Hypertension • Jaundice • Milky fluid from breasts

- Reduced resistance to some infections
- Weight gain*

- Phlebitis (thrombosis of superficial veins)
- Strokes
- Tumours of liver (adenoma and very rare primary cancer)
- Venous thrombosis with or without pulmonary embolism

Notes:
1. The order is alphabetical in each list. The different effects obviously vary enormously in their relative importance. Use Index to read more about each.
2. ?s and parentheses around an item mean conflicting research so that some doubt remains about whether, or to what extent, the pill causes the effect. Brackets on their own mean the pill can have real but quite opposite effects in different women: e.g. some pill-takers report increased pre-menstrual tension, others increased libido, allergies can improve or worsen.
*3. *These may seem good effects to some underweight women.*

that some women report loss of libido on the pill, for instance, but others report improvement: so loss of libido is in brackets, because it is difficult to be sure what the net (overall) effect would be in a large group of pill-users.

Fig. 6.1 shows somewhat more clearly, because the facts are known from the RCGP Study, how frequent certain of the good and bad effects are, and by how much the pill increases or reduces their rate of occurrence. The figure applies to older high-dose pills (now rarely used), so all the rates for modern pills are believed to be lower—but not very different.

Benefits and risks

If you have read right through Chapters 4 and 5, you are now perhaps surprised if not overwhelmed by the number and variety of non-contraceptive effects of the pill. You may well be wondering why anyone ever takes it. But suppose that you had instead been reading a very comprehensive account by a casualty surgeon of all the injuries and long-term complications which have been linked with road accidents—would you not similarly be wondering why people ever go anywhere by car? Yet all the different injuries due to cars added together are still uncommon enough to make it worthwhile for most people to use cars. Similarly, all the serious injuries which have been linked with the pill added together are uncommon. Indeed it would be a safe bet that most readers of this book will not know personally any family affected by a tragedy linked with the pill—whereas they probably know more than one which has suffered from a road accident. In spite of years of involvement with family planning, I am not aware of a case of a heart attack

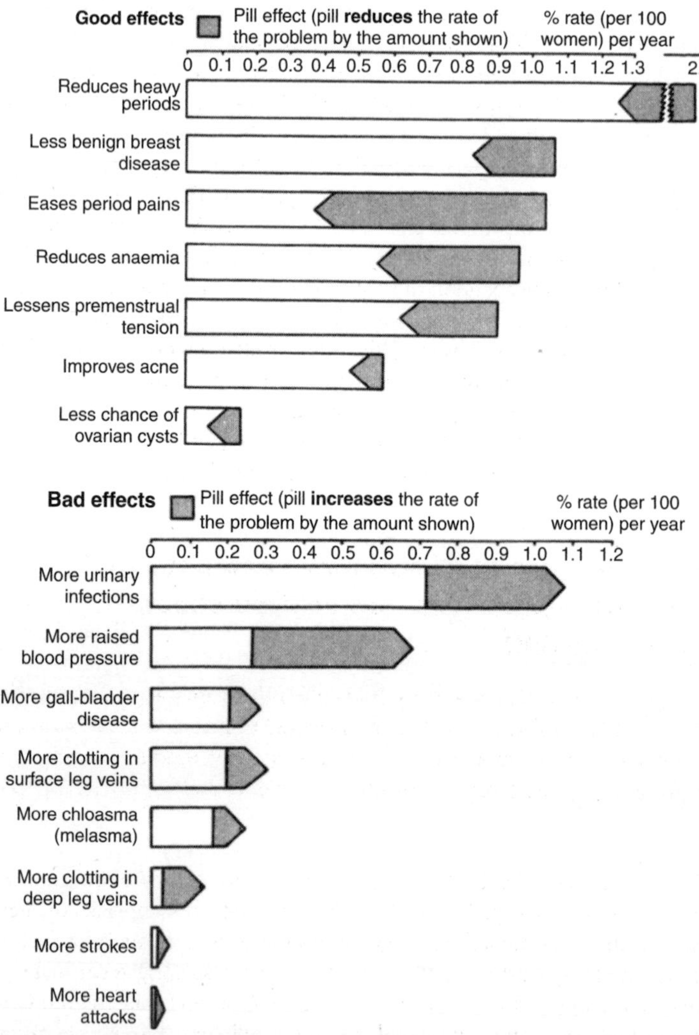

Fig. 6.1 The effect of the pill on the rate of occurrence of some selected conditions (RCGP Study)

Note: All rates shown are the rates of attendance at the doctor's surgery and/or hospital admission for each condition.

or stroke occurring in any woman to whom I had personally prescribed the pill (though I have been asked to look after one or two who had been prescribed the pill elsewhere after such an event).

By emphasizing the rarity of all the dangerous complications of oral contraception, the idea is to put things in perspective for the majority of actual or prospective pill-users. It is not by any means to shrug away the seriousness of the events if they do occur. Complications may be statistically rare, a risk often described as much less than 1 per cent, but it feels like 100 per cent to the person actually affected and her family.

If I came across such cases in my own practice, they would make me renew my efforts to promote the most careful possible use of the pill, as described in this book (see particularly the scheme on pp. 151–2). But they would not make me abandon the pill as an option, any more than sensible and sympathetic people after witnessing a tragic road accident would refuse ever again to travel by car. What they would do is everything in their power to help those involved, and they might then resolve to drive extra carefully in future, and to promote road safety.

You cannot lead your life without some risks, and when it comes to things like family planning, doing nothing can be risky too!

Why—in spite of all its known and potential unknown health risks—might you choose to use the pill?

The pill is as effective as any method currently available, short of sterilization. It is highly acceptable and unrelated to intercourse. It is almost 100 per cent reversible. These advantages are not unique, though, and apply also to injectables, implants, and the IUD and LNG-IUS (pp. 215–26).

The pill has beneficial effects. These are too often forgotten. They are listed in Table 6.1 (pp. 126–7). The improvement in symptoms of their cycle such as dysmenorrhoea and heavy periods is something that is appreciated by nearly all pill-users. There are also long-term benefits such as the lowered risk of cancer of the ovary and endometrium. One way of looking at all of these benefits of the pill is as 'side-effects of *not* being on the pill'!

If the frequency of a very rare event is increased several times, that is still a rare event. Fortunately, the serious conditions whose rate is increased by the pill, like heart attacks and strokes, are extremely rare in women of child-bearing years. So even if their rate is increased, that still makes them rare events. Suppose the pill increases the frequency of something by a huge amount, say ten fold (a relative risk of 10). If the annual rate in non-users was one in 100 000, this would mean 10 cases in pill-users (i.e. nine extra). But if the non-user rate was 10 in 100 000 there would be 100 cases per year in pill-users. So the same relative risk factor of 10 means 90 extra cases in the second example but only nine extra cases in the first. The extra cases are the so-called *attributable or excess risk*, and better convey the real importance of the pill effect. It is because the diseases are so rare, making the excess risk so low for young ages, that the relative risks, which are anyway much less than 10 (mostly around 2–5 for instance for the various circulatory diseases), can be accepted.

All the problems that are blamed on the pill happen also to women who have never had an artificial hormone in their lives, and, as far as diseases of the circulation are concerned—which are among the most important risks—to men too. The average man is up to three times more at risk of circulatory disease, just because of his sex, than the average woman before her menopause. So if your partner of the same age is not scared about just being a man, perhaps you (especially if free of risk factors) can be relaxed about being a pill-using woman.

Risk estimates are averages, and do not necessarily apply to subgroups. Please look back to p. 75 and see how there, in the discussion on heart disease, I showed how the various estimated risks multiplied worryingly with each other and with the pill. But the opposite is also true: anyone without risk factors must have a much lower risk than average.

Consider this analogy. Insurance companies always require a high premium from students when they try to insure their cars; yet some of those students are very much safer drivers than the average (and may prove the fact in due course by having no accidents at all in the next 20 years). They always were safer drivers, but the risk estimates by the insurers had to be based on all kinds of students, including those who are irresponsible, who drive under the influence of drugs or alcohol, and so on. *To some considerable extent—not altogether—those for whom pill use is especially risky can now be identified.* One way of putting it is: 'The pill is reasonably safe, but some women are "dangerous".' This is not to apportion 'blame': all it means is that they are themselves at risk already through one of the risk factors, and that that is the main problem. Such 'less safe' women can be empowered so they set out to remove the extra risk if they can (stop smoking, lose weight, etc.); or use another method; or ensure they are better monitored. For the remainder, the 'safe women', the pill is probably even safer than the overall estimates would suggest (like a car is safer for those safer drivers than for all students).

Table 6.2 Reduction in hormone dose given since combined pills were first introduced

	Amount used then (1960–62)	***Minimum* of same hormone used now (2004)**
Dose of estrogen (ethinylestradiol)	150 mcg in Enovid 10	20 mcg in Mercilon, Femodette, or Loestrin 20™
Dose of progestogen (norethisterone)	10 000 mcg in Ortho-novum 10	500 mcg in Ovysmen™, Brevinor™

Earlier risk assessments were based mainly on research on higher-dose pills than are now in general use. Table 6.2 shows how dramatically the doses have been lowered since the pill first arrived. Among the modern ultra-low-dose combined pills, which remain highly effective against pregnancy, it is possible to use more than seven times less estrogen. And as much of the same progestogen used to be taken in one day, in Enovid 10, as is now taken in one month!

Risks can be lowered, but they can never be entirely eliminated. It is important to understand that, even if you follow all the known guidelines for increasing the safety of pill-prescribing—including careful aftercare with those essential checks on headache history and blood pressure—trouble could still strike.

Pregnancy is fairly risky: the pill is very effective against pregnancy, so the risks of the pill may not be so worrying when the avoidance of pregnancy is taken into consideration. In the past, this point has sometimes been made too strongly, and various graphs and diagrams were produced which suggest that non-use of the pill is more dangerous than it is. But the main point still stands—that when considering methods which are not so reliable against pregnancy as the pill, we have to add together two things:

1. the risk (if any) of the method itself;
2. the risk of the pregnancies which will occur in a proportion of women due to failure of that method.

No guarantee of safety can be given to any sexually active woman, whatever method of family planning she uses, or if she uses no method at all and keeps becoming pregnant. Pregnancy itself, whether its outcome is a baby or an abortion or a miscarriage, still carries some risks even in countries like Britain or the USA, and far more in many less developed countries (Fig. 2.1, p. 20). One way or another, for women sex is dangerous. This is Nature's unfair sexual discrimination.

In fact, in the real-life situations of the RCGP, Oxford/FPA, and Walnut Creek studies the death rate due to pregnancy in the non-pill-users was extremely small. This shows that on average the women concerned, or their partners, were reasonably careful using alternative methods of family planning and they had good medical care during their pregnancies. Neither of these facts is necessarily true for other women whose circumstances are different—especially in many developing countries where there is appalling, unacceptably high mortality through pregnancy and labour without modern facilities. Worldwide one woman dies that way each minute.

The main conclusion then is that *the risk of death, whether from the method or from pregnancy if the method fails, of all the recommended methods of birth control is low, and below the risk of child-bearing* if no method is used: except for older pill-users who smoke. This is even more true wherever medical care for pregnant women is poor, and wherever, as tragically happens in many countries, unsafe illegal or back-street abortion is widely practised. Even in countries like Britain, young women are definitely exposed to less danger, particularly if they do not smoke, in any given year if they take the pill than they would be if they were to have a baby.

Few who want a baby are put off by the known medical risks—nor should they be. So your own decision about the pill can similarly be based more on other points, such as convenience and the fact that it almost eliminates the *fear* of an unwanted pregnancy.

Even the highest estimates of risk due to the pill are of the same order as many other risks many of us take every year. Most of us are extremely vague and uninformed about the relative risks of daily activities. Smoking is a good example—accepted as 'normal' yet truly lethal (pp. 79, 80).

Many people accept dangers similar to or much greater than those of the pill in their occupations, spare-time activities, or hobbies. Some of these were shown in Fig. 2.1 (p. 20) and Fig. 6.2 here (which is a repeat of Fig. 4.1) gives some intriguing estimates derived from the *British Medical Journal.* A one in a million chance of death is very small. But the time to reach it can be very short. The longest time to reach that rate in the Figure is for young non-smoking healthy pill-takers.

Can you think of anything you could do which is completely safe? We've already mentioned the built-in risks of love-making for absolutely every woman: these are further increased by the sad statistic that in any week of the year there will be two women in the UK who are murdered by their lover or ex-lover. How about eating? Surely that's safe? In the USA approximately

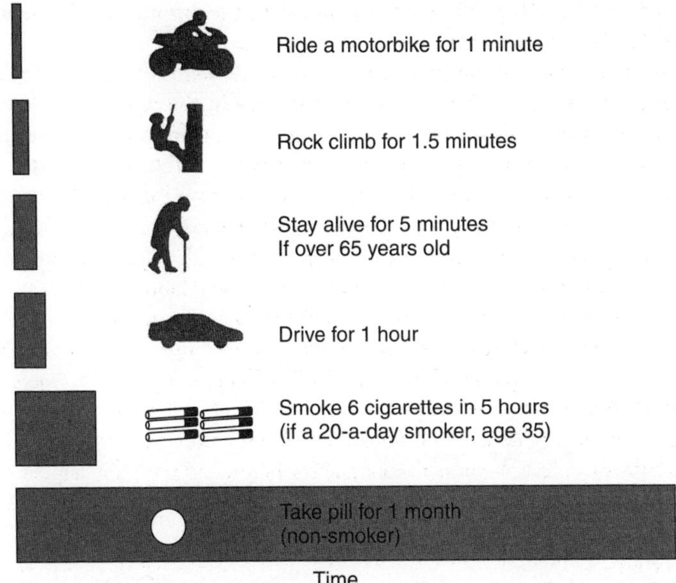

Fig. 6.2 Time required to have a one-in-a-million risk of dying

Adapted from Minerva, British Medical Journal *(1988) and from* Pharmacoepidemiology *(1994).*

3000 people die each year from accidentally inhaling food, usually a piece of steak. One would think that keeping household pets is a safe enough hobby—yet the Brompton Hospital in London has recorded at least three deaths from allergy to hamsters.

And what about unknown risks? There are many chemicals to which we are exposed every day which have never been studied as intensively as the pill. Tens of thousands of powerful chemicals from industry and intensive farming pollute our environment, the water we drink and the air we breathe, and also get into our food. The dose of each is tiny, but *nobody knows just how much or little effect they could have on our health, either alone or in combination.* Sperm counts have shown a marked decline over the past 50 years, possibly because of environmental pollution. And how about the chemicals that are added to much of the food we buy? These are perhaps essential if they are preservatives but often—with their mysterious E-numbers—they are just for colouring. They have not been nearly as intensively studied as the pill has been for their safety in humans. They might or might not very slightly increase the rate of all kinds of diseases. They could be at least as dangerous—or as safe—as the pill. The point is we just do not know. Taking risks is quite simply part of life: or as the car-sticker puts it, 'Living is hazardous to your health.'

I am not trying to argue here that two wrongs make a right, or rather that hundreds of wrongs make a right. Obviously there is no room for complacency about the risks of the pill. They should be reduced to the absolute minimum—and in the long run we hope the pill will be phased out and replaced by an entirely risk-free method (see Chapters 9 and 10). But right now, after considering the pill's advantages and convenience, given the methods available, the balance sheet of risks and benefits comes out favourable to the pill for many women (in their own informed opinion).

The effect of the mass media on people's thinking about the pill

The strange thing, as I have said, is that many people are quite illogically not at all bothered by known serious risks, such as smoking cigarettes, and yet are terrified by other dangers which are definitely not as great. Unbalanced press and TV publicity is often to blame.

It is well known that good news is not 'news'. For example, one of the good effects of the pill is the definite reduction in the chance of getting cancer of the ovary. When this was first shown convincingly, the silence of the media was deafening! By contrast the FPA switchboards were jammed and journalists produced numerous column-inches of copy during the 'pill scares' about thrombosis involving the leg veins and lung back in December 1969 and during the 'third-generation' scare in 1995 (see p. 69); about heart attacks or other arterial diseases in 1977; and about breast cancer in 1983 and again in 1989. Some of the research which triggered these stories included important good news which was overlooked. Instead, the headlines were so alarming that a large number of users all over the world were frightened into stopping the pill altogether, often half-way through a packet and without taking alternative precautions. In the UK alone it is estimated that, in 1970 for example, about 20, 000 babies were born as a result, not to mention the pregnancies which were terminated (abortions). A similar outcome followed the 1995 'pill-scare' (p. 69).

Conclusions

Four final points. First, *coincidences do happen*. Becoming ill sometimes is part of being human. Some people are inclined to blame on the pill every illness or symptom which occurs, in a past or present user. But the logical implication of that is that never-users must never get ill at all and presumably would live for ever!

Secondly, the risk of death or serious illness, though perhaps the major concern, is certainly not the only factor to consider when deciding between methods of family planning. As just one example, it has been shown by several experts that one of the very safest ways of birth control from the point of view just of avoiding death is to use a simple method of family planning like a spermicide—not usually recommended for use alone—and then, whenever a pregnancy occurs, to have an early legal abortion without a general anaesthetic. The facts are quite correct: there is no death rate using the simple method, and the death rate from the several abortions that would be necessary if this policy were followed would also be very low. Many readers of this book may be horrified and disgusted by this suggestion; others might feel less strongly but would agree that this is simply not the right way to go about things. Planning regular abortions is not family planning. Most women would feel very uneasy if this approach were seriously recommended to them. I use this example chiefly to show that in the real world risks are not necessarily the most important factor which people consider when deciding what they themselves are going to do.

Thirdly, if one day a new contraceptive medicine which affects the whole system like the pill is devised, it will be worth considering the saying 'better the devil you know than the devil you don't'. In other words, we now know a lot about the pill; a similar amount of knowledge will inevitably take a long time to emerge during use of a new drug. It may perhaps be said of such a new drug that it is believed to have no unwanted effects on the circulation or on breast cancer. That could be true, but then it might eventually prove to have more serious effects somewhere different in the body. 'Newer' is not necessarily 'better'.

Finally, in spite of what I have just said, as we saw earlier there are still many gaps in our knowledge about the pill itself. There are two very individual ways of reacting to this with the pill or any other drug. One person may say *'what we do know gives me no evidence of danger'*, but another may react to the same information with *'what we don't know gives me not enough evidence of safety'*. Absence of proof of something (whether good or bad about a drug) is certainly not proof of absence of something.

A good example of what I mean can be found on pp. 191–2 of this book. A microscopic amount of progestogen gets into the breast milk if a woman is on the POP while breastfeeding. There is so far nothing to suggest that this could harm the baby in any way. I myself would say 'there is no evidence that this harms the baby' and therefore I do prescribe this kind of pill at the request of a breastfeeding mother, after discussing the arguments with her. But others might react by saying 'there is no proof that this is entirely harmless to the baby' and choose another method until after weaning; this is an equally true statement, just the other way round. It is a bit like the difference between calling a whisky bottle 'half full' rather than 'half empty'.

The point is that we are all having to use our own judgement, to decide on the basis of the *same* present and absent facts. There are bound to be honest differences of opinion about whether and how pills should be used—at least until the facts become absolutely unarguable, which is a rare event in the whole of medicine.

Above all, and this goes back to Gwyneth's Foreword and why I wrote this book at all: *knowledge gives you power*—empowerment to exercise your own judgement and your human rights about any means that you choose, in order to have control over your own fertility. You are the boss!

7 Which women should take which pill?

The pill is reasonably safe, but some women are 'dangerous'.

(Chapter 6, p. 130)

Who are these women, based on the book so far and especially the last three chapters, who for some reason are 'unsafe' or 'less safe' for the pill method? Let us start by considering the first group, those who in the WHO's scheme (pp. 26, 142) need to be put in category WHO 4.

Disorders or diseases that are WHO 4 ('do not use')

1. Past or present serious disease affecting the circulation

Past history of any form of thrombosis in any artery or vein, anywhere in the body (see pp. 69–77). The pill should be avoided whether the clotting occurred while previously taking the pill or not, and whether it occurred in a situation which makes clotting more likely, such as pregnancy or being confined to bed after an operation, or completely unexpectedly. All of these troubles are rare, but the least uncommon would be clotting in one of the leg veins (see pp. 69–71).

Any past history of brain trouble diagnosed as a stroke (see p. 76), whether thought to be due to blood-clotting or to bleeding in the brain.

Extremely severe migraine lasting for three days; any migraine treated with an ergotamine-containing drug; or any migraine with aura symptoms (pp. 83–8). Migraine with aura shows itself by short-lived symptoms (usually lasting about 20 minutes, but could be for an hour) starting before the headache itself and stopping just before or shortly after it starts. The most important symptom is a loss of field of vision on one side, often surrounded by a bright scintillating wavy line (see pp. 84–5 for more detail). Any woman with migraine of this particular kind should either never go on the pill, or discontinue if she is already on it when the attack happens.

The same applies if similar symptoms were ever to occur without a headache at all—this could either be a variant of migraine aura or because there is temporary interruption to the blood supply (ischaemia) of the brain; such attacks are labelled transient ischaemic attacks. The pill should be avoided whichever applies.

An illness or condition which makes any type of thrombosis more likely—meaning a 'large dose' of one of the so-called risk factors for disease of the circulation. These normally matter when more than one applies (see pp. 74–5), but one alone can be enough if it's bad. I believe that most experts would agree that the following women should avoid the pill:

- A woman with one of the known *abnormalities that increase the risk of blood-clotting*. Like the blood fat problems below, these can run in families. As discussed in the next section on risk factors, these should be tested for if a parent or brother/sister suffers unexpectedly from any kind of thrombosis under the age of 45. There are also some abnormalities that can be *acquired (not born with) through connective tissue diseases* such as SLE (see below).
- A woman who has a known problem of *high or abnormal blood fats*, which promote coronary thrombosis or stroke. She may be on a special diet and possibly drug treatment for it already, since it often runs in families. If a close relative (parent or brother/sister) has suffered a heart attack or stroke under the age of 45, blood fat tests should be arranged before starting the pill: usually done while fasting (i.e. before breakfast).
- A woman with *severe diabetes*, who already has signs of damage to the arteries, nerves, or kidneys, or changes affecting the eyes.
- A woman with *significantly raised blood pressure*, even when she is not on the pill. Repeated readings at or above 160 mm for the systolic or 100 mm for the diastolic pressures—explained on pp. 77–8—would in the WHO's and my view be too high both for starting and for continuing with the pill. If there is a past history of blood pressure going up very significantly on the pill, and returning to normal when it was stopped, this also means that the combined pill should be avoided in future.
- A very *heavy cigarette smoker* (more than 40 cigarettes a day), in my opinion. Short-term use of the pill by a woman in her 20's might just be permissible. See also pp. 145–6.

- *Age above 51*: not exactly an illness, but safer options are available which by that age (the average age of the menopause) are equally effective. So it is hardly sensible to take the risks of the pill which do go up steadily with age.
- A *grossly obese woman*. The Body Mass Index (BMI) is calculated as weight/(height)^2: the person's weight in kilograms is divided by his or her height in metres, squared. A woman with a BMI of 40 or above should not take the pill whatever else applies.
- '*Complete*' *immobilization*: if you become suddenly bed-bound due to illness, accident, or major surgery, or even if only a leg is completely fixed in plaster after a fracture, the pill should normally be avoided or stopped. Less extreme immobility such as having to use a wheelchair (see below) is normally WHO 3 not 4.
- *Planned major surgery*. You should stop the pill for four weeks before and at least two weeks after you are fully mobile after any planned major operation (meaning one lasting more than 30 minutes with at least one day's confinement to bed thereafter) or most surgery to the legs, especially orthopaedic surgery. (Recent research indicates that a minimum of two weeks before the operation may be enough.) Varicose vein treatments, whether by injections or surgery, also mean stopping the pill (see p. 73). The main thing is to check with the surgeon if the risk of the complication of leg thrombosis is known to be linked with the planned operation or treatment or the confinement to bed which may follow. If it is not, then there is no problem (see next section pp. 146–7).
- A woman suffering from *angina*. This means heart pain, of a type which is usually described as a constricting feeling around the chest, and perhaps going up the neck or down the arms, which is brought on by exercise. If this diagnosis has been given to such a pain, it means that the heart muscle is being temporarily supplied with too little blood. This happens because the coronary (heart) arteries are already affected by atherosclerosis, i.e. hardening of the arteries. So to reduce the chances of an actual coronary thrombosis, which would block the arteries altogether, the pill is certainly best avoided by any woman who has been told she has angina.
- *Structural heart disease* (meaning significant heart valve trouble or so-called shunts and septal defects). If the woman is under the continuing care of a cardiologist, and the heart's anatomy has not been completely restored to normal by surgery, these are usually WHO 4. The question to ask the doctor to check with your cardiologist is: 'Is there is an added risk of thrombosis?' Also important here are diseases called *pulmonary*

hypertension; an irregular heartbeat problem where clots can be formed called *atrial fibrillation*; and any *cyanotic heart disease* (meaning the patient's lips are blue all the time).

- After surgical removal of the spleen if the *number of platelets* (p. 67) *is way above normal* ($>500 \times 10^9$/L).
- A woman suffering from the rare so-called *connective tissue diseases*, such as SLE and polyarteritis nodosa, and some *blood diseases*—leukaemia, polycythaemia—if there is already an increased likelihood of thrombosis (see above). (If not the pill might be permitted, in group WHO 3, see below).

The above conditions are such that the single risk factor is strong enough on its own. More commonly, the decision to avoid the pill is based on combinations of risk factors. If two or more of the factors apply then the woman should avoid the pill completely.

2. Present disease of the liver—whether or not connected with the pill

If you are still suffering from the effects of damage to your liver after any kind of *liver illness causing jaundice* (commonly caused by infectious hepatitis), or from a drug reaction or overdose, then the pill, like alcohol, should be avoided. This is normally for three months after the relevant blood tests have become normal. Further tests of liver function may be advised after a month or so of pill-taking.

The type of *cholestatic jaundice* described on p. 92 is so likely to recur if it previously occurred on the pill that it would be sensible to avoid it (WHO 4, but if it only happened in pregnancy this could be WHO 3).

The disease *cirrhosis* of the liver, a rare condition involving the liver known as *acute porphyria,* and a couple of *exotic disorders affecting the excretion of bile* (*e.g. Rotor syndrome*) all contraindicate the pill.

A history of any one of the very rare *tumours of the liver* (see p. 118) means using another method of contraception for the future.

Finally, for gallstones see pp. 92–3. (A change here: WHO 3 or even WHO 2 now once they have been treated.)

3. Past history of actual cancer of any type which might be aggravated by the hormones of the pill

The pill should be avoided in case the hormones were to make the cancer more difficult to cure. This rule particularly applies to those very few women of child-bearing age who have had cancer of the breast. The treatment of most gynaecological cancers (cervix, endometrium, or ovary) involves removing the uterus (hysterectomy), so there is then no need to use the pill for contraception. Otherwise it is best if any woman who has had cancer of any type takes the advice of the specialist looking after her, and avoids the pill until she is given the 'all clear'. See p. 187 for the possibility of using the POP.

4. Recent abnormal bleeding, other than at period times, from the uterus: until its cause has been found

The reason for avoiding the pill here is that any vaginal bleeding which is not clearly connected with periods—especially if it happens after intercourse—must be diagnosed as quickly as possible. This is to rule out disease of the uterus, commonly non-malignant growths called polyps, but very, very rarely cancer. As irregular bleeding of the type known as breakthrough bleeding can occur on the pill, if this rule were not followed there is a risk that the diagnosis would be delayed, because the bleeding might be thought to be a side-effect of the pill. However, once the gynaecologist has definitely ruled out a serious cause for the abnormal bleeding, they will almost certainly then be happy for you to take the pill.

5. Actual or possible pregnancy

Here the main reason for avoiding the pill until pregnancy has been ruled out—that there is a possible risk, though if it exists it must be very, very small, that pill-taking during pregnancy might damage the baby (see pp. 102–3).

6. Past history of any serious condition occurring or worsening in a previous pregnancy, and/or known to be affected by sex hormones

This is because the pill in some ways mimics pregnancy. The nasty skin rash now called *pemphigoid gestationis* (see p. 107) and *chorea* (see p. 89) are two examples.

In previous editions, *recent trophoblastic disease* (explained on pp. 117–18) was put in WHO 4, but it is now in the next section (p. 149). Indeed most bad pregnancy conditions, once there has been full recovery after delivery—even severe toxaemia, or the so-called HELLP syndrome, or pregnancy cardiomyopathy—are WHO 2, rarely 3 at most, and not now in the WHO 4 category. If in doubt, discuss with your doctor.

7. Important medical condition occurring on the pill in the past and considered to be due to it

High blood pressure which definitely seems in a particular case to be related to taking the pill has already been mentioned above. This category also includes other conditions which can be found in Chapter 5, if your doctor feels that the pill is very likely to blame: for example, the severe skin rash *erythema multiforme*, which may be due to an allergy to one of the hormones contained in the pill.

8. Unconvinced that the pill is right for you

If you or your partner cannot feel confident about using the pill after discussing things with your doctor, or reading a book like this, then obviously you should avoid it. A doctor may perhaps insist there is no medical reason why you should not take it, but you should always have the final word.

Notice, by the way, that several of the above reasons for avoiding the pill are not necessarily permanently WHO 4.

What about where caution applies rather than prohibition? It will help, first, to repeat here (Box 7.1) the WHO's excellent 1–4 scale (first shown on p. 26, where there is also an important 'disclaimer' in italics).

Box 7.1 WHO Classification of eligibility criteria, for contraceptives, including the pill (plus this author's supplementary comments)

Group 1. A condition for which there is no restriction for the use of the contraceptive method, indeed it may be beneficial
'A' is for ALWAYS USABLE

Group 2. A condition where the advantages of using the method generally outweigh the theoretical or proven risks.
'B' is for BROADLY USABLE

Group 3. A condition where the theoretical or proven risks usually outweigh the advantages, so an alternative method is usually preferred. Yet—respecting the person's autonomy—if she accepts the risks and rejects or should not use relevant alternatives, given the risks of pregnancy the method can be used with caution and sometimes additional monitoring.
'C' is for CAUTION/COUNSELLING, if used at all

Group 4. A condition which represents an unacceptable health risk.
'D' is for DO NOT USE, at all

Source: www.who.int/reproductive-health

Though this framework is well agreed, exactly where to put each condition within it is something about which the judgement of experts varies. For example, for a primarily UK readership I sometimes have a different opinion to the WHO, whose audience includes many different countries. Opinions tend to be firmer about the WHO 4 conditions we have already considered above. They also must change as time goes by and more research is done. My own advice is different today from that in earlier editions.

Those who might use the pill after special consideration and perhaps with special medical supervision

This means women with risk factors or what used to be called relative contraindications.

As we have seen, the WHO now helpfully divides these into two groups, WHO 2 and WHO 3, while the 'absolute' contraindications (meaning 'do not use'), already listed above, are in WHO 4. Note that WHO 1 ('always usable') situations will not often be mentioned, since they apply to the vast majority of women—in other words, those left after the other groups have been considered.

What would be a WHO 2 risk? Smoking even up to 20 cigarettes a day by a 20-year-old is WHO 2, meaning the benefits well outweigh the risks and the pill would usually be offered upon request. Still better if she could become an ex-smoker (WHO 1), though! Diabetes in a young woman considerably increases the risk of disease of the circulation, and the pill might add on to this, normally outweighing the benefits. So an alternative would usually be suggested. But diabetes also increases the risks of pregnancy and delivery above the average. So, if no other acceptable method can be found, the pill could still be a reasonable choice for short-term use in an otherwise healthy diabetic after discussion and with careful medical supervision (WHO 3).

The important risk factors and conditions are listed below (WHO 2 unless otherwise stated).

1. A family history of venous thrombosis with or without embolism (VTE)—p. 72—but normal blood tests

This means that the thrombosis or VTE occurred in a parent, brother, or sister under the age of 45, and means more if it happened in them 'out of the blue' and not because of a recognized cause like being immobilized. If available, blood tests for *hereditary* trouble such as Factor V Leiden should be done. If any tests show that the woman herself is especially prone to thrombosis—or if the tests are not (yet) available—she normally goes into the WHO 4 ('do not use') group already considered above.

If however the results are completely normal in her, she *cannot be completely reassured*, given that family history, because there are still some hereditary changes in the blood which modern testing still cannot detect. So she is seen as WHO 2 and may use the pill if she chooses—but it should be a LNG- or NET-containing one for the reasons discussed on pp. 69–71.

2. A family history of arterial disease: a heart attack (coronary thrombosis) or having a stroke—p. 76

This means again that the history was in a parent, brother, or sister under the age of 45. And here it only means something if the relative him- or herself was not a heavy smoker, a diabetic, overweight, or suffering from high blood pressure—because those well-known risk factors would be quite enough to explain the attack, rather than anything hereditary. But if the family history was 'out of the blue' then tests for fasting blood lipids (fats) should be arranged. If they show levels which the lab says make the woman herself specially prone to heart disease or a stroke, then she should avoid the combined pill altogether (WHO 4) or *might* be allowed it on a WHO 3 basis. POPs and other progestogen-only methods would be fine, however (see Chapter 8 and pp. 222–6).

If the levels of the various lipids they test are normal in the woman herself, then despite the family history she can be pretty confident there is no hereditary problem and the pill is acceptable (WHO 1).

Also tell the doctor if there is any tendency in your immediate family to have *raised blood pressure*.

3. Diabetes (WHO 3)

Diseases of the circulation are already more likely in diabetics, so in my view it is preferable to avoid any extra risk in the same direction (i.e. WHO 3). Women who have diabetes severely already are in WHO 4 (see above). However, some young diabetics who are free of any signs of complications of the disease do take the combined pill (see p. 159 for which brand they might choose) because they need maximum protection against pregnancy. (Indeed WHO itself differs from me, calling pill-use WHO 2 for such women.) There may be no satisfactory alternative. If so, they occasionally need to increase their insulin dose and they should naturally be seen at frequent intervals by a doctor. It is even more crazy for diabetics to smoke than it is for other people: and if they do they certainly should not use the pill on top (WHO 4).

Otherwise they should be on the lowest possible dose of pill, probably an estrogen-dominant one with only 20 mcg of estrogen, or even better the POP or a non-pill method of contraception (see Chapter 10). They should be on the combined pill for as short a time as possible. They will probably be encouraged to have their babies as young as their circumstances allow. Then they will most likely be advised to transfer to another method of contraception or perhaps be sterilized as soon as they complete their family.

Women with a strong family history of diabetes, or who are overweight, or who had the very mild blood test changes of diabetes in pregnancy, or who gave birth to a baby weighing more than 4.5 kilograms all come in WHO 2 and need to be carefully observed on the pill. Sometimes a special 'glucose tolerance test' may be arranged. But the main thing by far, if any of those factors apply to you—or if you have PCOS (p. 98) which has connections with diabetes—is to beware of putting on weight!

4. High blood pressure (WHO 2 or 3, rarely 4)

With high blood pressure (BP), everything depends on the actual levels (see pp. 77–8). Readings up to and around 140 systolic/90 diastolic will normally indicate just the need for frequent check-ups (WHO 2). If you have higher levels (WHO 3) your doctor may advise you to change pills or switch, perhaps to the POP (Chapter 8) or an injection or implant. But as we saw above, values above 160/100 mean WHO 4, 'do not use'. It is important to remember that a rise in BP may sometimes be an early warning sign of a circulatory disease (see p. 78). So if there are other risk factors already (e.g. in a smoker), even a small rise can be important.

A past history of raised BP during pregnancy (toxaemia) is WHO 2, even with a normal BP now, because the RCGP researchers (p. 65) showed an increase in the risk of heart attacks, especially in smokers (WHO 3). However, the extra risk due to pill-taking in smokers (they could not show an extra problem with the pill in non-smokers) did not seem to be still worse with that pregnancy history. So, and this is also true with a past history of kidney disease, the pill is an option (WHO 3); but with caution, strong advice to cut down/out smoking, and more frequent checks of the BP during early months of use.

5. Cigarette smoking and age (WHO 2, 3, sometimes 4)

This is discussed fully on pp. 74–80. The 'bottom line' is that smokers (ordinarily in WHO 2, according to how many they smoke) must stop the combined pill at 35 (at which age they are in WHO 4). Light smokers are allowed by the WHO, but not usually in the UK, to continue to use it into their 40s; but it's always WHO 3, meaning another method definitely would be preferred.

Non-smokers, if 100 per cent free of all the problems listed here, may continue to take combined hormones if they so wish (see pp. 159–60 for discussion of which one to choose), because of the pill's advantages to them, and voluntarily to take the small increasing risk of circulatory diseases which does occur with increasing age, right up to the menopause. So non-smokers free of all other risk factors here but above the age of 35 are in group WHO 2 for the pill, but should stop it above age 51. See also p. 115 for another factor they should take into account—breast cancer.

6. Migraine (WHO 2, 3, sometimes 4)

The problematic migraines 'with aura' are fully discussed on pp. 83–8 and Fig. 5.1. They mean WHO 4. But even migraines without those special pre-headache eye symptoms are a reason for a little caution (WHO 2), and this goes up to WHO 3 if aged above 35 or with any other single risk factor. Sufferers need to be taught the symptoms to look out for which would mean taking prompt advice (see pp. 84–5).

7. Excessive weight (WHO 2, 3, rarely 4)

Excessive weight increases the risk of both venous and arterial thrombosis, so it means WHO 2 if the BMI (see Glossary) is above 25, and WHO 3 from 30–39. If the pill is used at all above a BMI of 30, the venous thrombosis risk takes priority and a non-estrogen-dominant-type pill (meaning one containing LNG or NET) should normally be used (pp. 155–6, 159).

8. Life circumstances in which the risk of leg/lung thrombosis is increased (WHO 3 or 4)

Immobilization in bed, such as after an accident. Immobilization means stopping the pill at once, since being immobile in bed, perhaps in a plaster cast, increases the risk of leg thrombosis. Even having just a limb immobilized increases the risk of thrombosis locally in that limb, so the pill may need stopping even then (WHO 4).

Disabled women who are *confined to a wheelchair* may be permitted to take a non-estrogen-dominant (LNG or NET), preferably 20 mcg, combined pill provided they are not also overweight, and with special care and counselling (WHO 3).

Surgery. *The main thing for you is to check with the surgeon if the risk of the complication of leg thrombosis is known not to be linked* with the planned operation (unlike the ones on p. 139). Unless your surgeon or gynaecologist tells you otherwise, it is perfectly in order for you to continue on the pill (WHO 2) right up to the time of most kinds of minimally invasive or 'keyhole' surgery procedures done as day cases, such as female sterilization by laparoscopy. Apart from those done *on the legs*, (arthroscopy) and those causing immobility through pain afterwards, these all count as minor operations.

Emergency major operations. Being on the pill will, of course, never stop you having a life-saving major operation such as for appendicitis. In such a case, you must inform the surgeon if you are on the pill. Heparin (blood-thinning) treatment may be required. (This can also be used [WHO 3] in cases where there has been an oversight and someone has actually come into the hospital for a planned major operation without realizing they should have switched to another method.)

As the POP or Cerazette (see p. 190) and Depo-Provera™ (see pp. 222–3) do not contain estrogen and are not thought to affect clotting factors to any important extent, they can be continued up to and after major or leg operations. Indeed either could be ideal to tide you over the whole time on the waiting list, in hospital, and until you restart the ordinary pill. This would normally be on the first day of your first period at least two weeks after you are able to walk around. An advantage of the injection (as well as its excellent effectiveness) is that the combined pill could be restarted any time, without necessarily waiting for its 12 weeks of effectiveness to come to an end.

Travel to high altitudes. All women travelling to above 2500 metres and especially above 4000 metres should be informed about the risk of altitude sickness. This happens in some people unpredictably and is not caused by the pill, but in its most severe forms thrombosis can happen. Then being on the pill might in theory make things worse. So as a general rule the pill is perhaps best not used (WHO 3). Yet it is not ruled out and it could be only WHO 2 in a healthy Himalayan trekker if she planned always to follow the golden rule which is to 'climb high but sleep low'.

See also p. 72 re dehydration; and re long-haul plane journeys.

NB. An extremely important point about the above eight situations is that these risks multiply together. If more than one applies then you usually move to a higher category—for example, WHO 3 going to WHO 4 if a currently healthy diabetic also smokes, or is overweight. But now we move on to consider other WHO 2 and 3 conditions which are not necessarily connected with circulatory disease.

9. Chronic (long-term) diseases (unless otherwise stated these are WHO 2, sometimes WHO 3)

There is obviously no space to consider them all here, but if you look in the Index you will find that a number, such as *diabetes* and *Crohn's disease*, are discussed elsewhere.

Gallstones treated medically in the past could recur within the bile duct system, so it would normally be best to avoid the pill in future—but this is now WHO 3, not 4 as in previous editions (see p. 92). The pill should be entirely usable on a WHO 2 basis if the treatment was by removal of the gall bladder, but check this with your surgeon.

Otosclerosis is now placed in WHO 2: no increase in the number of patients with this trouble was shown among pill-takers in the RCGP Study and other studies.

Some women who have diseases which cause very heavy periods, or who perhaps because of disablement have difficulty in coping with naturally rather heavy periods, positively benefit from the light withdrawal bleeds that the pill gives.

If women with the allergic and auto-immune disorders considered on p. 109 go on the pill, the result is often unpredictable, so close medical supervision is essential. Melanoma (see p. 118), most cancers, Hodgkin's disease, multiple sclerosis, myasthenia gravis, and sarcoidosis are examples of illnesses which are now believed to be neither worsened nor improved by the pill. But more research is needed, into these and others too numerous to mention.

If you have a long-term illness, the main rules are:

- Discuss the whole matter with your doctor, who should consider particularly whether there is summation—that is, an additive or multiplying effect between effects of the disease and of the pill. Thus if the disease is one making thrombosis more likely anyway, special blood tests may be necessary and the pill's slight effects in the same direction will usually put the disease into WHO 4, or in lesser cases WHO 3. In the latter, as usual, it is a matter of balancing known and potential unknown risks of the pill in your total situation against those of pregnancy and the pros and cons of alternative methods.
- Be sure that you are carefully followed up by a doctor or specialist who knows the full story.

10. Sickle cell anaemia (WHO 3)

This is a type of anaemia which affects only black people. There are two forms of the condition and the milder one, which is pretty common, called *sickle cell trait*, definitely poses no problem for pill-taking (WHO 1). But in the past patients with the rarer *sickle cell anaemia* were told the pill must be avoided (WHO 4). Patients with this disease have painful attacks (so-called crises) from time to time, during which damaged red blood cells block up tiny arteries in the body. Theoretically these attacks might be worsened by estrogen in the pill, promoting thrombosis and thus turning temporary blockages of the microcirculation into more permanent ones. However, other evidence suggests that the progestogen of the pill might have good effects.

Since pregnancy is particularly dangerous in this condition, and the pill prevents that so well, many experts including WHO now definitely allow a low-dose, non-estrogen-dominant (p. 157) pill to be used, after full discussion. This makes it WHO 2 rather than WHO 4. However, in the UK it is more usual to prescribe Depo-Provera (see p. 222). Research reported in 1982 showed this injectable contraceptive can be positively beneficial to women with sickle cell anaemia, by reducing the frequency of their painful crises.

11. Recent trophoblastic disease (WHO 3)

This is explained on p. 117. Because of the risk of a rare cancer following it, in the UK (but not many other countries) it is still recommended that oral contraception should usually be avoided (WHO 3), but *only* until the special follow-up tests of hCG hormone levels are completely normal. After that the pill can be used in the normal way (WHO 1).

12. Scanty or very irregular periods or their absence (amenorrhoea) (WHO 1)

There used to be anxiety about this and taking the pill. But now—after any investigation that may be needed has been done—if this applies to you and you do not yet want a baby, do not be surprised if the pill is recommended. You may be short of estrogen and the pill is an excellent source of that along with contraception. Or, if you have no need for contraception, estrogen from hormone replacement therapy may be offered.

In teenagers, starting the pill should always be delayed until periods have appeared. Otherwise there are no proven special medical risks at this age. See also pp. 100–1, 105. Following use of—but *not* caused by—the pill, lack of egg release and therefore of periods for six months to a year or longer does occur in a few women (see p. 101). Some may require special treatment in order to achieve a pregnancy, but the success rate in good centres now approaches 100 per cent. Such women can be strongly reassured that the pill has not caused their problem.

13. Present disorder of the pituitary gland (WHO 3)

This is a cause of infertility and so a rare reason for even thinking about going on the pill. The woman concerned should already be seeing a specialist (see pp. 103–4), and once treatment begins pregnancy is very possible. WHO has not yet classified this; UK experts allow use of the pill but only while taking the treatment supervised by a specialist.

14. Severe depression (WHO 2)

A history of really bad depression which required treatment for a long time with drugs for 'nerves' means caution with the pill. But unplanned pregnancy can be very depressing; and the Oxford/FPA Study showed (in 1985) no link at all between the pill and severe depression or other 'serious' psychiatric illness (see p. 81).

15. The use of enzyme-inducing drugs—especially treatment for tuberculosis and epilepsy (WHO 3)

The drugs which may cause problems and what to do are fully discussed on on pp. 44–8. The main thing is to make sure that any doctor who prescribes or re-prescribes you the pill knows what, if any, other medicines you take; and if you are about to start any new treatment, to remind the doctor or nurse that you are a pill-taker. In the short term, extra contraceptive precautions may be needed. If treatment is long term, as with epilepsy, although there is a way of continuing on the pill (p. 88), switching to another method (as always with WHO 3) would generally be better.

16. Previous failure of the pill (pregnancy while taking it) (WHO 2)

The answer, especially if you keep missing tablets, may be another method altogether, especially a 'forgettable' one such as the injection or implant, or an IUD or the IUS (pp. 222–6). But your very ability to get pregnant by missing an occasional pill (lots of people do forget and get away with it) may mean you are someone whose metabolism gets rid of the pill hormones from your body extra rapidly. So to improve your 'margin for error' I often recommend tricycling the pill (see pp. 29–31), which means having fewer of those pill-free breaks from pill-taking which are times of potential weakness as a contraceptive. This is explained on pp. 37–41.

17. Abnormal cervical smears under observation or treated (WHO 2)

See p. 116. The pill may definitely continue to be used at the woman's choice during investigation for an abnormality in a cervical smear test, or following successful treatment whether by the laser or large loop excision or a cone biopsy (removal of the affected skin under anaesthetic). All experts are agreed that attending without fail for the follow-up smears as instructed (usually annually) is the first priority. This gives such safe monitoring of the situation that, if a woman wants to continue taking the pill, she may certainly do so (WHO 2). Or she might decide after full discussion to use a male or female barrier method in future (as well, or instead): this would have the advantage of protecting the cervix from the cause of the abnormal cells. The choice is up to her. It would be even more important for her than for other women to discontinue smoking (see p. 116).

18. Breast cancer in one or more close relatives, or benign breast disease (risk factors) (WHO 2 or 3)

Women in these categories are at some increased risk. After careful discussion of the pros and cons (pp. 114–15), the pill is usable. But given the increasing risk for everyone above the age of 35, usually not above that age (see pp. 121, 189).

A prescribing scheme

First, before moving to the actual choosing of a pill, I recommend the following scheme. It would help if all those involved would use this as their basis, both for first prescribing *and* for ongoing re-prescribing:

1. Women to whom something applies from the first list above on pp. 137–43 (WHO 4 'do not use') must avoid or stop this method, *but* they should not go away empty-handed! There are numerous new choices now. Usually all of them are still options when the pill is

WHO 4, since it is primarily the estrogen that must be avoided (see Chapters 8 and 10). But some new ways of taking *both* hormones (like rings and patches) also contain that hormone and so would still be WHO 4.

2. Women in Groups 3 and 2, pp. 143–51), if they don't choose to avoid/stop the pill, should use an appropriate selected brand under special medical supervision. This may mean:

   - being seen at the clinic or surgery more often than usual
   - being told if there is anything special to look out for (e.g. to do with their migraines, p. 86) so as to return earlier if necessary
   - sometimes having special tests done
   - it also means being ready to switch to another method of contraception should some disease they have worsen, or a new risk factor appear—such as newly raised blood pressure.

3. All pill-takers, especially those who are first starters or with risk factors, should use the appropriate pills with the lowest acceptable amount of body impact of both hormones (see pp. 155–7)—and have their use periodically reassessed (see pp. 121–3).

4. All pill-users should be monitored. This means being seen regularly by a trained person who can answer their questions, and mainly check:

   - their blood pressure (see pp. 77–8) and
   - their pattern of headaches, especially migraines (see pp. 83–8)
   - any symptoms that bother them
   - any new illnesses they have developed or medicines prescribed.

   These are (almost) the only aspects of long-term pill follow-up that matter, but they matter very much! Other things might be done as part of well-woman care, but they are not particularly to do with the pill.

NB After a while being seen six-monthly (p. 245), healthy pill-takers who are WHO 1 for the method, without any risk factors, are now often seen only annually, being given 13 packets at a time. However, every pill-user should still be able to contact a trained person at short notice should a symptom arise—whether it is an annoying or irritating one, or a more worrying one such as those in the list on pp. 50–1. This would sometimes be for a change of pill or a change of method, but more often just to be reassured about something.

Which pill? Is there one suitable for you?

What is available?

Table 7.1 (please refer, and note the important footnotes) lists the many varieties of pills, including POPs, which are currently available in the UK. You can use *Equivalent names worldwide* in the appendices, to match with the brands used elsewhere in the US and Canada; or alternatively visit www.ippf.org.uk for the formulations and equivalent names of all the hormonal contraceptives that are in use anywhere, in all other

Table 7.1 Ultra-low-dose combined pills with less than 50 mcg of estrogen available in the UK

Name of pill	Dose of estrogen (ethinylestradiol) (mcg)	Name and dose of progestogen (mcg)	Remarks
Group A		drospirenone (DSP)	
Yasmin	30	3000	
Group B		norgestimate (NGM)	EVRA is similar (p. 172)
Cilest	35	250	
Group C		gestodene (GSD)	
Minulet Femodene Femodene ED	30	75	
Femodette	20	75	
Tri-Minulet Triadene	30, 40, 30 [32.4]	50, 70, 100 [79]	Doses are for 6 then 5, then 10 days, respectively.
Group D		desogestrel (DSG)	
Marvelon	30	150	Nuva Ring is similar (p. 172)
Mercilon	20	150	
Group E		levonorgestrel (LNG)	
Eugynon 30	30	250	
Ovranette Microgynon 30 Microgynon 30 ED	30	150	
Trinordiol Logynon Logynon ED	30, 40, 30 [32.4]	50, 75, 125 [92]	Doses are for 6 then 5 then 10 days, respectively.

Table 7.1 *(Continued)*

Name of pill	Estrogen (mcg)	Progestogen (mcg)	Remarks
Group F		norethisterone (NET)	
Norimin	35	1000	
Binovum	35, 35, [35]	500, 1000 [833]	Doses are for 7 then 14 days, respectively.
Trinovum	35, 35, 35 [35]	500, 750, 1000 [750]	Each dose for 7 days.
Synphase	35, 35, 35 [35]	500, 1,000, 500 [714]	Doses are for 7, then 9, then 5 days
Brevinor } Ovysmen }	35	500	
Group F (cont.)		norethisterone acetate (See n. 2)	
Loestrin 30	30	1500	
Loestrin 20	20	1000	

Notes:

1. *Each group uses a different progestogen. All are 21 day regimens.*
2. *Within the body, all the progestogens in pills in Group F are largely converted into norethisterone.*
3. *The pills which are bracketed together have identical formulas, and the main difference is that they are marketed by different firms. Dianette is discussed on p. 158.*
4. *Average daily doses of phasic pills are in square brackets.*
5. *Every Day (ED) versions have seven blank or dummy tablets of lactose for the no-treatment days.*

countries of the world. One main estrogen called ethinylestradiol (EE) is used everywhere, but there are several different progestogens.

The only apparently higher-dose pill, Norinyl-1™, remaining on the UK market is really not so. After conversion in the body, the 50 mcg of mestranol estrogen that it contains actually turns into about 35 mcg of the same estrogen (ethinylestradiol) that is in all the other pills. So since its progestogen is norethisterone in a dose of 1000 mcg, it ends up very nearly identical to Norimin™ (see its doses in Table 7.1), and is really another 'low-dose' product.

Pill ladders

See Fig. 7.1. The pills from Tables 7.1 and 8.2 have been brought together in this figure. Those which provide the same progestogen in each of the Groups A–F have been arranged in ladders. They are ranked one above the other 'on the rungs'. Within any one ladder, the ranking order is clear, as you can see by checking the doses in Table 7.1. Between-ladder comparisons are much less reliable, due to the difficulty there is in assessing the 'potency' of progestogens. The recommended pills are below the second horizontal line, and below them—'at ground level' so to speak—are the POPs.

The main message of Fig. 7.1 is that, like all ladders, the lower down you are, the less risk.

How much safer are the modern very-low-estrogen pills and the POPs?

Although we still do not know for sure which is the 'best buy' among all the pills, the research available strongly suggests that, as far as risk is concerned, the lower the dose of both hormones being taken, the better. Actually, as we saw in the previous chapter (Table 6.2, p. 131), the amount of both hormones in pills taken for contraception has diminished most dramatically since they were first introduced—without any important loss of efficacy. The estrogen EE is still accepted by all experts to be the main

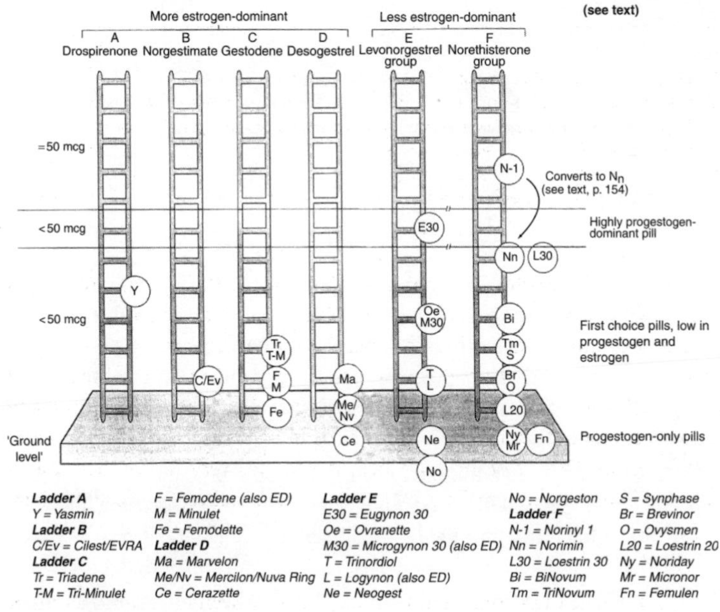

Fig. 7.1 Pill ladders

Note: Dianette uses a seventh progestogen—cyproterone acetate (CPA)—and is in the estrogen-dominant category. It is not shown here as it is primarily used for treatment, not contraception (see p. 158).

hormone connected with the small risk of thrombosis. But progestogens are also relevant to potential health risk, chiefly it is thought by interacting or modifying what the estrogen does.

But lowering the doses could increase the risk of failures and does lead to a bit more breakthrough bleeding in some women (see pp. 9, 164). An attempt to deal with this problem was the introduction in the 1980s of the new so-called 'third-generation' progestogens, the first two examples of which were desogestrel (DSG, as in Marvelon and Mercilon) and gestodene (GSD, used in Femodene™ and Femodette). They were potent so could be used in very low doses themselves along with the desired lower doses of estrogen. They produced good contraception and bleeding control and also less of the unwanted effects on blood fats (lipids) (p. 63) which had a high profile at the time. A win–win situation, it was thought, because it was not believed that these new progestogens could increase the pro-thrombosis effects of the lowered dose of estrogen.

Then, as discussed on pp. 69–71, along came the 1995 'pill-scare' which, now that the dust has settled, showed that some progestogens can indeed affect the estrogen. At one fell swoop we were all told (initially) that seven popular brands—Mercilon, Marvelon, Femodene, Femodene ED™, Minulet™, Triadene™, and Tri-Minulet™—should no longer be used! Fortunately the CSM relented and (as you can see from Table 7.1 and Fig. 7.1) they all, rightly, do remain on the market. Please read those pages if you have not done so yet. The main conclusion from all that, about all the pills available now, is that they are in two main groups of progestogens, shown in Fig. 7.1:

- a smaller group with two progestogens, LNG and NET, that seem to be the 'different' ones, able to oppose the estrogen in its (unwanted) effects on thrombosis—but also in its (usually wanted) good effects on greasiness of hair and skin and acne. Since even tiny risks are best made smaller still, the first pill chosen normally comes from this group (most commonly Microgynon or its ED equivalent, in fact)
- a larger 'estrogen-dominant' group of products, using the progestogens DSG, GSD, NGM, and DSP. There is a fifth progestogen in this group which is not among the ladders in Fig. 7.1—only because it is on the market as a treatment, not as a 'routine' pill (p. 158). Yet it (cyproterone acetate) does have the same contraceptive effects as the others and can be a useful option. Pills containing all these are sometimes chosen from the start for some reason, e.g. if acne is a big problem, but they are more normally tried second, when the first choice has not suited (for that or any other reason).

Progestogen-only pills, in Chapter 8, not only have no estrogen (so the 1995 CSM letter story doesn't apply), but they also have less progestogen than most combined pills. So they ought by rights to have the lowest health risk of all, and are shown at the bottom of the ladders in Fig. 7.1.

What do we know about norgestimate, the progestogen in Cilest?

At the time of the 1995 'pill-scare' there were no good data, so the CSM letter in 1995 (p. 69) which advised doctors not normally to use DSG- or GSD-containing products left Cilest (which contains the usual estrogen EE combined with NGM) a bit 'in limbo'.

Now it's an interesting fact that 20 per cent of NGM actually turns into the 'second-generation' LNG, by metabolism in the body. Thus, all Cilest users actually finish up with about 55 mcg of LNG as well as other progestogenic products coming from the other 80 per cent of the swallowed NGM. Based on the story on pp. 69–70 above, this suggests that there is some counter-action of the estrogenicity of the 35 mcg of EE in Cilest.

In practice, pending more research, Cilest appears to act as a moderately estrogen-dominant pill, and so is useful for mild acne or to maintain the benefit after acne has been treated. See also p. 72 re EVRA™.

And how about Yasmin and Dianette?

Yasmin tablets all contain 3.0 mg drospirenone (DSP) with 30 mcg of EE. DSP differs from other progestogens in pills because:

- it is an *anti-androgen*, and the combination is also estrogen-dominant (p. 156), making it a good alternative to the well-known Dianette (see below) for the treatment of moderately bad acne and the PCOS
- it is a weak diuretic, meaning it makes the kidney get rid of more fluid from the body. This makes it a useful second choice to try for some minor side-effects, particularly if there is fluid retention such as bloatedness and cyclical breast enlargement; also arguably for a pill-taker with *mildly* raised blood pressure.

Last, and this definitely is least, what about Yasmin being good for losing weight? Sorry to disappoint, but the initial idea that it was a specially good pill for weight was not confirmed. All modern pills are good in that way (p. 65). The apparent advantage was due we think to Yasmin users having just 'wee-ed out' more of their body water! Also, not having LNG or NET in it, this would not be a good pill for anyone who already has a high BMI (p. 159). So Yasmin should really only be tried, in a person with a

BMI of <30, when there is a history suggesting fluid retention as the reason why there was weight gain with another pill.

Where does Dianette feature now?

This is another anti-androgen plus estrogen combination (cyproterone acetate, CPA 2 mg with EE 35 mcg). It is licensed for the treatment of severe acne and moderately severe hirsutism (p. 107–8) in women.

But practically everything else, good and bad, about ordinary (estrogen-dominant) pills in this book applies also to Dianette.

There has been no good head-to-head comparison of Yasmin and Dianette, but each has been compared with (and found to be slightly better than) Marvelon for controlling acne. So we can consider them similarly effective. Both are estrogen-dominant products and need careful assessment of VTE risk factors: though an increased VTE risk compared with the LNG pill Microgynon has only been shown so far for Dianette.

In the official Summary of Product Characteristics (SPC) data sheet it is recommended that 'treatment is withdrawn when the acne or hirsutism is completely resolved'. So you will usually be encouraged to switch after about one year. My patients often find that Marvelon is well able to control milder acne either from the beginning or once it has first been controlled by Dianette (or Yasmin, in fact). If there is a relapse, why not try Yasmin as its SPC allows long-term use? Or, your doctor may agree to your going back on Dianette for a while longer.

So, finally, which pill should I choose?

Starting the pill? All marketed pills may now be considered as options from the start (see Fig. 7.1). Your own choice, after a proper discussion, of a DSG or GSD or any other estrogen-dominant product from Fig. 7.1 must be respected. As already explained (p. 70), there is only a very tiny possible difference in VTE risk between the two groups of pills—amounting roughly to the risk of driving for two hours in an entire year. If you accept that, your choice may then be based just on your having some spots of acne, on a friend's recommendation, or perhaps the need for better control of your bleeding cycle.

Ordinary first-time users? Despite the above first point, *a low-dose LNG or NET* product should, in my view, remain the *usual* first choice. This is because it's still worth avoiding a two per million risk when there's no special reason not to do so. (Consider also starting off with the more easily remembered 28-day or ED pill-type, see p. 40).

In the UK, since it is seen as 'second-generation' (a now outdated term), usually gives good cycle control, is well tolerated, and costs less than most brands, most commonly the first one tried is the formulation called Ovranette™ or Microgynon. But if you start out with one of these or a NET one (e.g. Loestrin 30) and later develop any side-effects, once again it's your choice to switch. As always, 'the informed user should be the chooser'.

In the presence of a single WHO 2 or 3 risk factor for venous thrombosis—if the pill is used at all—a LNG or NET product is preferred. We do not have a 'Microgynon 20' product in the UK, but Loestrin 20 is sometimes useful in cases like this, where high BMI or immobility are a concern.

The official SPCs for the relevant pills in the UK say that in this group of women—for example, someone with a high BMI of over 30, but not over 39—the 'third-generation' DSG/GSD products should not be used (implying this is WHO 4).

I would agree with that, when the pill is being used just for contraception. But it is sometimes used for more than that, for treating someone with a medical problem. In that case a different risk–benefit balance may apply. For example, a young woman with a BMI of 34—which does indeed make her more at risk of VTE—might also have severe acne due to the polycystic ovarian syndrome (PCOS), p. 98. Her extra benefit from therapy over and above contraception might well in my view justify the small extra risk of VTE due to her risk factor. So she might decide that she is prepared to take, say, Marvelon or Femodene, or, if her acne needs something more, Yasmin or Dianette. All these would be on a WHO 3 basis.

NB. In my view all these brands, which are in the estrogen-dominant group of pills in Fig. 7.1, are likely to share with each other that tiny increased VTE risk compared with, say, Microgynon, even though this extra risk has only been established so far for Marvelon (with DSG) and Dianette (with CPA). This is because they don't have LNG in them, with its special effect of opposing EE, reducing EE's thrombosis problem but simultaneously explaining why it's not the best pill for acne (see p. 69–70).

Women without a high BMI but with a single definite arterial WHO 2 or 3 risk factor, like some diabetics; or women whose sole WHO 2 factor is being above age 35 (p. 74). Maybe, they should consider starting with—or might later change to—an estrogen-dominant-type product, but if so a specially low EE one with only 15–20 mcg (e.g. Femodette, Mercilon, or the NuvaRing™ when it is available). This is still controversial.

The thinking here is that these pills lead to relatively 'better' blood lipids (p. 63) and this *might* be a help to women who are, for example, slightly older and who, without any pill, already have an increased risk of heart attacks or strokes through their disease. Research has not proved this, and also suggests that if there is any advantage of the more estrogen-dominant group of pills, it certainly can only be among pill-takers with those arterial risk factors, including smoking. (You will recall that *unless* one of those is there, there is no extra arterial risk from the pill (see p. 74)). Any advantages in these arterial risk cases from switching and so not continuing to use a low-dose LNG- or NET-containing pill have *not* been established.

What is clear is that the primary reason a well-informed woman should ever choose, or change to, a more estrogen-dominant pill brand is for the control of side-effects; and that then, on her say-so, the very small risk difference (p. 70–1) means it's absolutely fine to do that. Yet if such a non-LNG, non-NET product is chosen, the prescriber ought officially to write in the case notes that the pill-taker taker does clearly understand that the UK CSM continues to advise that she could have *an even lower* risk of *venous* thrombosis (if she instead used a product which does contain LNG or NET).

Phasic pills: triphasic or biphasic brands

Phasic pills are included in almost everything I have said about the pill so far, since the actual hormones they contain are not different. All are low-dose varieties in which the ratio of the progestogen to the estrogen is not fixed, as normally, but is made to change at least once during each 21-day course of pills. There is a stepwise increase in the progestogen dose at each change, so that there is less in the first phase than in the second (biphasic pills), or in the second and usually the third phases (triphasic pills). There are eight brands in all (details in Table 7.1), one of which (BiNovum™) is biphasic and seven are triphasic (one being ED, p. 29, 153, 161).

*Although like all combined pills the phasic types take away the menstrual cycle (see pp. 13–17), the hormones are given in a way which does somewhat imitate the normal monthly variations. There is no evidence this is better for general health. But under the microscope a more 'normal'-looking lining to the uterus does develop, and comes away better during each 'period' (withdrawal bleed). So, although Trinordiol™/Logynon™ gives a smaller dose of LNG hormone than Ovranette/Microgynon 30, leading to less possibly adverse effects on body chemistry, that formulation tends to give a better bleeding pattern, at least in early cycles:

With phasic pills, treatment starts as usual on the first day of your period, with no extra precautions. Always take the pill phases in the correct order!

Logynon ED has a special starting system (see p. 33), very like that for Microgynon ED and Femodene ED (pp. 29, 40, 153), and explained in the PIL leaflet with each foil pack. Each contains: 21 small active pills in 3 rows (6 light brown, 5 white and 10 ochre-coloured), then 7 larger white inactive tablets.

- The first Logynon ED pill in the foil pack is marked 'start'.
- There is also a set of 7 self-adhesive strips, each starting with a different day of the week. Peel off the strip that starts with your starting day. For instance, if your period starts on a Wednesday, use the one that starts with 'Wed'.
- Stick the strip along the top of the foil pack so that the first day is above the pill marked 'start'. You will now see on which day to take each tablet and will have contraceptive protection at once.
- After you have taken all 28 daily pills (during the inactive larger white ones you will have your 'period'): fix a new sticky strip to the next pack and take the pill marked 'start', on your same start day.

If transferring from another pill higher up a ladder, or if you are in any doubt about the relative strength of your new pill, it is best to follow the rule on pp. 47–8: i.e. immediate transfer from the last pill of the old packet to the first of the phasic pill, again with no extra precautions.

Now for a summary of the main pros and cons of these pills.

Advantages of phasic pills

1. There is little effect on most substances measured in the blood. But this is now also true of most other ultra-low-dose monophasic brands giving a fixed dose.
2. They are almost 100 per cent effective, like other pills, if taken regularly (but see 1 below).
3. There is usually good control of the bleeding pattern—especially in some women who have great difficulty with all other products.
4. They are particularly 'good' at giving a definite 'withdrawal bleed', and some women like to see a good flow.

Problems of phasic pills

1. There is a reduced margin for error if women forget pills in the first week of a pack, after the 'contraception-free' time.
2. It is probably a bit easier to get confused and hence to make pill-taking errors, as there are two or three phases (or even four in ED versions) to

take in the right order. What is more, unhelpfully some versions do not have the day of the week against the tablet. There is some evidence that failures are actually more common as a result.

3. Explaining how to use them takes a bit more of the doctor's or nurse's time.
4. Some women complain of premenstrual symptoms, such as breast tenderness, during the final phase of pill-taking.
5. Headaches and other symptoms which can be brought on by hormone fluctuations may become more frequent.
6. A very few women transferring from fixed-dose pills do not like the heavier bleeding (the mirror of advantage 4 on p. 161), and sometimes it is more painful.
7. They are not suitable for tricycling (see pp. 29–31), and even just postponing a period is more complicated than with fixed-dose pills (p. 31 describes the usual very easy way to do this, by taking two packets in a row). With a phasic pill (except Synphase, whose third phase is identical to the first) that might well not work; the switch from the higher progestogen dose of the last phase to the low dose of the first phase tends to cause withdrawal bleeding. So there are two options (Fig. 7.2):

   - *take extra pills from the last phase of a different packet.* This will give a maximum of 10 days' postponement with Trinordiol/Logynon, for example, using the yellow tablets; or seven days using the third phase of Trinovum™ (which can conveniently be snapped off);
   - *interpose a packet of the next higher brand up the same ladder in Fig. 7.1.* You should make an 'instant' switch from the phasic pill to the fixed-dose brand—i.e. no days without pill-taking till the end of a 42-tablet sequence. This should give at least six weeks free of bleeding.

   Example: The very next day after her last TriNovum pill on, say, a Monday, Mrs Jones takes the first tablet (marked Tuesday) from a Norimin packet. Three weeks later she takes the last of the Norimins on her usual finishing day, a Monday, and expects to bleed during the seven-day break thereafter. Then she simply goes back to her usual brand, on her usual starting day, taking the Tuesday tablet from the first (white) section of another TriNovum packet. Contraceptive protection continues uninterrupted, though a day or so of breakthrough spotting *might* happen towards the end of the Norimin pack used for the postponement.

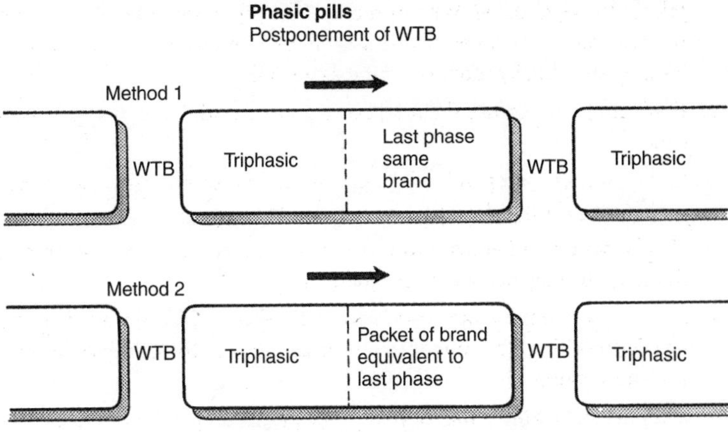

Fig. 7.2 Two possible methods for short-term postponement of withdrawal bleeding (WTB) by women using phasic pills

Note: The brand 'equivalent to the last phase' will be a monophasic pill with a (near-) identical formulation, e.g. Microgynon/Ovranette in the case of the triphasic levonorgestrel pills Logynon/Trinordiol. See Table 7.1 pp.153–4.

If in doubt, discuss this with a doctor or nurse. Obviously you must omit the 'dummy' inactive tablets if postponing periods on an ED version of a phasic pill.

All in all, phasic pills are not necessarily ideal for everyone: yet they do form a useful addition to the available range.

Tailoring the pill to you

Doctors have in the past produced elaborate schemes from which they claimed to be able to choose the right pill for each woman's hormonal make-up. Unfortunately, they never really worked, chiefly because of too little information on the effects of different formulas; and also because of the variation between women, in the way their bodies absorb and react to the pill's hormones. For example, complaints like nausea, vomiting, breast discomfort, menstrual cramps, and delay in return of periods post-pill all tend to be commoner in underweight women (though weight is not otherwise a useful guide as to how strong a pill to give).

Regardless of weight, on comparing different women at a set time after taking the same brand of tablet, very different blood hormone levels have been found. Furthermore, relatively high levels of hormone (in this case the estrogen) have been found in those pill-takers who developed high blood pressure. A likely conclusion is that many unwanted effects, both serious and 'minor', are connected with having unnecessarily high blood hormone levels—caused either by unusually efficient absorption or inefficient elimination of the hormones. But the problem of BTB or spotting on the other hand seems sometimes (not always, see Box 7.1) to be linked with quite the opposite: too low blood levels reaching the womb's lining.

Since it is impractical to measure blood hormone levels routinely, and low levels do have the problem of leading to more irregular bleeding (see p. 165), doctors have tended in the past to give some women more

Box 7.1 Problems with the bleeding cycle: breakthrough bleeding (BTB) on days of pill-taking

It is important to eliminate other causes of BTB before it is blamed on pills. The following checklist is helpful:

- *Disease*, e.g. Chlamydia (see Glossary), can cause a blood-stained discharge. If so, there needs to be treatment of both you and any contacts.
- *Disorders of pregnancy* that cause bleeding (e.g. recent miscarriage).
- *Default*: i.e. missed pills; the resulting BTB may start two or three days afterwards, but can be very persistent thereafter.
- *Drugs*: primarily enzyme inducers. Cigarettes can also be the cause, enough to explain the BTB problem.
- *Diarrhoea and/or vomiting* (diarrhoea alone has to be incredibly severe before it could make the pill fail).
- *Duration of use too short*: i.e. assessment too soon (minimal BTB, which you do not mind too much, often settles after two to three months' use of any new pill brand). The opposite possibility is during 'tricycling' (see pp. 29–31), namely that duration of continuous use has been too long in that woman for that way of taking the pill, and the lining of the womb begins to come away with bleeding or spotting: in which case 'bicycling' of two packets in a row, then a gap, may be the answer.
- *Dose*: after the above have been excluded, it is possible to: try a phasic pill if you are on a monophasic; increase the progestogen component (or estrogen if Loestrin 20, Femodette, or Mercilon is being used); or try a different progestogen.

Modified from E. Sapire, Contraception and Sexuality in Health and Disease (New York: McGraw-Hill, 1986, 1990).

hormone than might have been necessary. To make this less likely, in general, and there are exceptions, new prescriptions should start with a brand of pills from near the bottom of one of the ladders. This policy will avoid giving any woman who tends to have high blood hormone levels a stronger pill than the lowest available—which would be more than enough for her. Those with low levels should still receive adequate protection against pregnancy, but might get problems with their bleeding pattern. These can be managed, along with other side effects, by forewarning, and by following the scheme of Figs. 7.3 and 7.4. Note carefully the footnotes to Fig. 7.4 and do be tactful as you discuss the next move each time with your doctor.

If the first pill does not suit, which should be the second choice?

Problems with the bleeding cycle: bleeding on days of pill-taking.

There can be a number of different explanations for this problem (Box 7.1). If you started taking the pill just after an abortion or miscarriage, the bleeding could have a special cause and you should turn at once to p. 35. Otherwise, one reason for this so-called breakthrough bleeding is that there is too low a level of pill hormones in your blood, and therefore too little is reaching the lining of the uterus. Although you might therefore need a change of pill there are a number of important different causes to be worked through first: see Box 7.1 and follow through the questions and suggestions in Fig. 7.3*a*.

Fortunately, while this is being sorted, contraception should be maintained throughout—so long as you are *never* a 'late restarter', never lengthening your pill-free time (see pp. 37, 39–40).

If you are in the first 8–12 weeks of taking any particular pill, it is well worth persevering, as improvement can be expected. Otherwise—and whenever bleeding is a persistent or unexplained problem, or it occurs with love-making—you should see your doctor soon. They need to eliminate potential gynaecological causes for bleeding by examining you and doing some tests. One quite common and potentially serious example that should be tested for is infection with Chlamydia (see Glossary). Or there could be a polyp at the entrance to the uterus. Any treatment necessary would be simple and minor, often just as an outpatient. But if Chlamydia is found, it is a STI so in addition any sexual contacts (either of you or of your partner) will need treatment too.

But usually there is no gynaecological explanation. After eliminating vomiting or the taking of an 'enzyme-inducer' medicine as the cause (see Box 7.1), the problem can then often be solved by a change of pill. You might shift to using one of the phasic pills (see pp. 160–3); or otherwise try moving 'up the ladder' to another pill containing the same hormones as

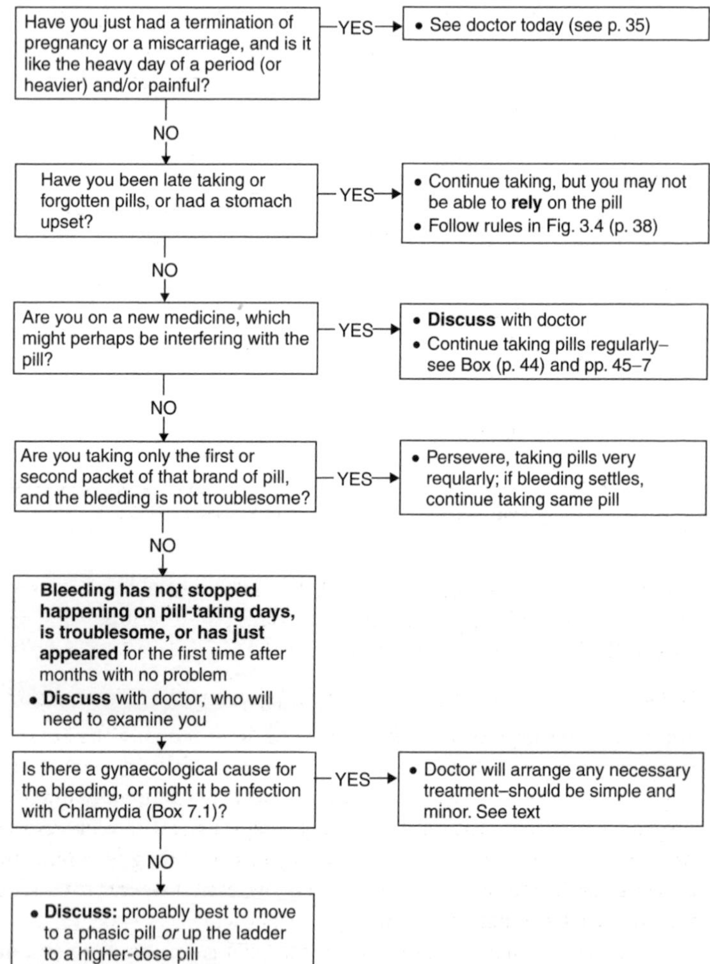

Fig. 7.3*a* Which pill? Bleeding patterns (BTB)

Note: See Box 7.1 -usefully referred to along with this Figure.

the one which you are presumably finding satisfactory except for this bleeding problem. For example, if you were to develop breakthrough bleeding or spotting with Ovysmen or Brevinor in Ladder F, your doctor

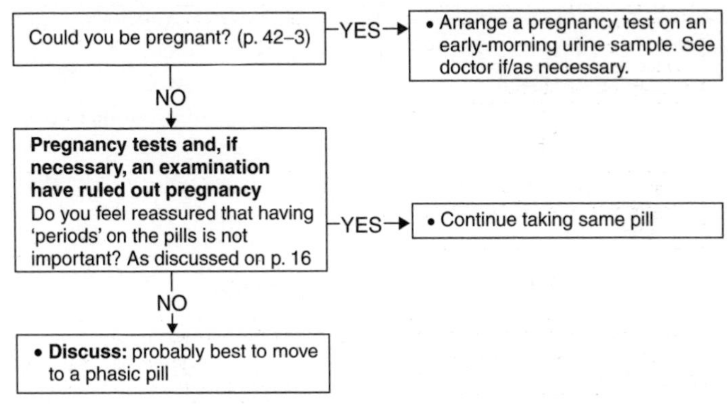

Fig. 7.3*b* Which pill? Bleeding patterns (no WTB)

Note: See Fig. 7.4, note 1!

*Very important: if only one 'period' is missed and there is no reason to suspect failure of the pill, do not delay—start the next cycle of pills on the usual day (see pp. 42–3).

might suggest Norimin or Loestrin 30. A smoker with a bit of acne who might have first been tried on Mercilon could go on to Marvelon, or be tried with Cilest or Femodene/Minulet from a different ladder (B).

Problems with the bleeding cycle: no bleeding during the pill-free week.

You should now refer to Fig. 7.3*b*. Have you forgotten any pills? Or has something else happened recently, like a bad stomach upset early in a packet, which might have reduced your protection against pregnancy? If there is any doubt, pregnancy must be ruled out by one or perhaps a series of urine tests and probably an examination (see pp. 42–3). If you start getting symptoms such as nausea or pain, or miss two periods in a row, even if you are sure no pills were missed it is important to have a pregnancy test.

Once the explanation of pregnancy has been ruled out, then you may like to stop and think whether it really bothers you whether you get bleeding between packets of pills or not. Some women are keen on not bleeding and take steps to avoid it anyway by tricycling or using Seasonale (p. 30).

The fact is that no pill-user ever has real periods anyway. The bleeding which you think of as a period is entirely artificial (see pp. 14–16) and caused by you when you stop taking pills for seven days in each 28 days. If the loss of the pill hormones does not cause a bleed, it just means there was no blood to come away. So far as we know, either no bleeding, or the passing of a little dark-brown discharge rather than blood, mean nothing as far as your health is concerned; and nor do they indicate any risk to your future fertility (see pp. 101–2). In fact, if you were to transfer to a barrier method, I can almost guarantee that your periods would come back with no more delay than the average pill-user who does have cyclical bleeds.

If this reassures you, you could, if you wish, stay on the same pill as long as you want to use this method. Otherwise the answer once again, with the approval of your doctor, may be to try first a phasic pill and then perhaps the brand on the next available rung up your particular ladder.

What about side-effects which are nothing to do with the bleeding pattern?

Please refer now to Fig. 7.4. If you have a symptom which could perhaps be serious (see the list on p. 50), or if you are not quite sure that it is not one of those, you should contact your doctor today and take no further pills unless the doctor says that you may.

There are many other less serious but annoying non-bleeding side-effects that pill-takers may get: nausea, weight gain, breast symptoms, headaches which are not 'migraine with aura', mood changes and depression, acne—and there are others in Chapter 5 and listed on p. 126. Doctors (who often tend to be rather 'bossy' by nature!) usually call these 'minor' symptoms. But they can seem pretty bad to those affected.

If such side-effects continue beyond the two or three courses of pills which are often necessary to give your body a chance to get used to any particular brand, or much sooner if you find the symptom cannot be tolerated, then there are two possibilities. First, you could ask to move further down your current ladder provided there is a pill brand available which contains even less hormone (always follow one of the rules on pp. 47–8 if going down a ladder). Second, if:

- there is no room for you to go down more rungs on a particular ladder, or
- doing that causes breakthrough bleeding, or
- it seems possible that your side-effect is due to a particular progestogen

then the other 'trial-and-error' possibility to discuss with your doctor is a 'sideways shift'. This means moving to a different ladder altogether and starting to take a pill which contains a different progestogen combined with the EE estrogen. Many women find one of those estrogen-dominant non-DSG/GSD brands useful here, as well as for bleeding problems. There needs to be a good range of pills from which to prescribe, since experience

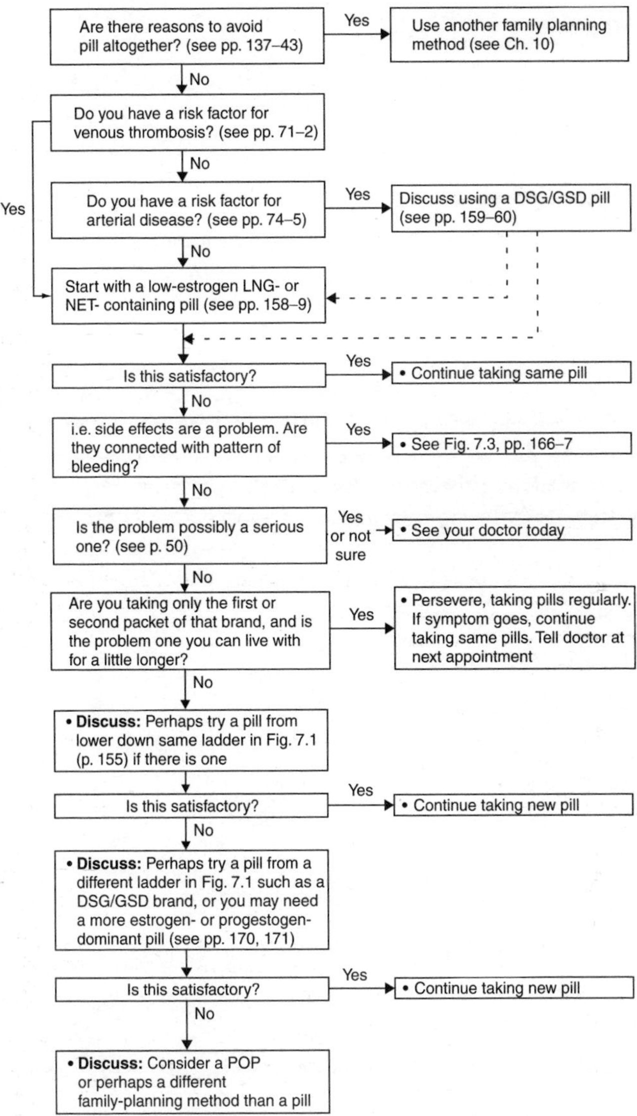

Fig. 7.4 Which pill?

Notes:

1. 'Discuss' means discuss next visit with doctor *or nurse*: they will not take kindly to being *told* by you what to do next.
2. If moving down a ladder, start the new packet without any break (see pp. 47–8).

with the pill has always shown that what suits one woman does not always suit another.

See Boxes 7.2 and 7.3 for some more specific (though not fully scientifically proven) guidelines. These may sometimes be helpful in deciding which pill to try next.

Are the side-effects actually caused by the treatment given?

In a research study from Mexico, 147 women who had recently had a miscarriage and (reportedly) did not mind too much when they again became pregnant, were given tablets which they thought were some kind of contraceptive. In fact, however, they were all—and the ethics of this are very questionable—given nothing more than placebos (dummy tablets of milk-sugar plus starch). These 147 women were then followed for a total of 424 woman-months. During only one-third of these months of observation were there no symptoms reported. Decreased libido was reported in 30 per cent of the months; dizziness in 11 per cent; indeed no less than 31 different effects of the 'no treatment' were reported!

Other studies in which placebo tablets were used in comparison with other drugs, and where the volunteers were men, have similarly shown that dummies can 'cause' numerous symptoms.

Box 7.2 Some conditions linked with relative estrogen excess may be helped by a more progestogen-dominant pill (LNG or NET Type). (See Index)

- nausea
- dizziness
- feelings of bloating/cyclical weight gain due to fluid retention
- vaginal discharge (no infection present)
- some cases of breast pain with enlargement
- some cases of lost libido without depression, especially if taking an anti-androgen (Yasmin or Dianette)
- growth of breast lumps
- growth of fibroids
- endometriosis

For any of the above problems it is often worth trying a pill with the lowest possible dose of estrogen combined with relatively more progestogen. Lowering the estrogen (e.g. Ovysmen to Loestrin 20) is one possibility, otherwise Microgynon 30/Ovranette would be appropriate. Rarely, Eugynon 30 might be tried, especially tricycled to control endometriosis.

Box 7.3 Conditions linked with relative progestogen excess may be helped by a more estrogen-dominant pill. (See Index)

some cases of

- dryness of vagina
- sustained weight gain
- depression/tiredness
- loss of libido along with depressed mood
- breast tenderness
- acne, and greasiness of skin and head hair
- unwanted hair growth (hirsutism)

There may be other causes of all these problems; but among the low-dose combined pills the most estrogen-dominant formulae seem to be Marvelon, Ovysmen/Brevinor, and Cilest. Yasmin and Dianette are usually even more successful in moderately severe cases of acne or hirsutism. Caution is needed, as estrogen dominance may go with a slightly higher risk of VTE, especially if the woman is overweight.

The reason for mentioning this research is not to suggest that women imagine the problems they have with the pill, which can be real enough, as already described in this book. However, it must be clear that the pill could sometimes be blamed for things which are not really caused by any effects of its hormones. If women are very anxious about possible health risks of taking the pill, or if their doctor or nurse is in a hurry and fails to inspire them with any confidence, it seems that they are more likely to complain of such problems as dizziness, headaches, and mild depression. On the other hand, women who see somebody who inspires them with confidence, who answers their questions and is reassuring, and checks by examining them that all is well, are much less likely to complain of symptoms from the pill, to keep changing brands, or to discontinue it altogether.

In the RCGP Study, no less than 27 per cent of the pill-users stopped the method in the first year while still feeling the need for contraception. No fewer than 199 symptoms or diseases were given as the reason for giving up the pill, and in only a fraction is there any convincing evidence of them being a true effect of the pill. A further very relevant fact is that about one in five of these women who stopped the pill while still planning to continue avoiding pregnancy in fact became pregnant within the next year. Perhaps more should consider the progestogen-only pill—see Chapter 8–or, nowadays, one of the new ways below to take the combined pill's hormones.

New combined pill-type methods: new routes of delivery for hormones

EVRA skin patch: the transdermal route

This is an innovative skin patch delivering EE with norelgestromin, the name for the active progestogen hormone produced in the body out of the NGM contained in a tablet of Cilest. Indeed, in an oversimplified way, you can say that using EVRA is a bit like taking 'Cilest through the skin', since the daily skin dose produces blood levels in the range of those after a tablet of Cilest, though fluctuating much less.

Each patch is worn for seven days for three consecutive weeks followed by a patch-free week, during which the bleed happens (often starting later than with the pill and lasting till after the day you must put on the next patch). If wanted, bleeds can be easily postponed by just skipping a patch-free week (very like with pills, p. 31).

Like any version of the combined pill containing estrogen, it might still cause rare serious side-effects such as thrombosis.

Although too new a product to have yet been assessed by WHO, in my opinion all the WHO 4, 3, and 2 conditions (pp. 137–51) and most of the practical management advice in earlier chapters about the pill apply also to EVRA, with some obvious minor differences. It seems to be relatively estrogen-dominant, and has bleeding and non-bleeding side-effects very like Cilest itself—plus about 2 per cent of women in the trials had local skin reactions bad enough to make them give it up. Breast discomfort, vaginal spotting, and period pains were commoner than with the combined pill it was compared with (the pill called Trinordiol in the UK).

The patch sticks really well, even in hot climates and in the gym or when bathing or showering. In the trials, overall 1.8 per cent of patches fell off and 2.9 per cent became partially detached. Its effectiveness (see Box 7.4) was similar to the oral pills overall—the failure rate being less than one per 100 woman-years. Interestingly, one-third of the few failures happening occurred in the 3 per cent of users who weighed above 90 kg. This apparently reduced effectiveness makes the patch WHO 4 ('do not use') for such women, who would mostly be at least WHO 3 for VTE risk at that level of BMI anyway.

EVRA needs to be disposed of properly to avoid potential water pollution by its hormones: sealing it with the sticky label provided.

Box 7.4 Ensuring EVRA is effective

- Avoid use at all if your body weight is greater than 90 kg.
- In a 2002 study, patches, when compared with pill-taking, seemed to help younger women to follow the correct instructions, though this has not yet been proved by fewer conceptions. The patch could therefore be useful for those who find it difficult to remember a daily pill, especially as if the patch-user does forget, there is a two-day margin for error for late patch change (i.e. it still works up to nine days). However:
- As with the ordinary pill it is *essential* never to lengthen the contraception-free time, which is the patch-free time. If this interval exceeds eight days for any reason (either through late application or the first new patch detaching and this being identified late), I advise extra precautions for the duration of the first newly applied patch (i.e. for seven days). This should be after immediate emergency contraception as well, if the woman had sex during the preceding patch-free days.
- Absorption problems through vomiting/diarrhoea, and taking the antibiotic tetracycline by mouth, do not affect this method's effectiveness, but:
- During any short-term enzyme inducer treatment (p. 44–6), and as usual for 28 days after this ends (p. 48), additional contraception is advised (as for COCs) plus elimination of any patch-free intervals during this time. For the present, EVRA is only recommended for long-term use during such treatment if the user is prepared to continue always using condoms as well.

NuvaRing: transvaginal combined hormonal contraception

Already available in some European countries and the USA, this is expected in the UK in 2005. It is a combined vaginal ring which releases etonogestrel, which is the active substance in the body after swallowing DSG. It gives a dose of 120 mcg along with EE 15 mcg per day, so thus ends up very like 'vaginal Mercilon'. It is normally retained for three weeks and then taken out for the withdrawal bleeding during the fourth week. Once again, at the woman's choice this bleed could be missed by putting in her next month's ring straightaway, with no break.

Most men don't notice NuvaRing during love-making, but if preferred it is optional to remove it during sexual activity—for up to three hours without having to use extra precautions. This should be long enough for most people!

Once again, for the time being we must assume that it has about the same risk as Mercilon has of serious side-effects like thrombosis. Moreover, all the WHO 4, 3, and 2 conditions and most of the practical management

Box 7.5 Ensuring NuvaRing is effective

- Expulsion was a problem for some women, especially those who had had babies. This occurred mainly during the emptying of bowels or bladder, so the women therefore easily noticed this and could take steps to avoid the method failing.
- As with the COC, it is still absolutely essential never to lengthen the contraception-free (ring-free) interval. If for any reason this exceeds eight days, I advise extra precautions (e.g. condoms) for seven days. Emergency contraception should also be added if there was sex during any ring-free time that was more than eight days.
- Absorption problems, vomiting/diarrhoea, and broad-spectrum antibiotics like tetracycline have no effect on this method's efficacy.
- If there needs to be enzyme inducer treatment, additional contraception and missing the ring-free intervals are both still advised, as for EVRA (see Box 7.4).

advice about the pill earlier in this book must be presumed to apply to NuvaRing (in my opinion—not yet assessed by WHO). It appears to be relatively estrogen-dominant, with a minor side-effect rate very like Mercilon itself.

We first used a very similar product in studies at the Margaret Pyke Centre back in the 1980s and it was very popular, with excellent control of the bleeding pattern and once again a failure rate seemingly as good as well-taken pills. See Box 7.5.

Combined hormonal injectables

The 'pill by injection', known as Lunelle™ in the USA, is a monthly combined injectable giving monthly bleeds. It uses medroxyprogesterone acetate plus an estrogen (estradiol cypionate). Its arrival in the UK is likely to be delayed for several years yet, at least until a planned self-injector system is perfected.

8 The progestogen-only pill

Progestogen-only pills (POPs), previously known as 'mini-pills', are completely different from the pill we have been discussing so far. They contain no estrogen at all. They can be a logical choice if you like the idea of pills and:

1. if reducing the health risk of your method to the absolute minimum is particularly important to you;
2. if you are an older woman with a 'relative' contraindication to the combined pill from the list on pp. 143–51;
3. if you have a side-effect problem which has not been dealt with by following the suggestions of Fig. 7.3 (p. 169);
4. while you are breastfeeding a baby.

What are POPs?

First let us be clear what POPs or mini-pills are *not*. They are *not* specially low-dose versions of the combined oral contraceptive (COC), which is the longer name we will use in this chapter for the pill that has been the subject of most of this book so far. Even ultra-low-dose combined pills still contain both the hormones estrogen and progestogen. Progestogen-only pills represent a completely different method of contraception.

Because the word 'mini-pill' causes confusion, I shall just call them POPs. However, there has been a new development since the last edition: the arrival of Cerazette™ (see pp. 177–8) whose main action is different. So from now I will try to make a clear distinction between:

- Cerazette and
- 'old-type POPs' (the rest)
- the POP or POPs—unqualified (all of them, meaning Cerazette included).

Unlike combined pills, POPs are taken every day while contraception is needed, including during periods. They contain no estrogen and the progestogen itself is generally also in a lower dose than in combined pills. Just as with COCs, an overdose of POPs can cause no serious harm to an adult or child. It is believed that POPs are even less likely to harm your health than COCs—though the POP has never been widely enough used for us to be able to answer fully many of the questions about it.

How do they work?

Table 8.1 shows that old-type POPs do not rely entirely on stopping release of the egg. As a result, most periods that a woman gets on this pill, unlike those on the COC (see pp. 14–15), are natural ones. They are due to the loss of the natural progesterone and estrogen from the ovary reaching the lining of the uterus, as the corpus luteum comes to the end of its usual limited lifespan—about two weeks after egg release.

POPs often operate by interfering with the passage of sperm through the mucus at the entrance to the uterus (cervix). The slippery mucus which is normally released under the influence of estrogen is altered by the artificial progesterone and becomes a scanty and thick material which is an effective barrier to the sperm. This happens whether or not the POP prevents egg release that month. When the POP stops conception this way it's a bit like a barrier method of family planning which is taken by mouth.

Old-type POPs do also interfere with egg release, in about half of menstrual cycles studied, and even more in long-term use and among older users. When this happens it makes the method even more effective, of course, but it also causes either erratic bleeding patterns or complete absence of the periods (see below).

How effective are POPs?

If taken very regularly, POPs are capable of giving excellent protection. The failure rate ranges from 0.3 per cent to 4 per cent per 100 woman-years (see pp. 13–14 for what this means). The lowest failure rate is in older women (over 35)—indeed, for women over 40 it really is just as effective as the COC.

This pill is, therefore, especially suitable for the older woman who is a really good pill-taker. It is also good during breastfeeding (see p. 191), when the combination is again about as effective as being on the COC pill.

Table 8.1 How POPs prevent pregnancy

	Combined pills	**'POPs old-type'**	**Old-type POPs with breastfeeding or Cerazette on its own**
1. Reduced FSH therefore follicles stopped from ripening and egg from maturing	++++	++	++++
2. LH surge stopped so no egg release	++++	++	++++
3. Cervical mucus changed into a barrier to sperm	+++	+++	+++
4. Lining of uterus made less suitable for implantation of an embryo (uncertainty, whether this effect is sufficient alone to stop a conception)	+	+	+
5. Uterine tubes perhaps affected so that they do not transport egg so well (uncertainty about this also)	+	+	+
Expected pregnancy rate per 100 women using the pill method consistently for one year (compare use of NO METHOD = 80–90)	<1	1–4	<1

Notes:

1. The more +s the greater the effect.

2. The old-type POP disturbs or prevents egg release (effect 2) in over half of all POP users increasingly with increased duration of use. Women with regular cycles are more likely to be relying on effect 3.

3. Note the difference during breastfeeding (or if Cerazette is the POP, although equivalence to COC not yet proved, see p. 178).

What is Cerazette? How does it work, and how effective is it?

This useful new product 'rewrites the textbooks' about POPs. It contains 75 mcg of the progestogen desogestrel (Table 8.2). It is taken every day like other POPs. But studies show that it is able to stop egg release in 97 per cent of cycles and would therefore have to rely on the mucus-block described above only about 3 per cent of the time—instead of the 50 per cent or so that POPs do.

Table 8.2 POPs available in the UK

Name of pill	No. in packet	Name and dose of progestogen (mcg)	Remarks
Group D		desogestrel	
Cerazette	28	75	Blocks egg release more often than the other POPs
Group E		levonorgestrel	
Neogest	35	37.5	Plus in addition 37.5 mcg inactive progestogen
Microval } Norgeston	35	30	No extra, inactive hormone—therefore preferred to Neogest
Group F		norethisterone	
Micronor	28 }	350	
Noriday	28		
Group F (cont.)		etynodiol diacetate	
Femulen	28	500	Converted to norethisterone in the body

Note: Groups contain the same progestogens as the groups with the same letter in Table 7.1 and Fig. 7.1.

This makes it very unlikely not to be much more effective than old-type POPs, and indeed its reported first-year failure rate in consistent users not also breastfeeding is *well under one* per 100 women. It's not possible (because the comparative study has not yet been done) to say that it is actually as effective as the COC. But even if it were a little less effective per tablet, so to speak, it has a compensating advantage: the user never takes any contraception-free seven-day breaks which, as we saw on pp. 37–40, tend to weaken the COC method.

POPs in overweight women

There was a suggestion in some research that the old-type POP, like EVRA and some other methods—but fortunately *not*, it seems, injectables, modern implants, or the levonorgestrel-IUS (pp. 222–4, 224–6)—may be more likely to fail in overweight women. Therefore if women weigh over 70 kg (11 stone), and this applies regardless of their height, the UK FPA in its publications and leaflets has for some years warned of a possibly increased failure rate—and there has been some uncertainty what to do about it.

Rather than get into the slightly muddy waters of giving heavier women two tablets a day, as has been the policy of some, Cerazette (one daily) would now be my first choice among POPs for normal young women who weigh over 70 kg. This is because anovulant hormonal methods (those that primarily stop egg release) have generally been found not to lose their effectiveness to any important extent as weight goes up, at least to 90 kg.

How about breastfeeding? Or being over age 45?

If any woman fully breastfeeds and is seeing no periods, until her baby is six months she has a method with only a 2 per cent failure rate (see Fig. 10.3, p. 213). If she also takes even the old-type POP her combination is very close to 100 per cent.

The reason for mentioning older age in the same paragraph is that above age 45 fertility potential is also much lower. So old-type POPs should be adequate to give nearly 100 per cent contraception in both these groups, and there would be no need usually for (the more expensive) Cerazette.

How should POPs be taken?

Meticulously!—is the short answer. Definitely not a method for the forgetful, though Cerazette is expected to be more forgiving (see below). The sperm-barrier effect on the cervical mucus reaches its maximum about four or five hours after each pill is taken. As the commonest time for love-making is around bedtime, you may have heard the idea that the very best time to take old-type POPs is at, say, 7 o'clock in the evening. But that is not necessarily an easy time and the idea is out-of-date anyway. Pill-taking can be at any time of day, a time of your own choosing.

More important than the precise time is the regularity with which you take your old-type POP at the same hour of each day. The mucus effect seems to be lost if you are just three hours late, i.e. just 27 hours since the last tablet. Not easy, so I strongly recommend POP-takers set a dedicated alarm on their mobile, say, or an alarm watch in their handbag! But really regular pill-takers can, find it gives good effectiveness, and even better if they use Cerazette.

How do I start taking this type of pill?

You take your first tablet of any POP on the first day of a period, and start each subsequent packet immediately following the last tablet of the one before. With a day 1 start, no extra contraceptive precautions need be taken. Similarly, no extra precautions are required if the POP is started on the day of a *miscarriage* or *termination of pregnancy*.

After *delivery of a baby*, this pill does not increase the risk of blood clots (thrombosis). So it *can* be started straight away. However, extra bleeding or spotting can be caused by an early start even if you breastfeed and expect no periods: so it is usually better to start on about day 21 after the delivery. No extra precautions are required, even if you do not breastfeed (see p. 35). Another option: if periods have not yet returned and another pregnancy has been ruled out by a urine test, start the POP any time. In that case allow seven days for the full build-up of the contraception before having unprotected sex.

From and to the combined pill

From the COC to the POP

Take the first pill from the POP packet the day after the last combined pill. As there is some 'carry-over' of the latter's contraceptive effects, it is then unnecessary to use another method initially as well.

From the POP to the COC, or another family-planning method

It is best to have the first packet of the combined pill ready, and to transfer directly to it on the first day of your next definite period, perhaps before you have finished the final POP packet. This is also the best time to stop if you are transferring to a method like the condom or the cap. The reason is that waiting to the end of your POP packet might coincide with egg release, at the most fertile time two weeks before the next period—not a good time for changing methods.

If you do not see any periods at all (see below), then you could wait until the end of your current packet before taking the first COC, or starting another new method. Either way you can assume continuous protection against pregnancy.

What if I forget to take or vomit one or more POPs?

There is a lot less 'margin' with old-type POPs than with the COC. If you are more than *three hours* late in taking the POP (see below for Cerazette) then:

- you should take the one(s) you have missed but *also*
- *abstain or use another method for two complete days (48 hours), during which you have taken two daily tablets correctly.*

Should you vomit a newly taken pill within two hours, similar loss of protection must be assumed:

- replace the vomited pill (or pills, if it was a long vomiting attack)—take tablets from the end of your current pack, or a spare one, so you can keep the days of the week of your pill-taking right
- *abstain or use another method for 48 hours, during which you have taken two daily tablets correctly.*

Diarrhoea on its own is no problem unless it is exceedingly severe.

Important note: the two-day part of the rule just given is new, and follows the recommendations of the WHO and the 2004 FPA leaflets. It replaces what is now seen as unnecessarily cautious seven-day advice which has been current since before the time of my last edition (1997), and is actually what I used to recommend back in 1991! The contraceptive effect on the mucus (see Table 8.1) takes only a few hours to build up.

What advice for users of Cerazette, and during full breastfeeding with old-type POPs, about pill-taking and missed pills?

The above rules are far too cautious:

- with Cerazette and also
- when breastfeeding as this makes old-type POPs so much more effective (see p. 179, 191).

We know that Cerazette primarily blocks egg release and relies very rarely on the sperm-blocking mucus effect. Initially; it had not yet officially been approved for any lengthening beyond three hours of the time before that single delayed pill triggers the need for added precautions. But now (July 2004), new research has shown that the leeway if a Cerazette pill is missed can be 12 hours. If you are *more* than 12 hours late in pill-taking, follow the advice at the top of p. 181: to use an extra method for 2 days.

Cerazette has a major advantage that unlike old-type POPs it can be offered to the kind of young and highly fertile users for whom we would have previously not even suggested a POP. Realistically, despite the tricks I recommend, like setting a mobile phone alarm, busy or maybe slightly 'scatty' individuals are sure to miss some POPs by up to three hours. But even if they do not follow the missed-pill rules to the letter, the point is that with Cerazette they are much more likely to get away with it, i.e. not conceive. It has more *margin for error.*

When would I need to discuss taking emergency pills? (EC, pp. 54–8)

If you have missed an old-type POP for more than three hours but made love without condoms during the next two days—which is the time it might take for the mucus barrier to get fully restored by the POPs—then:

- within the *next 72 hours since the sex,* it would be safest to *take emergency pills.* This should as usual be along with:
- *condom use for 48 hours during which two daily POPs are taken and they have time to restore the mucus barrier (p. 176).*

However, if you made love after you had similarly missed a *Cerazette* or an *old-type POP during full breastfeeding,* I suggest you take advice from your doctor- or nurse-provider. While we wait for more research information I personally would only consider emergency pills—on top of the usual 'extra precautions for 48 hours' advice—if the gap between tablets was over two days. This would be the same as being more than a whole day late with one tablet.

If you are breastfeeding, once you begin to rely mainly on the old-type POP because your baby is being weaned and coming off the breast, the previous (three hours late) advice above about EC would be safer. It is better to be safe than sorry.

What about interactions between POPs and other medicines?

Ordinary antibiotics, we can be absolutely sure, are not a problem with this pill. This is because progestogen blood levels are not dependent at all on that recycling process from the large bowel (p. 44), which happens only with estrogens.

But the medicines called enzyme inducers that can make the liver work better to eliminate both the COC's hormones from the blood also reduce the effectiveness of the one hormone in POPs. So extra precautions *do* need to be used during short courses of such treatment (and for seven days thereafter).

Women with epilepsy or others who have to be on a drug long-term from Box 3.3 (pp. 44–5) should preferably use another method, such as an injectable (pp. 222–3). But if nothing else suits, two old-type POP or Cerazette tablets a day might sometimes be recommended to restore effectiveness.

In all of these circumstances—missing pills, stomach upsets (vomiting or diarrhoea), the use of interfering drugs—your loss of protection against pregnancy is more likely and more immediate than with the combined pill. Except during breastfeeding, you are also more likely to get irregular bleeding, which is in any case a commoner problem on any POP.

What if I am late for a period?

As a general rule on this pill, whatever your periods do, coming early or late, or not at all, do not stop taking the tablets unless advised to do so by a doctor. Irregular bleeding and no bleeding are, simply, the main side effects. But if you go six weeks with no period, and especially if you see no bleeding during the four weeks after you know pills were missed or after a stomach upset, you might need to arrange a pregnancy test on an early morning specimen of your urine, to be on the safe side.

If the test shows you are pregnant, you should stop taking the pill. If the result is negative, you should take advice as to whether and how often it should be repeated—no need of course if you then get a period. Fortunately the tiny dose of progestogen in the POP is even less likely than the ordinary pill to harm an early pregnancy (see pp. 102–3, 191).

What if I continue with no periods and am shown not to be pregnant?

In some women, even the small amount of hormone present in the POP can be enough to stop egg release, and this is even more likely with Cerazette. It means two things: first, the base of the brain (the hypothalamus) and pituitary gland are being made inactive by this low dose of a single hormone in the same way as happens in any woman who is taking any combined pill.

So no egg release means you are as protected against pregnancy as if you were on the combined pill. But second, *on the progestogen-only pill, no egg release means no periods.* Why not? The reason, of course, is that on the POP you do not (*and must not*) take the pills in a cyclical way, with the regular seven-day break in each 28 days. That is what causes the 'periods' (more correctly called hormone withdrawal bleeds) on the combined pill (see pp. 14–16).

If then you get no periods at all on the POP, no eggs are being released: so you are actually much better protected from pregnancy than any other woman also using this pill who goes on seeing regular periods and is therefore being continually reassured!

Of course this is true only if you continue to be unfailingly regular in taking your pills, and even then only if tests and perhaps an examination have proved that the method has not let you down. It is a bit muddling that the same situation—i.e. absence of periods—could mean *either* that you are already pregnant *or* that you are extra safe against pregnancy. It can also be rather worrying and puts some people off the old-type POP method. But if the same situation of no periods at all happens with Cerazette, the pregnancy explanation is so very unlikely it makes the worry much less.

How reversible is the POP?

As the dose of hormone is so low, return of fertility with all POPs, including Cerazette, is rapid. Indeed if continuing to avoid a conception is vital afterwards, becoming fertile again must be assumed to be almost immediate.

After stopping this pill, your fertility should be just the same as it would have been at your (now a bit older) age if you had never taken it. Remember though, that at least one in eight of all couples experience delay or may need some treatment before they achieve a pregnancy.

If while taking the POP you go on seeing periods, this is almost a test of fertility, as it probably means that, in spite of taking the artificial hormone, you are able to continue to have egg release and natural periods.

What, however, if while taking the POP you have no periods at all? Well, all this means (if you are shown not to be pregnant) is that, while on the POP, your own menstrual cycle has been put in the same 'resting' situation as it is in any *average* woman taking the ordinary COC. The POP has done the same temporary inactivating job on the base of your brain (hypothalamus), pituitary gland, and ovaries as the combined pill does to everybody: no less, and no reason to suppose more, or any kind of threat to your fertility. This pill does after all contain only a very small amount of a single hormone. So when you discontinue taking the POP your periods and fertility will be the same as they would have been at your current age had you never taken a single pill.

If after stopping either the POP or the COC or any other method your periods do not return for six months or more, this is a different matter. The cause should be sought by appropriate examinations and tests.

What about side-effects of the POP?

Though little research has been done, what we do know about unwanted side-effects is reassuring when compared with our knowledge about the combined pill. Any important increase in *cancer risk* is believed unlikely (though that's not *proven*).

Blood pressure seems to be unaffected, unlike with the combined pill. It often falls on transferring from the COC to the POP.

*Research into *body chemistry* has shown that the factors involved in blood-clotting seem to be quite unaffected on any POP. They also return to normal if a woman transfers to it from the combined pill. This is usually explained by the complete absence of the artificial estrogen, ethinylestradiol (EE), which, you will recall, is the main ingredient causing the thrombosis problem with the COC. And although Cerazette does contain DSG (a 'third-generation' progestogen), the 1995 'pill-scare' was about *combined* hormones: no adverse effect is expected in the complete absence of EE.

In general, the metabolism and systems of the body seem to be affected less by this pill than even the lowest-dose COCs in Fig. 7.1. Part of the reason is that the woman's own ovary usually carries on producing at least some *natural* estrogen, which counteracts unwanted effects of the (albeit tiny) dose of progestogen.

So the POP is an excellent kind of pill and would be much more widely used if only it did not tend to cause an *erratic bleeding pattern—which is still the biggest problem with Cerazette too.* Although some of the bleeds which happen are periods caused the normal way, the progestogen can, and often does, affect the bleeding mechanisms of the lining of the uterus. So, although, as already explained, there may be complete absence of bleeding for months on end, it is equally possible for periods and other bleeds to become more frequent; longer or shorter than before; very irregular; or relatively regular with frequent and unexpected extra bleeds from the lining of the uterus in between the periods. This is the major problem of the method. But forewarned is forearmed and many women adjust very well after a month or two to their new bleeding pattern, or find that it improves. In the studies of Cerazette before it was marketed, there was a useful trend for the more annoying frequent and prolonged bleeding to lessen with time: at one year around 50 per cent of the women had either only one or two bleeds per 90 days or no bleeds at all (which they liked).

Other symptoms of the menstrual cycle, such as *premenstrual tension*, are very variable, depending on how much the cycle is altered by the POP. They are usually unchanged, but in different women they can be either worsened or improved. In the Oxford/FPA Study more women stopped the POP for *breast tenderness* than stopped the combined pill for that reason.

A much smaller proportion of women than is found on the combined pill complain of things like *weight gain*, *loss of libido*, *headaches*, and *dizziness*. As with the combined pill, these symptoms are usually only a problem in the first two or three months, and it is worth persevering at least that long, as they could well disappear. A few women also complain of *acne*. Pain caused by *cysts on the ovary* of the type described on p. 97 can occur with all POPs, including Cerazette, though more often such cysts give no symptoms. Unlike the combined pill, POPs make them more likely to be formed.

Finally, if a pregnancy does occur during use of the old-type POP, it seems it may be more likely to be in the wrong place—particularly in the uterine tube. This is known as an *ectopic pregnancy*.

Ectopics are rare, but serious, as the pregnancy cannot continue normally and may eventually break into a blood vessel. It starts with severe pain in the lower abdomen, usually on one side or the other, not coming and going like normal menstrual cramps. If the cause is an ectopic, the period will generally be a few days overdue, or you may have had what seemed like a prolonged and lighter-than-usual period. However, even without that history, when in doubt you should see *and be examined by* a doctor. If you have a positive urine pregnancy test and they feel it possible that the pregnancy is in the tube—it can often be very difficult to be sure—then you will be referred to the nearest hospital for further tests and possibly an operation if required.

Even in POP-users the actual cause of virtually all ectopic pregnancies is not the POP: it is damage to a tube by an earlier pelvic infection, most commonly with Chlamydia (see Glossary). Since on the old-type POP (unlike the combined pill) egg release can still occur, a sperm may manage to get through the barrier of altered cervical mucus and fertilize an egg; and then, because of the damaged tube (which you can't blame the POP for), the early embryo may get stuck and grow there rather than on the wall of the uterus. So it is that, although ectopics are overall *less* likely in POP-users than among women not using contraception, among the very few failures that happen the old-type POP is less good at stopping that kind of pregnancy from resulting.

This is a POP problem which is definitely not shared by Cerazette: because of its very strong ability to stop egg release, it is equally as good at stopping ectopics as womb pregnancies. So it is a better choice than an old-type POP if someone has already had one ectopic in the past, to reduce the risk of having another.

Who should avoid the POP?

As a generalization, WHO 4 conditions and diseases for the COC are normally only WHO 2 or 3 for the POP. Both of these categories mean that the POP can be used if it seems right in the particular case, relative to the risks of alternative choices, and with added discussion and supervision—particularly if WHO 3 applies.

Although there is no research that proves that any *past thrombosis* makes users of the POP more likely to have another, a past history of thrombosis is still often described as a reason for not taking POPs (WHO 4). But many doctors, myself included, strongly disagree with this policy because this is a totally estrogen-free contraceptive (see pp. 67–8). We call such a past history WHO 2 and are very prepared to prescribe old-type POPs or Cerazette.

WHO 4 conditions for old-type POPs and Cerazette are few

- Any *serious side effect on the combined pill which was not clearly due to estrogen*, e.g. past liver tumour, allergy to progestogen itself
- *Breast cancer if recent* (see below)
- *Undiagnosed bleeding*
- *Actual or possible pregnancy*

The last two are WHO 4 only until they are properly diagnosed and may be temporary. And:

- Note that, since it contains no artificial estrogen (EE), the POP does not have to be stopped during immobilization or before major or leg surgery.

WHO 3 conditions

- *Breast cancer*: if in remission, with no problems for years (the WHO says five years) past. The hospital specialist should be consulted about this; and I would more usually recommend a method like the IUD (pp. 216–17), where there would be no question as to whether it might reactivate the cancer (given lack of proof either way with the POP).
- *High risk or past history of thrombosis in an artery* (due to concern about slight unwanted effects on blood lipids [fats])
- *Enzyme inducer medicine treatment* (pp. 44–5): another method is preferable, but (in my opinion) compensating by taking two POP tablets a day is also reasonable in some cases.
- *Cysts on the ovary of the type discussed on pp. 97, 186, if history of pain.*

- *Acute porphyria* (p. 140), unless the woman has had a previous bad attack brought on by sex hormones (then WHO 4)—very rare
- *Past ectopic pregnancy*: in my opinion, this is WHO 3 for old-type POPs, but WHO 1 for Cerazette (see above), which like the COC or injectables should prevent any recurrence

WHO 2 conditions

- *Past venous thrombosis or risk factors for VTE* (see pp. 187 above, 71–2)
- *Risk factors for arterial disease* (pp. 74–5)
- *Almost all long-term diseases*, including liver damage with abnormal blood test levels; but might be WHO 3 if the disease (like bad Crohn's, p. 92) significantly interferes with the POPs being absorbed

Which POPs are available?

The kinds of POP available in the UK are as shown in Table 8.2, and also in Fig. 7.1, where they are shown as at 'ground level', because they contain so little hormone. If you live in another country, you can refer to www.ippf.org.uk to compare the locally available brands of POP.

Any of these pills may prove satisfactory. If you develop a problem with the cycle or any other side-effect with one POP, and still wish to use the method, then it is certainly worth switching to one of the others (including either from or to Cerazette). At the moment this has to be done very much on a trial-and-error basis. If you persevere, the menstrual pattern normally becomes acceptable after a few months. If you get no periods at all this is not a problem (see pp. 183–4).

Who might consider using the POP? And which POP?

The short answer to the first question is:

- recent mums who want to *breastfeed* and prefer a pill method (p. 191 below) as the POP does not lower the amount and quality of breast milk like the COC does, and
- anyone who is considering taking a pill at all!

A POP would be the obvious choice if maximum safety against health risk is particularly important to you. A lot may depend on how well you manage to live with an unpredictable menstrual cycle, which is the number one difference between all POPs and the COC. Because of this snag, the POP really comes into its own as an (early) second choice when there is a reason for not using the COC (but a pill is wanted).

From the lists on pp. 137–51, in my experience the POP is particularly valuable for:

- *when there are risk factors for using, or side-effects on, the COC. Weight gain, nausea, mood problems and depression, and headaches* all seem to be helped by this move. *Family history of breast cancer* can also be why some women choose a POP rather than a COC (p. 151)
- women who have *migraine with aura*
- *blood-pressure problems* on the COC pill
- *diabetics*, not only because it cause less health risk for them than the COC but also because they are particularly good at remembering to take it within that narrow 'window' of 24–27 hours: they can time it along with an insulin injection. But there are other good choices too, like an IUD or the IUS (see pp. 224–6)
- *overweight with a BMI over 30 and especially 40 and above* (usually using Cerazette, pp. 178–9)
- smokers, especially *over the age of 35*
- *other older women, especially non-smokers around the menopause* (usually using an old-type POP, p. 190).

How do you find out when you have reached the menopause?

If the older POP-user has no periods, it can be quite difficult to know if the menopause has actually happened, though a blood test can sometimes help. A low value of the hormone FSH from the pituitary gland (Fig. 1.5, p. 12) suggests that the lack of periods is just because of the POP (pp. 183–4) and that you still need to take it! High values of FSH are suggestive of being at or around the menopause, especially if you have hot flushes as well. Unfortunately the rule is that the only proof that you can no longer conceive is after a whole year without periods when no hormones are being taken! That may seem a very long time, but very late ovulations can still occur in some women of this age, even when the periods seem to have stopped.

So the POP can be stopped and another simple method—a sponge or foam would be enough (p. 214)—used for one year. If you hate that kind of method, another option I find some women like is simply to keep taking the (old-type) POP till age 56. This is a safe thing to do healthwise, and 56 is five years after the average age of the final period. So if you stop the

POP then—and your own periods don't, against the odds, come back—you can be sure your ovaries have completely stopped working.

Incidentally, HRT, which may be prescribed for symptoms around the menopause, should not be relied on as a contraceptive. The dose system is different from that used in any kind of contraceptive pill, and pregnancy is possible—unless of course you had definitely reached the menopause first, before the treatment started. If you need HRT treatment before the menopause and are an absolutely healthy, slim, and migraine-free non-smoker, careful use of a 20 mcg estrogen-containing pill like Femodette or Mercilon may be best (see pp. 159–60).

If you have any queries, discuss this whole matter with your doctor or at the clinic.

More about which POP—and when to choose Cerazette

Cerazette, as we have seen, blocks ovulation much more regularly than old-type POPs, and yet as back-up it still has the mucus-blocking-of-sperm method. So I see it as highly unlikely not to be more effective and to have more margin for error than the others. However, it is not very different from the old-type POP for annoying bleeding symptoms in early months (though more often getting better later, p. 185); and it costs more.

So what's the 'bottom line' about which POP to choose? I see no special reason not to continue using old-type POPs:

- during full breastfeeding, and
- above age 45

since the efficacy in those two situations is already so brilliant (p. 176).

But I would recommend Cerazette instead for:

- *the young, fertile woman who wants a pill method, cannot use or does not want to use the COC, and wants or should have more effectiveness than other POPs*, especially if she thinks she might be at all forgetful. An important example of '*should have*' more effectiveness would be a young woman with complicated structural heart disease, as in such cases a pregnancy might be unusually risky. And a good reason for a COC-user to switch to Cerazette would be while waiting for major or leg surgery (p. 147).
- *a woman who might specially benefit from a method which blocks ovulation* (egg release), such as with a *past history of an ectopic pregnancy*. For the

same reason it also helps some women with some menstrual-type problems that are more usually treated by the COC, such as:

– *period heaviness or pain*
– *PMS*
– *breast tenderness*

(though the benefit is less predictable, because instead of getting what is desired with Cerazette—no bleeding at all—they need warning that they may get the usual POP side-effect of too frequent or prolonged bleeds)

- *a woman who weighs more than 70 kg* (pp. 178–9), given also that any POP is safer than a COC for women with a high BMI.

Breastfeeding: the main use of old-type POPs

Breastfeeding under certain conditions has a good contraceptive effect on its own (see p. 213). So it is not surprising that in combination with the old-type POP it is so remarkably effective. Indeed, provided your periods have not returned, the breastfeeding is practically 100 per cent, and your baby is not more than six months old (i.e. the lactational amenorrhoea method [LAM] applies), in my opinion the 'leeway' for needing to take two days extra precautions because of a missed pill can go up to 24 hours. This is the same as is now advised for the lowest-dose combined pills. Moreover, during full breastfeeding the emergency pill would very rarely be necessary for missed POP tablets (see p. 182).

The POP does not interfere at all with the quantity or significantly with the quality of breast milk. (The combined pill, however, often does, and most doctors now feel that it is illogical to use it during breastfeeding.)

How much of the POP does the baby get?

If a mother who breastfeeds does choose the (old-type) POP, in the UK she is usually advised to start on about the 21st day following delivery. However, since risk of conception early on in full breastfeeding is so low, the WHO prefers that mothers wait to start the POP till their baby is six weeks old (not later). Thereafter, a very tiny amount of the hormone in all POPs has been shown to get into the milk, the least being found in milk from women who use pills containing only levonorgestrel—meaning Microval™ or Norgeston™ in the UK. This transfer via milk to infant causes concern to some mothers. And yet, there is absolutely no evidence that this amount of hormone has ever harmed any baby. After more than two years of full breastfeeding, the infant of a mother using these POPs will have taken the equivalent of just one tablet.

To put this in perspective, if a breastfeeding woman smokes, a far greater number of potentially dangerous chemicals are swallowed by the baby.

If you plan to feed your baby yourself—and there is abundant scientific evidence that human breast milk is better for human babies than any kind of modified cow's milk—you might discuss the use of this type of pill during the months that you are breastfeeding. Your protection against pregnancy is as good as that of any woman on the combined pill. When you or your baby decide to cut down on the breastfeeding, and especially when your first period comes on, you may like to change to Cerazette, or back to an ultra-low-dose combined pill, or perhaps use an injectable or implant. This will give extra reliability when you lose the contraceptive effect of breastfeeding.

Or of course you could choose a completely non-hormonal method right through, such as an IUD or the sponge or condoms (p. 214, 216–19). *It's your call*—as contraception always should be!

9 What became of the male pill?

New hormonal methods for men

Why are we still waiting? The female pill (the pill) was much less slow to arrive. It makes one wonder: back in the early 1950s, was the pill a confidence trick by male chauvinist scientists? Was there a conspiracy, with pharmaceutical companies keen to make money, to unleash an untried chemical on the unsuspecting, docile, and passive female population? Out of all the money ever spent on contraceptive research worldwide, only an estimated 8 per cent is on male methods.

'What is sauce for the goose is sauce for the gander'. In other words, if we have a pill for the goose, why are we still waiting for a pill for the gander?

Would a male pill make a vas deferens?!

Apologies for the corny heading, but a woman must first have made that pun. I do a lot of lecturing to (mostly women) doctors and nurses about contraception, and at question time if someone asks 'Why don't we have a male pill?', someone else immediately puts their hand up to say 'If there were a male pill, who would ever trust a man to take it [regularly—if at all]!' After all, men don't 'carry the baby' (Fig. 9.1). What hope is there, given that even among women, who do, major contraceptive mistakes are not exactly unknown.

Can men be trusted? After much of my working lifetime in this business, I confess I am truly disgusted with my own gender sometimes: the sexual violence of some and the sexual self-centredness of many (though definitely not all) of the rest: The account below just about says it all:

> Among 98 male students aged 18–29 from two university campuses in Georgia, USA, who took part in a standardized interview about their use of condoms, 50 per cent reported ever experiencing condom breakage.

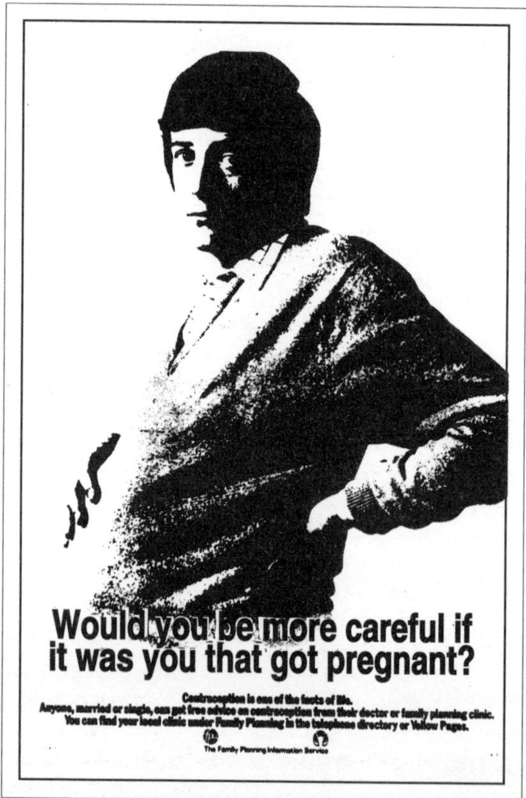

Fig. 9.1 Family Planning Association campaign poster (1970).

Among these 49 men, 15 (30 per cent) had at some time failed to disclose knowledge of a broken condom to their female sex partner, nine of them many times! Overall, 13.2 per cent of condom breakage episodes were never revealed to the partners. The reasons given were (n = number of individuals out of the 15):

- unwillingness to interrupt intercourse because orgasm was approaching (n = 6)
- wanting to avoid being blamed for the break (n = 5)
- desire not to make their partner anxious about the break (n = 4).

I was quite speechless when I first heard about this 1997 study. Its implications are devastating: for example, how many women never even know they ought to be seeking emergency contraception?

Then comes 'machismo', which includes a powerful myth in some parts of the world that equates fertility with virility and potency. This would stop many men from even taking badly any male pill! These ideas do seem to have influenced researchers, who have wondered whether there would be a demand for a male pill if it were invented.

Yet the assumption that all men wash their hands of birth-control matters is not in fact true. It takes all types to make a world and there are many men, especially within marriage or steady relationships, who show a lot more responsibility than might perhaps be expected. The best example of this is the remarkable increase in the number of vasectomy operations performed in so many countries, both developing and developed, in recent years. Given choices, men in many different cultures, like women, now frequently prefer their families to be small. In one survey in the USA, 65 per cent of the men stated that they would use a male pill or injection if it were available and not too expensive, and there are very similar findings in 2000 from countries as different as China, Scotland, and South Africa.

Research into male methods

Male contraception is biologically more difficult to achieve than female contraception. The main reason is that there is no single regular event like egg release which can be stopped. The manufacture of sperm is a continuous process throughout a man's life from puberty to death. So instead of just stopping one egg being released about 13 times a year, we have to interfere with a process producing 1000 to 2000 sperm a second—hundreds of millions of them every time a man ejaculates. As I say in my lectures, 'If each sperm could find an egg there would be enough for any fertile man to populate the whole of North America on a single occasion!'

Secondly, just as in the woman, any pill must not affect libido, must give extremely good protection against pregnancy, and be as free as possible from side-effects. There is a special risk here too that interference with the production of the sperm might be incomplete. So if one sperm were to be *damaged* by whatever the treatment might be, yet managed to fertilize an egg, this might result in the birth of an abnormal baby.

Yet another problem is that the manufacturing process takes a long time, about 70 days in the human male. Thus any male pill working on the manufacturing process will take at least two months to become effective. It also means that there must be a long recovery period after stopping the method. After some of the experimental methods have been stopped, more than the usual number of abnormal sperm have been seen. So if in the recovery period another method of family planning were inadequately used, again there is the fear (which will need more research to allay) of an increased risk of adverse effects on the baby.

Research has focused either on:

- stopping the production of sperm or
- inactivating or blocking them once produced.

Interference with the manufacturing of sperm

This can be done in two ways: indirectly by blocking the action of the hormones from the pituitary gland which normally stimulate the process, and directly by some drug acting on the testicles (see Fig. 9.2).

Indirect methods

These are similar in principle to the female pill. The pituitary gland of a man produces the very same two hormones that are so important in the menstrual cycle, namely FSH and LH. However, they are not produced in a cyclical way. In a man, FSH is the hormone which is directly involved to promote sperm manufacture. LH, on the other hand, stimulates special cells, also in the testicle, which produce the male hormone, testosterone. This hormone, as well as producing the special sexual characteristics of a man such as the deepening of his voice, the hairiness of his chin, and his sex drive, joins with FSH in the business of manufacturing normal fertile sperm.

So, if the levels of FSH and LH reaching the testicles can be made to drop, the process of sperm manufacture will cease. This can be done by 'negative feedback' which was explained on pp. 8–9. An obvious way of doing this is to feed the man with his partner's pill! This certainly cuts down the production of FSH and LH from the pituitary and hence interferes with manufacture of sperm. Obviously, however, it would rapidly produce some very unacceptable side effects on his whole masculinity.

One way out of that difficulty was to use a 'pill' or actually an injection plus implant to deliver a combination of a *progestogen with an androgen*, an artificial equivalent of testosterone. This would still block both pituitary hormones, and so switch off the man's own testosterone (Fig. 9.2), but the androgen from the contraceptive would keep his libido and drive going. Problems are that the doses need careful adjustment to avoid the drive turning into aggressiveness—and the amounts required are relatively higher than

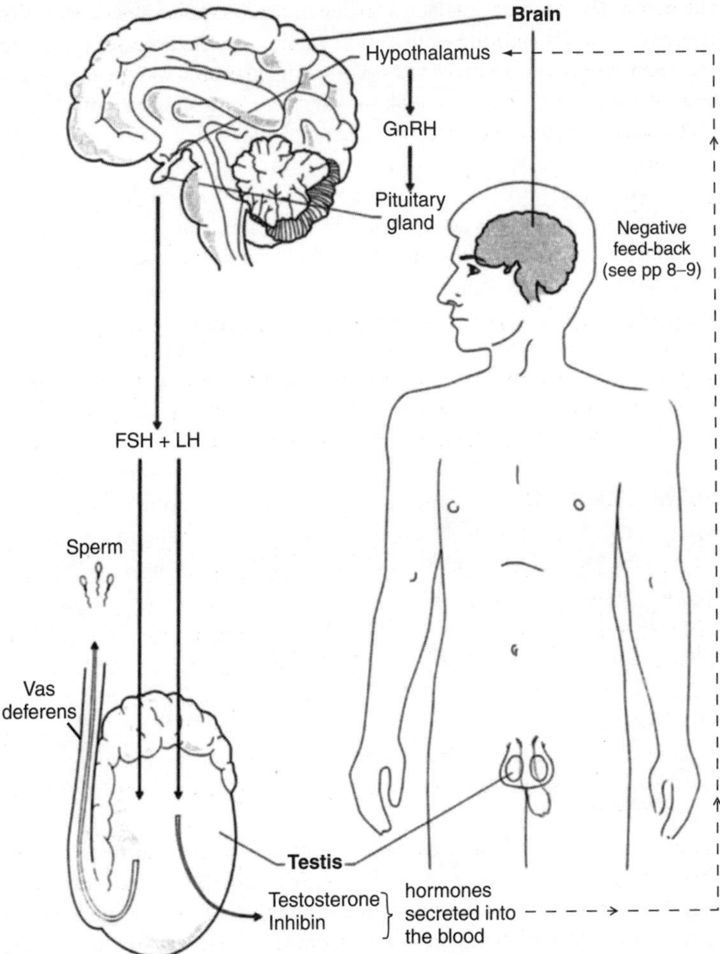

Fig. 9.2 How reproductive hormones work in men

Note: Testosterone, as well as having well-known effects as an androgen, can give negative feedback (see pp 8–9) to suppress FSH and LH. Inhibin feeds back to suppress FSH alone (see text p. 198).

in women. That means, so far, annoyingly frequent injections of the androgen (how many men will accept having a needle every single month?) and the results are variable: it does not always work in every man to stop sperm production completely. As with any drug there are fears about unwanted effects, especially on the liver, prostate gland, and the arteries through bad effects on blood fats. But there's some good news: the method does seem fully reversible, like the pill in women. The hope is to develop a long-acting androgen which would be released along with the progestogen in a combined way from implanted rods, like having three Implanon™ implants (see p. 223), and hopefully only needing to be implanted every year, or ultimately less often.

'Watch this space', as they say: some version of this method is quite likely to be available for your partner before this decade is out. One important advantage is that it's not going to be a male *pill* at all. If he says he is on it, you will be able to check on the implants for yourself, through the skin of his upper arm!

Other indirect methods are being tried without as much success so far, including using a synthetic blocking drug to stop the man's GnRH, which, as in a woman (pp. 4–6), comes down in pulses from the base of the brain (hypothalamus) to the pituitary gland, to release both FSH and LH. Synthetic versions of GnRH are researched in male volunteers as an injection or implant along with enough male hormone to balance the loss of testosterone production from the testicles. Success is going to depend on discovering more potent and longer-acting GnRH-blocking drugs than are available so far.

There is a complex natural substance in humans and other primates called *inhibin* (Fig. 9.2). If only it were not such a complicated molecule to synthesize, it would be theoretically ideal since it only suppresses FSH. Therefore it ought to leave alone the LH which controls a man's own testosterone production. A kind of magic bullet—but not yet!

Direct methods

Various drugs which directly damage the manufacturing process of sperm in the testicles have been tried in male animals and human volunteers. If only a reversible safe product could be found, a big advantage would be no reduction in the man's testosterone. Sadly, the experiments were abandoned in most cases because they were found to be too toxic or insufficiently predictable in their contraceptive effects.

A still ongoing saga is *gossypol*, a drug in this group. A report on the use of this substance appeared in the *Chinese Medical Journal* back in November 1978. Scientific workers in mainland China discovered during the 1950s that cooking with crude cottonseed oil could lead to infertility, and it was the men that seemed to be affected. The active ingredient was tried first in a number of different experimental animals. Then 4000 healthy men were put on regular gossypol treatment for up to four years. Close on 100 per cent of them became infertile as judged by sperm counts of zero or well below the usually accepted levels for fertility. Side-effects were said to be mild and uncommon.

So far, so good. Quickly dubbed the 'Chinese sperm take-away', at first it seemed a promising male contraceptive. But then serious side-effects emerged: the chief ones were feelings of great weakness, connected with a lowering of potassium in the body and irreversible infertility in as many as 10 per cent of the volunteers. It looked like a kind of irreversible chemical sterilization! But trials have continued with lower doses alone or in various combinations, or as a potential new spermicide.

Maturing of the sperm in the epididymis

The epididymis is a very long (7 metres), fine coiled-up tube, which forms into something about the size of a baby's little finger closely applied to the testicle (Figs 9.2 and 10.2). It receives the sperm leaving the production line from the testicle and its main job is to deliver at the other end, at the start of the vas, sperm which are now mature and able to swim. Several drugs have been found to interfere with this maturing process.

The great advantage of acting at this stage, if only a safe drug could be discovered, is that there would be a far more rapid loss and return of fertility than by any of the methods above which interfere with sperm manufacture. The treatment should affect within a few days only those sperm which are just ready for ejaculation. And when the drug is stopped, once any (perhaps damaged) sperm have been flushed out, the ones arriving fresh from the production line should hopefully not have been affected by it.

Derivatives of ordinary sugar, modified and containing chlorine atoms, had seemed very promising. In animal experiments they interfered with the fertilizing ability of already manufactured sperm, and when the treatment was stopped the animals were fertile again within a week. But none of them was safe enough to use in man: they are toxic to the bone marrow and nervous system. But the basic idea is sound.

Blocking the function of the vas deferens itself

Reversible 'chemical vasectomy'?

This probably sounds very far-fetched! But there are muscles in the vas which contract to squeeze the sperm and seminal fluid along it, so as to reach the penis whenever a man ejaculates. Researchers at King's College in

London (now working with us in fact, at the Elliot–Smith Clinic in Oxford) have discovered chemicals which can affect these muscle contractions; and their work raises the distinct possibility of producing a new product that a man could take just before intercourse.

If this method worked as envisaged, the vas would be prevented from contracting normally. So when the man ejaculated, the sperm-bearing fluid would be stopped from reaching the prostate gland (see Fig. 10.2, p. 206) on its way to the base of the penis. He would still ejaculate the (larger amount of) semen-forming fluid that normally comes from the prostate, and other glands called the seminal vesicles. Would he notice any difference in the amount of fluid produced? Probably not, as men who have had the usual surgical type of vasectomy do not have any problems there. Would intercourse still give him the same pleasurable sensations though? Maybe—after all, men following ordinary vasectomies say their enjoyment of sex is completely unchanged. This chemical vasectomy *might* feel different, though, and sadly, the lab work is still a long way from even producing the actual vas-blocking chemical to try out.

Other ideas involving the vas tube

These seem at least as far away from becoming regular options as the above, though a fair amount of work has been done, especially in India, on:

- reversible mechanical blocks and taps for the vas
- a delightfully 'wacky' idea of inserting into the vas a very low voltage battery and special switching. A low current does indeed electrocute the sperm—but my guess is it will be a very long time before your partner will be able literally to switch his fertility off and back on again in such a way!

Immune methods

This concept cashes in on the fact that some men are naturally infertile through having developed a kind of immunity with antibodies against their own sperm. Yet they are otherwise healthy in every other way, including sexually. Hence the idea of deliberately vaccinating men against their own hormones, like GnRH and FSH (Fig. 9.2).

Unfortunately a major problem with this, once again, is individual variation. What this means here is that some men would need ultra-frequent repeats of the booster injections for the immunity to become strong enough to work at all (impractical); while others might over-react to even one or two doses, so for them the method could be irreversible (unacceptable). Therefore progress here has been rather disappointing.

Conclusion

The fact is that the practical male methods available now, or likely to appear in the near future, remain, apart from withdrawal, simply the condom and vasectomy. My 'crystal ball' predicts that the more promising form of indirect method above, the one using a progestogen plus an androgen (initially with injections but eventually solely as long-acting implant(s)), might be the first to arrive, maybe by about 2010?

Let's hope so. Many women would like men to take more of a share in this matter of birth control, and plenty of men would like to be able to do just that. As making love itself is very much a sharing business, we badly need an adequately safe 'pill' for each sex—so that Mary could be on the pill, say for six months, followed by her partner Matt for another six months. By taking turns each would be exposed to half of any long-term risks of the methods.

But an *implant* or similar, which would be completely forgettable by Matt, and yet checkable by Mary, would always be better than any male pill!

10 Contraception: your choices

Can there ever be an ideal method?

Apparently, though you won't find it in the Bible, after God created Adam, He said to him: 'I have some news for you: two bits of good news and one bit of bad news. Which would you like to hear first?' And Adam said, 'The good news first please, God.' So God said to Adam: 'The first good news is that I am going to create for you an Organ. This Organ is called the Brain. With this gift of mine you will be able to think, and to learn, and to feel—and you can devise good names for all my other creatures.'

'Thank you very much,' said Adam. 'What's the other good news?' 'Well,' said God, 'I am going to create for you another Organ. This Organ is called the Penis. With it you will be able to give to your wife and receive back from her, much pleasure—and with my help, create children to follow you. You should teach them to be good stewards and care for all the other creatures I have made.'

'Thank you again,' said Adam. 'So, what's the bad news?' 'You will never be able to use both at the same time!' said God.

Fig. 10.1 shows, very approximately, some of the latest available information on current British usage of all the main methods of birth control. One conclusion must be that different couples make different choices: there is certainly no one ideal method.

What should we look for, anyway, in a method of birth control, present or future? Box 10.1 provides a useful checklist of what would be ideal. Given how true to life the above little story is—isn't there truly a lot of difficulty (in both genders) of getting the brain and the genitalia to work sensibly together?—items 1–5 are all vitally important things to aim for.

I wish it were not necessary to add number 10 to the list, but I think the point should be made. It is a sad comment on the relationship of many couples that they can sleep together yet be unable to trust each other. More specifically, a lot of *men* are not trustworthy about contraception

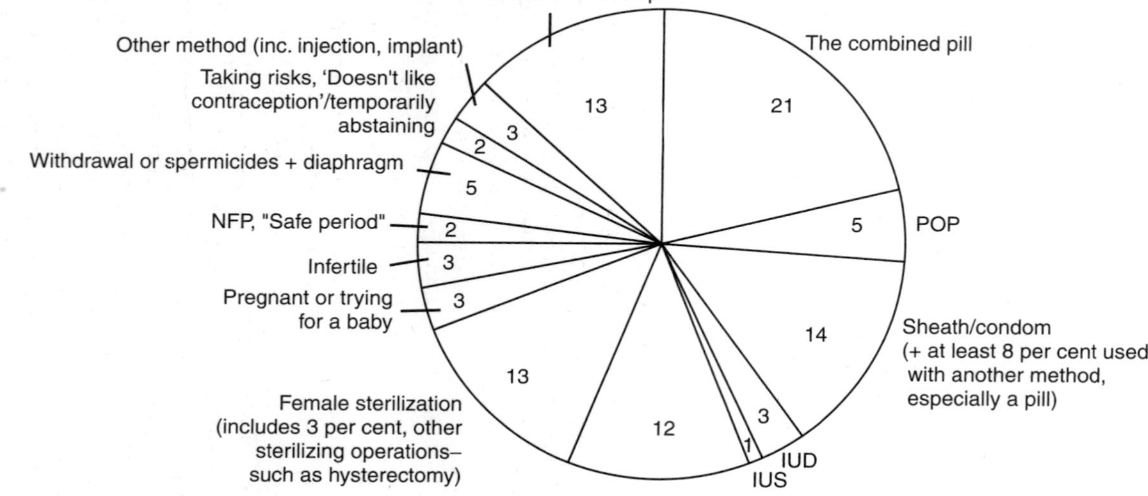

Fig. 10.1 How birth control methods are used in the UK

Derived from the Omnibus Survey of the Office for National Statistics from a random probability sample of households surveyed up to March 2002. (Adjusted by the author [JG] for respondents giving > 1 answer.)

Box 10.1 Features of the ideal contraceptive

1. 100 per cent effective.
2. 100 per cent safe, with no unwanted effects—both risky and nuisance-type.
3. 100 per cent reversible.
4. Convenient, independent of intercourse.
5. Effective after acceptable, simple, painless procedures(s), not relying on the user's memory—i.e. fully 'forgettable'.
6. Reversed by a simple, painless process under the user's control.
7. Cheap, based on simple technology, easy to distribute.
8. Independent of the medical profession.
9. Acceptable to every culture, religion, and political view.
10. Used by, or obviously visible to, the woman.
11. Giving one or more non-contraceptive beneficial side-effects, such as reduced menstrual problems and protection against STIs, particularly HIV/AIDS.

(see p. 193–4), or are just forgetful or careless. Either partner can be unreliable, of course, but only the woman ends up pregnant. An advantage of the condom is that it gives visual proof that it has in fact been effectively used.

Perhaps the last item in Box 10.1 is asking for too much, but we *are* talking about the ideal. For all its faults, the pill does help women who suffer discomfort or misery from their so-called 'normal' menstrual cycles. A method which was ideal in all the other ways listed in Box 10.1, such as a simple, painless, totally reversible method of female sterilization, might still leave some women less well off than on the pill, if they continued to have heavy, painful periods, premenstrual tension, and the like.

Fig. 10.2 illustrates the various stages or events in reproduction at which birth control methods either do now, or could one day, operate. The main points were described in Chapter 1, and Chapter 9 for the male; if anything is not clear, you may like to refer back to pp. 1–15. Any future method you hear about has to be based on detecting or interfering with one of the stages in Fig.10.2. It is a complex system, so it is never going to be easy to alter it without the possibility of unwanted spin-offs and side effects. This means expensive testing. Yet, given its enormous potential importance (see pp. 241–4), far too little money and scientific attention is ever directed to contraceptive research. In most countries drug regulatory committees have been created. They have the praiseworthy aim of ensuring that new medicines and techniques are as effective and as safe as can be. But in the contraceptive drug field their understandable caution plus fears about litigation have made development of new methods so

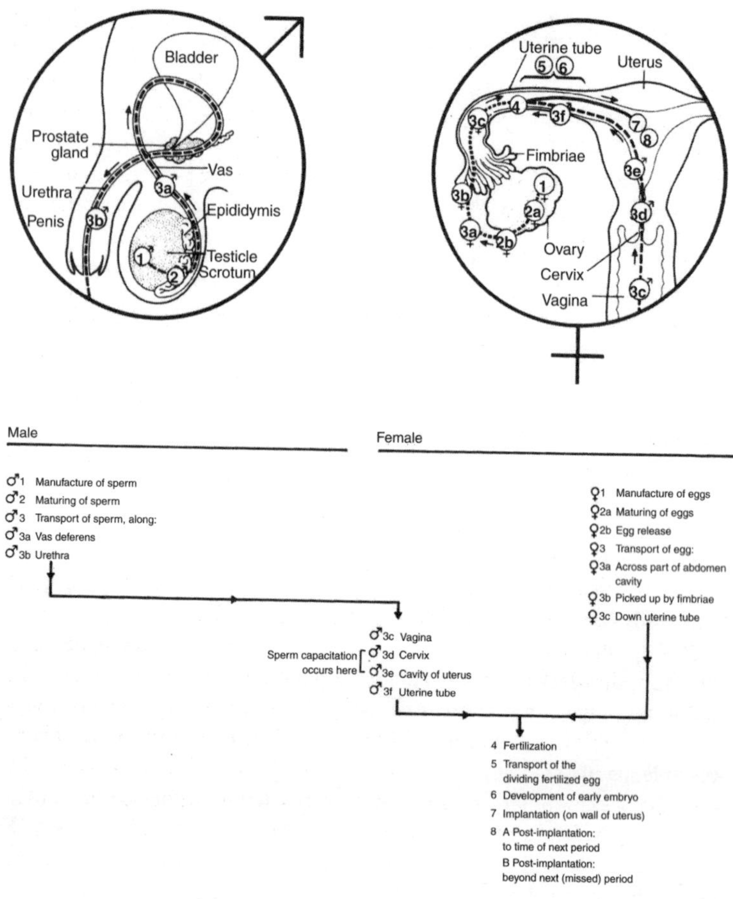

Fig. 10.2 The stages of reproduction

expensive and prolonged (15 years is the minimum) as to tend to stop it altogether.

You should always be sceptical when you read reports of 'breakthroughs' in contraception. Journalists often suggest that a brand-new method is just around the corner, when in fact it could be many years before it is cleared for general use, if at all. This can be irritating to many who find all the available methods unsatisfactory for one reason or another.

Many women feel that they were betrayed during the 1960s and 1970s over the problems of the original combined pill. Doctors are accused, sometimes but not always fairly, of doing too little to warn users that there could be long-term problems. (That is why, in part, I wrote this book.) It seemed at that time a magical method, a panacea, 'the pill of the Brave New World'. Time has shown up its drawbacks, but these have often been exaggerated, and unexpected benefits have also emerged. These lessons must be learned and applied when any new pill or other medical method comes along, whether for use by men or by women. Ethical considerations must also be confronted and resolved by each couple.

Some ethical aspects of birth control methods

A question which concerns some people is whether methods which are able to act after fertilization are in reality abortifacients (causing an abortion) and hence ethically unacceptable.

Just as the definition of death has had to be altered—it is no longer cessation of the heartbeat, but final death of the brain—so now that we have more knowledge of the processes of reproduction the definition of conception needs to be reconsidered. It is my view, along with many modern ethicists, that methods which sometimes work after fertilization (stage 4 in Fig.10.2) but before the completion of implantation (stage 7 in Fig. 10.2) are not causing abortions. They are correctly in the category of family-planning methods.

A complication for the debate is that when a woman does not become pregnant using a method that is *capable* of working in more than one way (see, for example, Table 8.1 on POPs, p. 177), it is usually impossible to know precisely why—i.e. which mechanism actually operated. Was it by stopping ovulation or by preventing the sperm from getting through to the egg, or was it by interfering later with the fertilized egg or embryo (which is believed to be a much weaker mechanism of action with the POP, but still might work when the others failed)?

*Research can prove that the pregnancy has been prevented from progressing *after* implantation (embedding in the wall of the womb), since hCG (see p. 6, 9) would then be detectable for a few hours or days thereafter, in a woman whose pregnancy was caused to fail at Stage 8A, because her next period nevertheless came on normally. This would be, indubitably, an early abortion, and unacceptable to most as a family-planning method. But there is as yet no study that has proved by some measurement during sustained use of a method, that a block to conception occurred before successful implantation yet still after fertilization (during stages 5 and 6 but before 7 in Fig. 10.2).

A most important point is that the fact that a method is *capable* of working in a post-fertilization way does not mean it necessarily ever needs to do so. Thus women who are conscientious COC pill-takers, never once lengthening their pill-free week even by an hour, or users of Depo-Provera (see p. 222–3), never being late with their next 12-weekly dose, can in my view be confident that their avoidance of pregnancy is entirely due to the block to ovulation (egg release) and maybe the mucus block to sperm (see pp. 12, 13). Those mechanisms are so strong that the back-up by blocking implantation will never be needed, even during years of use.

The question 'could my method be causing an induced miscarriage/abortion?' therefore arises primarily with all the intrauterine methods, all the progestogen-only methods *except* Depo-Provera, and of course with emergency contraception (see pp. 54–8). In my view the answer is still 'no' in all these cases even if they might, rarely or sometimes, operate by a pre-implantation but post-fertilization mechanism. But that depends on definitions, and specifically on accepting the definition of 'conception' as only being complete after implantation—as in my equation below.

Here then are my thoughts on the matter, after much deliberation. I address myself to those of any faith who would call themselves theists (as I am). The scientists of the 19th century who were believers said they were 'thinking God's thoughts after him'. How should theists today 'think his thoughts' about the earliest stages of human reproduction? Biologically, we now know so much more about *con-ception* (a word whose etymology is 'being with child'). But theologically, these are uncharted waters—there is nothing specifically relevant in texts such as the Bible or the Koran.

So I suggest we start from the 'chart' provided by the normal God-ordained events *in vivo*. To recap (p. 9 and Figs. 1.4b, 10.2), after fertilization there is cell division to produce an early embryo, technically known as blastocyst (a cystic structure forming a tiny fluid-filled sac). This reaches the uterus and begins to implant no earlier than five days after fertilization. If it implants successfully, its secretion of human chorionic gonadotrophin (hCG) enters the mother's bloodstream and prevents the otherwise inevitable failure of the corpus luteum, and the resultant loss of the blastocyst in the next menstrual flow.

So what is the status of the unimplanted blastocyst? Clearly while it is free in the uterine cavity, any biological scientist will tell us that it has a 100 per cent 'no go' status. As day follows night, it is a certainty that in a few days it will be flushed through the cervix (neck of the womb) and vagina, in a gush of endometrial debris and blood.

The only way the blastocyst can stop this is by getting its magic signal of hCG into the mother's bloodstream and so to the active ovary—and that requires implantation (see p. 9). The blastocyst's 'no go' status only changes to 'go' after hCG tells the corpus luteum to continue to produce essential estrogen and progesterone, and so stop the blastocyst being flushed away via the cervix at the next period. Until implantation, because the woman's body does not 'know' it is there, it has no more chance of life than the particular sperm and egg that made it, about five days earlier, in the tube. (Thereafter, it has about an 80 per cent chance of making it to term.)

Until then there is no proper two-way *relationship* with the mother.

Thirdly, best estimates suggest that up to 50 per cent of blastocysts do in fact fail to implant naturally. Now we know that God is omnipotent, omniscient, and omnipresent. Does he not also have (and I say this with the utmost respect), surely, 'omni-common sense'? How likely is it that a God with that attribute as well as the other 'omnis' would expect us to give the status, importance, and respect to this entity, with which Nature is so prodigal, as we rightly give to the potential unborn child *after* implantation (when there is a two-way relationship with the mother and, for the first time, there are above zero prospects of going on to term)?

From these considerations one can write an equation for the definition of conception as follows:

CONCEPTION	=	FERTILIZATION	+	IMPLANTATION
(being with child)		(crucial)		(also crucial)

Before implantation at Stage 7 in Fig.10.2 there is no true 'carriage', as the blastocyst is floating free in the cavity of the womb and certainly doomed so long as it stays there. So how can it be 'procuring a miscarriage' (i.e. abortion) to use:

- the emergency pill
- intrauterine devices and systems
- progestogen-only pills?

All of these do have anti-implantation effects, agreed, though they are mainly back-up mechanisms of action to their main effects.

Note that those who accept this interpretation can agree wholeheartedly, as I do, that 'life begins at conception'. But we understand that word as *not* being synonymous with fertilization (alone). It follows that we are willing to classify as methods of contraception those that might sometimes block implantation. This is also the UK legal position, established finally in 2002 by the Judicial Review on emergency contraception.

Two additional points:

- For those who retain the belief that any method which might *ever* act post-fertilization would then be acting as an abortifacient: even so they need not forego the chance to use hormonal emergency contraception after a single act of unprotected intercourse that was treated between day 1 and day 10 of a 28-day cycle. With that timing there can be a definite risk of conceiving if nothing is done. Yet although applied after intercourse, the method if it worked would have to be operating by stopping/delaying ovulation or by changing the mucus of the cervix to stop the sperm ever getting to an egg. (The hormones could not, so far as we know, have any appreciable effect on the endometrium—i.e. to block implantation—much later on in the cycle, well over one week after they were ingested.)
- Moreover, in sustained use of methods like the most effective modern banded copper IUDs, or the levonorgestrel (LNG) intrauterine system, the anti-fertilization effects of the copper (toxic to sperm) and of the LNG (preventing sperm-penetrability of the cervico-uterine fluid) are so strong that the back-up mechanisms which stop implantation are most unlikely ever to need to be utilised, despite years of use.

I shall have to leave it to you to decide whether you draw the line at fertilization (stage 4), or at the time of implantation (stage 7 in Fig 10.2), which would allow you to join me and most modern ethicists in classifying the IUD, the IUS, the POP, implants, and post-coital pills (and similar research methods not yet marketed) all as contraceptives.

What would be illogical, however, would be to accept IUDs and reject emergency contraception. Even though as I have just stated there is good evidence that copper IUDs (when they are there all the time) work mainly pre-fertilization, it would be impossible to guarantee that during years of use they *never* worked the implantation-blocking way. So it is a package: either you accept all these, including emergency pills and IUDs, as family-planning methods, following my argument here; or you have to say they are all off-limits in your case.

If doctors and patients are rather muddled on this subject, it is not surprising that the law in many countries is illogical and confused and the ethical arguments often generate more heat than light! The silly thing is, as we have seen, that the arguments boil down mainly to being about definitions. Perhaps the most important conclusions are that respect for life, for each other (whatever our varying views), and a proper sense of awe about the whole process of reproduction are all more important than rigid definitions.

Natural family planning (NFP)

Fertility-awareness methods

These are acceptable to the Roman Catholic Church and certain other religious groups who do not accept methods which are 'artificial'. But in addition many other women and their partners appreciate the approach at least some of the time during their sexual/reproductive years.

Present methods depend mainly on combinations of calculations according to the length of previous menstrual cycles; on taking and charting the early morning temperature; and on learning to recognize certain changes in the cervical mucus which usually occur before, during, and after the fertile time. If the woman cross-checks using more than one marker of ovulation, such as checking both mucus and temperature changes (the 'symptothermal' or multiple index approach), well-motivated couples can control their fertility well.

But sooner or later many fertile long-term users even of the best existing natural family-planning methods tend to be let down. The failure rate with 'perfect' use can be as low as one to nine women per 100; but in more typical use over the first year it rises to 20 per 100 women, and even higher in the real world with partners who come home drunk in the evenings. The difference is mainly caused by the long time of abstinence demanded by natural methods, usually at least 10 days each cycle, so people understandably 'break the rules'. And the methods are 'very unforgiving of imperfect use', as one researcher put it.

One of the prime objectives of new methods is to shorten the number of days of required abstinence, as well as improving accuracy of ovulation detection/prediction.

There are really two challenges for fertility-awareness methods. One detects egg release, and can be quite effective (because the egg dies quickly). The other tries to predict egg release. It is obviously more difficult to forecast than to detect a biological event; but the first so-called 'safe' phase, leading up to ovulation, will also always be less safe because of the remarkably good and unpredictable survival of those millions of sperm once they enter the uterus. Recently, *ultrasound scanning*—the same method that is used for checking the well-being of a baby as it grows in the uterus—has been used to watch the growth of the follicle on the active ovary, and to see the exact time of its rupture to release the egg. A really futuristic—and at present far too expensive—application of this method would be to issue women with mini-ultrasound-scan machines and teach them to observe their own egg release on their own TV monitors! More practical right now is testing of the *mucus*, *saliva*, or *urine*. The hormones of the menstrual cycle get into body fluids, and the changing levels can be measured.

Persona™

This personal contraceptive system tests the urine. It was first marketed in 1996 following years of research and is a very sophisticated micro-laboratory plus computer. It uses the first significant rise in natural estrogen to show the start of the fertile phase (a red light comes on when a test stick dipped in urine is put into the hand-held electronic monitor). The green light comes back on when the LH surge (see p. 9) is detected by the system in the urine on the test stick and sufficient time is allowed thereafter for egg survival. Its internal computer is clever enough to keep updating and therefore individualizing the data on which it bases its decisions as to the start and end of the unsafe time. It is claimed that only eight days' abstinence are usually required to achieve low pregnancy rates.

In the real world the manufacturer's claimed failure rate (six per 100 women or one in 17 in the first year of use) seems optimistic. Better results can be expected if unprotected intercourse is restricted only to the second 'green phase', after the egg is dead. But much worse failure rates are inevitable if a couple ever disobeys the red light. Although not cheap, many couples find the price acceptable for a method completely free of health risk. It also gives such a feeling of empowerment, particularly to the woman.

The fertility awareness approach is ideal for people 'spacing' their family (see Tables 10.1 and 10.2). Persona mainly makes it all more user-friendly; similar results can be obtained by conscientious well-taught couples using no gadgets at all apart from a good thermometer. For more details, including how you and your partner might visit a trained teacher in your local area to learn to use these methods well, visit www.fertilityuk.org. See also Further Reading (p. 265).

The lactational amenorrhoea method (LAM)

This is another very natural method which is not as widely publicized as I believe it deserves to be. It is fully explained in Fig.10.3. Notice that it has a very acceptable success rate of 98 per cent, so long as all three questions can be answered 'No'—which means not relying on the method beyond six months after the birth. Thereafter a progestogen-only pill or maybe a vaginal method might be chosen, added to not so 'full' breastfeeding. Or, for greater than 98% effectiveness, this could be your combination from early on, after the delivery (pp. 191, 124).

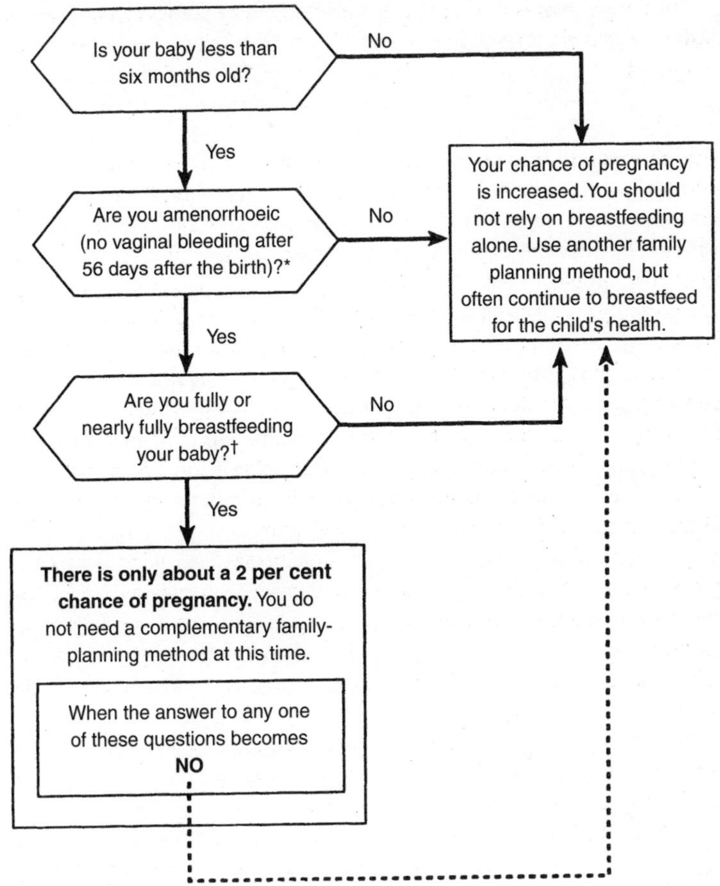

Fig. 10.3 The lactational amenorrhoea method (LAM)

**Spotting that occurs during the first 56 days is not considered to be menstruation.*
'Nearly' full breastfeeding means that the baby obtains almost 100 per cent of its nutrition from the mother alone, and certainly no solid food.

Which method to choose?

The final decision has to be your own: books and doctors can only answer your questions, so far as the facts are known, and maybe give you some unbiased advice. But it is up to you to weigh up all the pros and cons, in consultation with your partner, and decide which method will suit you both best.

Your own 'best' method will depend on many things, among them: how crucial it is that you do not get pregnant; how much medical risk you feel prepared to accept; and how the actual method fits in with your sex life. Table 10.1 summarizes the most important pros and cons of the main recommended artificial methods of birth control which are widely available, and may help you to make up your mind.

Non-hormonal contraception

No variety of *spermicide* is recommended for use on its own by normally fertile couples, even though in some countries they are heavily promoted by manufacturers who imply that they are much more effective than they are. They appear in many different guises: pessaries, foaming tablets, creams, gels, ovals, films, and foams, as well as the contraceptive sponge, which is primarily a carrier for the contained spermicide. The sponge's failure rate in the Margaret Pyke Centre study was 24 per 100 woman-years, too high for most young people to rely on; but it is nevertheless an adequate method for those with very reduced fertility (above the age of 50, or during breastfeeding for example), and so is being reintroduced to the UK in 2005.

Contraceptive foam (e.g. Delfen™) does find a useful niche as an *extra method* when fertility is already low for some reason: e.g. once again during breastfeeding or in the early months after the menopause (before the year has gone by which allows one to be sure that the ovaries have completely stopped egg release), or above the age of 51 anyway.

The foam can also be useful if a couple insist on using only the *withdrawal method*. It is a fact that some couples manage to use this successfully for many years, though we would always recommend use of some kind of spermicide *as well*. Even if it works, withdrawal is often reported as being a bit frustrating. But it's a great deal better than nothing—and always available, even at 4 o'clock in the morning!

The WHO now advises that neither male nor female condoms should be lubricated with a spermicide. This is because of:

- studies showing that the main substance used as a spermicide (called nonoxinol-9) can, when used exceptionally frequently within 24 hours as by commercial sex workers (CSWs), damage/irritate the vaginal skin and actually increase the risk of transmission of HIV.
- spermicides have anyway never been shown to improve the effectiveness of condoms.

But nonoxinol-9 is still approved for normal use with caps and diaphragms, contraceptive sponges, and alone as in Delfen (above)—since

Table 10.1 The main recommended and widely and available methods of birth control

A. Reversible methods

Advantages	Disadvantages
The ordinary combined oral contraceptive (COC) pill	
1. Extremely effective against pregnancy. Pregnancy rate in the range < 1–3 per 100 woman-years. 2. Independent of intercourse. 3. Beneficial effects, especially on problems and diseases connected with the menstrual cycle: e.g. period pain, cancer of the ovary and womb (see pp. 27).	1. Medical supervision required. 2. Needs a reasonably good memory to take the pills regularly. 3. Minor problems such as weight gain. 4. A slight chance of major problems such as thrombosis. 5. Unsuitable for women aged over 35 who are also heavy smokers. 6. Some of the possible long-term consequences are still unknown.
The progestogen-only pill (POP) (see Chapter 8)	
1. Effective against pregnancy. Pregnancy rate < 1–4 per 100 woman-years, the lower figure applying to Cerazette and to women above age 45. 2. Independent of intercourse. 3. Probably medically safer than the combined pill, as much less hormone is taken and estrogen-free. 4. Can be used by smokers aged over 35 and others for whom the combined pill is not recommended, or is proving unsatisfactory. 5. Good when breastfeeding, when it is nearly 100 per cent effective.	1. Medical supervision required. 2. Needs to be taken obsessionally regularly. 3. Minor problems, especially with irregular bleeding in the menstrual cycle. 4. Very slight chance of major problems.

Table 10.1 *(Continued)*

A. Reversible methods

Advantages	Disadvantages
Injectable (usually DMPA, Depo-Provera—see text)	
1. Extremely effective against pregnancy. Pregnancy rate < 1 per 100 woman-years. 2. Independent of intercourse. 3. Beneficial effects: mostly as combined pill, including protection against pelvic infection and cancer of the womb. 4. Especially good for sickle-cell anaemia. 5. Probably medically safer than the COC—estrogen free. 6. No tablets to take: one injection lasts for three months.	1. Medical supervision required. 2. Disrupts the menstrual cycle, causing irregular bleeding or stopping the periods. 3. The injection cannot be removed once given, so side effects may have to be lived with for a long time. 4. Delay in return of fertillity, though no permanent fertility problems. 5. Minor problems such as weight gain and mood changes. 6. Some of the possible long-term consequences unknown.
Contraceptive implants such as Implanon (see text)	
1. Extremely effective against pregnancy. Pregnancy protection < 1 per 100 woman-years. Lasts 3 years. 2. Independent of intercourse. 3. Beneficial effects, including protection against pelvic infection. 4. Probably medically safer than the COC. Estrogen-free. 5. Immediately reversible on removal, contrast injectables.	1. Medical supervision required. 2. Disrupts the menstrual cycle, often causing irregular bleeding. 3. Minor problems such as weight gain, breast tenderness, acne, and mood changes. 4. Some of the possible long-term consequences unknown. 5. Removal difficulties, rarely.

Copper intrauterine device (IUD) (copper-on-plastic device which is inserted into the uterus.)

1. Highly effective against pregnancy. Pregnancy rate < 1 per 100 woman-years, *banded* IUDs lowest.
2. Independent of intercourse.
3. Nothing to remember: nothing to take or use daily. Lasts 5–10 years depending on IUD (and to menopause if fitted above the age of 40).
4. No systemic effects, on the whole body.
5. Overall risk of death the same as or less than if the combined pill is used, and, unlike the COC, it becomes medically safer the older the user becomes.
6. Works as an emergency contraceptive as well (see p. 57)
7. Almost immediately reversible on removal.

1. Medical supervision required.
2. Insertion: can cause discomfort, + slight risk of perforation of womb.
3. The device may get expelled from the uterus into the vagina. This has to be watched out for.
4. May cause period cramps, and heavy or prolonged or unpredictable bleeding.
5. Has certain medical risks, among them miscarriage and ectopic pregnancy. Pelvic infection is only a problem if IUD-user is risking STIs through own or partner's lifetyle.
6. Because the infection problem mentioned at 5 can lead to damage to one or both of the uterine tubes and hence interfere with future fertility, not an ideal method for women who have not yet had their family. Particularly unsuitable for most women under the age of 20.

The LNG-releasing IUS, 'Mirena' (see text)

1. Almost 100 per cent effective, pregnancy rate < 1 per 100 woman-years.
2. Lasts for 5 years.
3. Independent of intercourse.
4. Nothing to remember; nothing to take or use daily.
5. Much lower incidence of minor and major side-effects on the body than any other hormonal contraceptive (no EE, plus lowest systemic dose of any LNG contraceptive).
6. Reduction in normal quantity of menstrual bleeding.
7. Reduced menstrual pain.
8. Almost immediately reversible on removal.
9. Possible protection against pelvic infection.

1. Medical supervision required.
2. Insertion: can cause discomfort. As with IUDs there is a *very* slight chance of perforation of the wall of the womb.
3. The device may get expelled. This has to be watched out for.
4. Despite less quantity of bleeding, may cause prolonged spotting, especially in early months.
5. Some mainly short-term medical side effects, like breast tenderness and acne (see text). Any protection against infection not complete—so still not ideal for most young women.

Table 10.1 *(Continued)*

A. Reversible methods

Advantages	Disadvantages
The male condom	
1. Effective if used with care. Pregnancy rate 2–15 per 100 woman-years; very much depends on the user. 2. Easy to obtain at odd hours. 3. Good for infrequent intercourse. 4. Lets a man take responsibility! 5. May also help a man who tends to climax too soon. 6. Visual proof that it has 'worked'. 7. No medical risks, no medical supervision. 8. Protects against STIs, including viruses like those causing AIDS and cervical cancer (safer sex). 9. Plastic versions (Avanti™, Ezon™) good if rubber allergy.	1. Needs very careful and consistent use, otherwise gives poor results. So often best combined with a medical more effective method AS WELL ('Double Dutch' approach). 2. Forward planning necessary, to have the condom available every time. 3. Not independent of intercourse. Seems a 'messy' intrusion into love-making for some. 4. Both partners may be aware that it is being used. Loss of sensitivity, much less with the newest designs. 5. Can slip off or rupture in use. 6. Rubber ones may be damaged by oil-based chemicals. Water-based lubricants and silicones OK.
The female condom, 'Femidom'	
1. Fairly effective, failure rate 5–15 per 100 woman-years. 2. Visual proof that it has worked. 3. No medical risks whatever. 4. No medical supervision required. 5. Believed to protect against picking up or passing on STIs. 6. Can be used ahead of intercourse, before complete erection.	1. Needs very careful and consistent use, otherwise poor results. 2. Forward planning necessary. 3. Not independent of intercourse. 4. Particularly intrudes during foreplay. 5. Needs care to avoid the penis entering beside the outer ring, with complete loss of effectiveness. 6. Can become pushed in.

7. Less likely to rupture than the male condom. 8. During the penetrative phase, sensations of intercourse more normal (this noticed more by the male). 9. Not damaged by any chemicals.	7. Can be noisy! (put some music on . . . ?) 8. Rather expensive.
The cap, used with a spermicide and put in by the woman to cover the entrance to the uterus. Diaphragm is the most commonly used cap 1. Moderately effective if used with care. Pregnancy rate 4–8 per 100 woman-years with careful use, but up to 10–15 otherwise. 2. More independent of intercourse than the condom. Can be put in as a routine ahead of time and should not therefore interfere with spontaneity. 3. Neither partner usually notices any loss of sensitivity. 4. If properly fitted and used, virtually no side-effects. 5. Protects against some STIs and (very probably) cancer of the cervix.	1. Medical (or more often nursing) supervision required, to choose the right size of cap and to be trained to use it properly. 2. Needs very careful and consistent use, and even then rather a high failure rate. 3. Forward planning necessary. 4. Seems a bit messy to some. 5. Diaphragm may increase the risk of bladder infections. Other types of cap may be preferable if this is a problem.
Natural Family Planning (NFP), including Persona—whose main advantage is greater simplicity in use 1. Moderately effective with consistent use. 2. No side-effects. 3. No hormones or other drugs, no devices, no procedures. 4. Acceptable to all religions and cultures. 5. Empowers women, who feel more in tune with their body rhythms and sexuality. 6. Actually benefits some couples' communication and relationships. 7. Can be used to plan as well as avoid a pregnancy.	1. Very unforgiving of inconsistent use, leading to poor results. 2. Requires long durations of abstinence to be fully effective. 3. No.2 means more commitment than some men are prepared to give—can cause stress to some couples. 4. Except Persona, NFP has to be learned from a trained teacher. It takes at least 3 cycles to learn. 5. Events such as illness, stress, and travel may make the fertility indicators harder to interpret.

Table 10.1 *(Continued)*

B. Methods which are not readily reversible

Advantages	Disadvantages
Sterilization in either sex	
1. Almost but not quite 100 per cent effective. 2. Independent of intercourse. 3. Nothing to be taken daily. 4. Medical supervision and possible problems mainly during the year of operation. 5. No known long-term medical effects of importance.	1. Not readily reversible—but pregnancy rates after reversal operations by experts can be better than 50 per cent. 2. An operation is required with more or less discomfort and inconvenience. 3. Not in fact 100 per cent, despite being so 'final'.
Female sterilization by blocking the uterine tubes	
1. Once a woman decides to be sterilized, she is less likely in later years to want it reversed than a man might do, because nature will sterilize her anyway around the age of 50 (the menopause). 2. The operation is immediately effective.	1. Medical risks of the operation are greater than vasectomy, though still small. Latest techniques using clips are much safer than before. 2. Usually requires admission to hospital and often (not always) a general anaesthetic. 3. Late failures a long time afterwards are more common than after vasectomy. 4. If the operations fails, which it very rarely does, there is a risk of ectopic pregnancy. 5. Psychologically, though illogically, women may feel no longer so feminine because they cannot have babies.

Vasectomy (male sterilization) by blocking the vas deferens 1. Almost completely safe medically. 2. Can be done under local anaesthetic in about 10 minutes, as an out-patient, almost anywhere. 3. There is a ready check of success by doing sperm counts.	1. Occasional short-term local complications of the operation, such as swellings or infection. Lowest risk if 'no scalpel' method used. 2. It takes three or more months for the sperm to be eliminated and the operation to become effective. Even then, *late* failures do rarely occur. 3. Especially if they remarry, more older men than women will wish for a reversal operation (see the point about the menopause, above). 4. Psychologically, though illogically, some men may feel 'threatened' by the operation, and may seem to overcompensate needlessly to show how manly they still are. 5. Some remotely possible long-term effects still unknown, but available human evidence is very reassuring.

Note: Only condoms (male or female) realistically offer safer sex (protection against STIs, including HIV/AIDS). Even men who have had vasectomies must remember this!

with less frequent use (than in those CSWs) the vagina seems able to recover adequately between applications.

Barrier methods of family planning such as the condom and the cap with spermicide have been criticized for their messiness, but this has been much exaggerated. And even if partly true, it is worth pondering the following comment made by a woman journalist: 'But women's lives are messy; it is messy to bleed once a month; it is messy to give birth; sex itself is not for the fastidious.'

Hormonal contraception

Three non-pill methods listed in Table 10.1 require a bit more highlighting.

Injectables

Depo-Provera is the name for the progestogen injection which utilizes depot medroxyprogesterone acetate (DMPA for short), given in a dose of 150 mcg into a muscle (usually the buttocks) once every 12 weeks. It is brilliantly effective since it mainly works by blocking ovulation, like the pill. Its failure rate is in practice lower even than the COC because there are no tablets to forget. It seems very safe medically, with so far no deaths proven to be caused by it. That clearly means it is even safer than the COC, though no one can say it is risk-free.

1. *Cancer.* Experiments showing that beagle bitches develop breast cancers probably have no relevance to humans since the beagle bitch has a high tendency to develop breast tumours, even under the influence of her own natural progesterone. WHO research has shown a strong protective effect against cancer of the lining of the womb, and no proven increase in the risk of any other cancer (though for breast cancer, there is still the *possibility* that DMPA is like the COC, pp. 110–15).
2. *Reversibility.* This used to be a worry, but research from Thailand where the method has been very popular gives good evidence that there is complete return of fertility on stopping DMPA. Women take about four months longer after their first missed dose to conceive than after stopping other methods, and a few might take well over a year—but do eventually. Forewarning is essential, and the couple might need to do some forward planning about when they stop for a wanted conception.
3. *Other problems.* The main problems are *excessive and irregular bleeding*, often but not always going on to absent periods; and *weight gain*, which can be very marked and unpredictable in some women. Everyone should be forewarned about these side-effects, also about the fact that *DMPA cannot easily be removed* if any side-effects do develop.

The possibility that DMPA may increase the risk of osteoporosis through long-term lowering of blood estrogen levels is still uncertain, and being studied. In my view this potential problem should be discussed after five years of use. Many women will then decide simply to change to one of the many new alternatives available, such as an implant or IUD or IUS. Others, who have no special risk of the osteoporosis problem, may say that they are comfortable to continue, understanding how safe DMPA is in almost every other way (definitely safer than the pill, very acceptably safe though that is!). If so the discussion is noted, and the issue simply kept under review during follow-up.

DMPA has been very controversial, with accusations that it has been used in a racist way; also that women have received it without adequate counselling about its known or possible unknown risks. Wherever that has been true, that is an indictment of the doctors or other providers concerned, not of the drug. In the UK it took 30 years from its discovery before it received a licence as a first-line method: in other words, a method which may and usually should be discussed and offered to anyone asking about contraception.

Contraceptive implants

Norplant™consisted of six implants, Jadelle™ in some countries has two implants, but in the UK we now have Implanon. The length of a matchstick but only 2 mm wide, this is put just under the skin via a special needle under local anaesthesia (Fig.10.4). Trained clinicians can insert this with minimum discomfort in about one minute, and remove it in two minutes: a great advantage compared with Norplant.

1. *Advantages.* In some ways it is like DMPA, with even greater effectiveness (less than one failure per 1000 women in the first year); but with

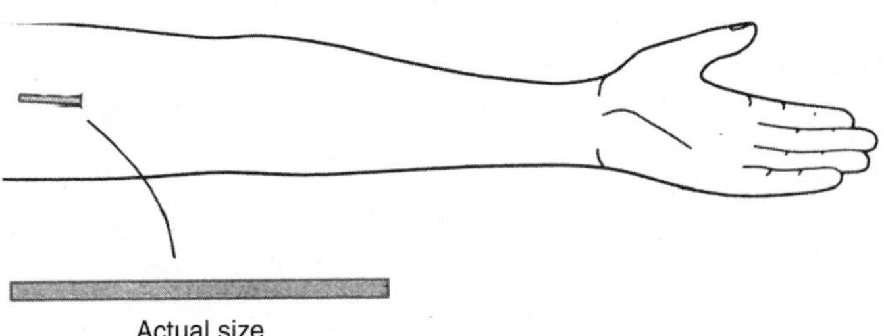

Fig. 10.4 Implanon capsule implanted in the upper arm

a much longer potential lifespan of three years. Yet it can be reversed quickly at any time if side effects occur or for a wanted pregnancy. About 40 per cent of users get no periods at all, which many like, and that seems to be acceptable—without the question-mark about osteoporosis that there is with DMPA.

2. *Disadvantages.* The biggest problem with Implanon as with most progestogen-only methods is irregular bleeding: up to about 20 per cent of users get unacceptable frequent or prolonged bleeding. This can sometimes, but not always, be helped by two to three cycles of Mercilon. The bleeding problems do not settle so predictably as with Mirena (below).

The levonorgestrel-releasing intrauterine system (LNG-IUS, or just IUS), marketed as Mirena™

As shown in Fig.10.5, the IUS is a T-shaped system releasing just 20 mcg per 24 hours of LNG from its special reservoir, through a rate-limiting membrane. This is sufficient for contraception over at least five years.

Its main contraceptive effects are local, by changes to the cervical mucus which block sperm and by suppressing the lining of the womb. This is why it also reduces bleeding and pain (see below).

1. *Advantages.* Mirena is brilliantly effective at its main job, with a failure rate of only two per 1000 women in the first year of use. Return of fertility is rapid and complete, so it is like a fully reversible alternative to

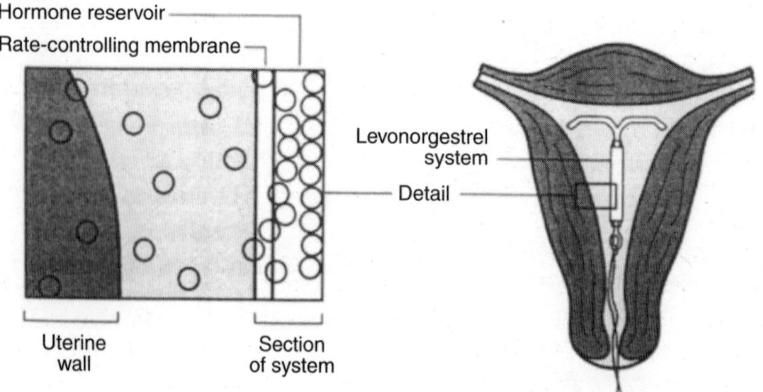

Fig. 10.5 The levonorgestrel-releasing IUS (Mirena)

being sterilized. It is very convenient and provides most of the good points of both the pill and ordinary copper IUDs, but without most of the disadvantages of either.

Users of this IUS can expect a dramatic reduction in amount and, after the first few months, in duration of their periods. Dysmenorrhoea (period pain) is also generally improved. Mirena is the method of first choice for women with heavy periods and tending to get anaemia, who do not want the pill: a much easier option too than hysterectomy.

Mirena may be used with careful supervision by many young women who would not be good candidates for conventional copper IUDs. Like them, however, the IUS is recommended for use chiefly by women who have had one or more children.

2. *Disadvantages.* Like any intrauterine contraceptive, Mirena has to be inserted, which can be uncomfortable (you should be given painkillers, and the choice of local anaesthetic if you prefer). It can be expelled, and, like with IUDs, there is the usual very small risk of perforation (see p. 217).

A more common problem is the likelihood in the first months after it is fitted of bleeding, which, though much smaller in amount than before, may be very frequent or continuous and can cause considerable inconvenience. Later on amenorrhoea (absent periods) is very commonly reported. For both of these effects, particularly the first, 'forewarned is forearmed': meaning good counselling in advance of the fitting. It is well worth persevering, as the 'trickle' nearly always stops and then you either have light bleeds about once a month, or nothing at all! Because estrogen levels are not low, the absence of periods is pure gain—as described for absent withdrawal bleeding and the pill on p. 16. It is a positive benefit of the method.

Though this method is mainly local in its action, some LNG hormone does get into the blood. This amounts to about the same as taking two or three POPs a week. So some women who are extra sensitive to hormones can still get hormonal side-effects such as acne and breast tenderness. If they happen at all, these can be expected to improve over the first few months. And the good news is that weight gain has not been shown to be a side effect of the IUS.

3. *Your choice.* The IUS is a major advance, and I still call it the greatest advance in the field of contraception since the pill! If only it were much cheaper it would be particularly suitable for women of the developing world, because it would offer the additional advantage of preventing anaemia—very common there, due to malnutrition, parasites, and loss of iron through periods and supplying iron to too many babies. It seems to fulfil most of the criteria in Box 10.1 (p. 205) for an 'ideal' contraceptive.

It approaches 100 per cent reversibility, effectiveness, and even, after some delay, convenience. After the initial months of frequent bleedings and spotting, the usual outcomes of either intermittent light periods or nothing are very acceptable to most women. It does not provide protection against sexually transmitted viruses like HIV, of course, nor complete protection against the causes of pelvic infection like Chlamydia. But the bad side-effects are few and generally in the category of 'nuisance' rather than dangerous. It has special benefits for women with heavy or painful periods.

In short, we have here a really valuable new choice for women, especially those who have either WHO 4 or WHO 3 problems with other methods such as the combined pill and the conventional copper IUD.

For a summary of the pros and cons of the IUS, in comparison with the copper IUD and with other choices, see also Table 10.1.

How to plan your family planning

Some people will use only one or two methods of family planning throughout their lives; others will 'ring the changes' between the various methods, as shown in Table 10.2. The best choice of method is likely to vary with time, or according to what I call 'the seven contraceptive ages of woman' (actually eight, as you see!). But this table is just a guide: the choice of a method of contraception is a very individual thing and no one method is ever ideal and best for everyone, even within a particular age category. Not all the satisfactory options are even mentioned. The scheme only represents the 'state of the art', based on the methods available in 2004.

Table 10.2 is meant to represent an ideal scheme, so it is assumed that the woman concerned will be a non-smoker and will, if she can, breastfeed her children. It is also assumed that she or her partner will use whatever method is chosen responsibly and consistently, and that they are fundamentally monogamous. (If not they will need to use condoms regularly *as well* as the medical methods mentioned.)

Once your family is complete, sterilization of either partner can seem the ideal because it is so safe medically and so effective against unplanned 'afterthoughts'. Vasectomy is more effective and much easier to do. But with so many relationships failing these days, the banded copper IUD (p. 216) and especially the Mirena IUS may be better choices for many couples, in future. The IUS is ideal for many in the fifth, sixth, seventh 'ages' of Table 10.2: by having one inserted a great many women may be able to avoid either having a hysterectomy or even one of the less scary new techniques of uterine ablation which have been developed. It is also being increasingly used for a form of HRT, in combination with estrogen by any chosen route.

Table 10.2 The 'seven' contraceptive ages of woman

Age	**Suggested method**
0 Birth to puberty	No method required. Responsible sex and relationships education (SRE) is essential, *started and carried on by parents* and continuing through schooling.
1 Puberty to marriage (or the equivalent)	Either (a) a barrier method, with emergency contraception back-up available; (b) the combined pill/similar combined options (i.e. skin patch EVRA or perhaps NuvaRing) or Cerazette/injectable/implant: outside of mutual monogamy always with a condom; or, if acceptable, (c) abstinence until the person's final life-partner be found. The choice depends on factors like religious views, perceived risk of STIs, and the frequency of partner changes and of intercourse.
2 Marriage (or equivalent) to first child	First choice probably a pill, but could be one of various patches/rings/injectables/implants followed by a fertility awareness method for some months before 'trying' for the first child.
3 During breastfeeding	Either LAM, or POP or any progestogen-only method or a simple barrier method plus the breastfeeding. IUD or IUS, male or female injectable, or implant likely to be appropriate only if a longish gap is expected between pregnancies.
4 Family spacing after breastfeeding	Continue with any method started during 'age' 3, or shift from an old-type POP to Cerazette/the combined pill/injectable/implant for greater effectiveness. Later, a banded copper IUD or IUS is progressively more appropriate, for a combination of the least long-term health hazards, efficacy, and reversibility.
5 After the (probable) last child	The first choice is an IUD or IUS, depending on whether periods are troublesome; other possibilities are any POP, or (if free of arterial or venous factors) a combined hormonal method, or injectable/implant according to choice.
6 Family complete, family growing up	First choice still as 5: banded copper IUD, or the IUS if periods at all heavy or painful. According to choice, vasectomy would be generally preferable to female sterilization as it is more effective and easier to perform.
7 Perimenopausal (not sterilized)	Contraceptive hormone replacement therapy, perhaps, such as the IUS plus estrogen patch or implant. It is important to recognize that, at this age, a weaker contraceptive (e.g. foam or sponge) may be fully effective when combined with very reduced fertility.

If you are a completely healthy, slim non-smoker with no migraines, remember that there is now also the definite option of staying on the combined pill right through to the menopause.

Whatever reversible method is used, it should not normally be abandoned until one year after the very last menstrual period (and if this was under age 50, two years is recommended). Pregnancy during this time is not entirely unknown following an unexpected delayed egg release (see p. 189)!

Some people really have difficulty in finding any method at all that suits them. Contraception can then be the source of a lot of tension and frustration. Occasionally a workable solution may be found if the partners, so to speak, share the contraceptive load: for instance, sometimes using the male and sometimes the female condom ('his night', then 'her night'!).

Conclusion

Looking back over this chapter, and over the whole book, it is impossible to avoid one conclusion. A lot of the time in family planning we, and for the most part unfortunately that means women, are having to 'make the best of a bad job'. While we can hope for a successful outcome to some of the ongoing research, we have to lead our sex lives now, with the methods actually available now.

If you do decide to take the pill, and currently this is the most effective personally controlled reversible method, make sure it is an informed decision which seems right to you and is not influenced by pressure from anyone else: your partner, the media, let alone any doctor. Remember condoms, maybe as well, for safer sex! And if you decide the pill is not for you, be sure to use some reliable alternative. Sex and birth control are matters which affect your body; they are your responsibility and require your decisions. That about says it all.

11 Postscript

Throughout this book I hope I have made it abundantly clear that no doctor or other worker in this area of reproductive health should ever push his or her own views, including moral/ethical views, on those who come for advice about controlling their fertility. But they can reveal them when appropriate. Readers of this book may be interested in what underpins my life and work.

Population matters: without sustainability there is no tomorrow

I have often been called a 'driven' man. What drives me is an intense concern, ever since that lecture I attended in 1959 (see Preface), that we continue so seriously to neglect all those who will come after us on this small planet. In 1959 there were only 3000 million people on earth; now we have 6400 million and the number rises by 1.5 million each week. Given each person's natural desire for a comfortable lifestyle, and the hard fact that the only way to obtain that is to consume resources and create pollution (see the equation below), this puts the planet's environment under intolerable pressure (see Box 11.1).

According to the regularly updated Living Planet Report of the Worldwide Fund for Nature (WWF), the 9000 million humans who will (barring the catastrophes we wish to avoid) be around in 2050 will need to use around 100 per cent more resources than the whole biological capacity of the planet! So where will we find, in less than 50 years time, a second or even third world, so we can properly care for so many people? Why a third? Because WWF's calculations are *without* having dealt with that open sore, that infamy of grinding poverty that blights so many billions of our 'neighbours' overseas; and certainly *with* so much habitat destruction as to cause the mass extinction of tens of thousands of plant and animal species, on land

Box 11.1 Take an apple, to represent planet Earth.

Slice the apple into quarters.
Throw away three of them.
These represent the oceans of the world.

Q: What fraction do you have left? (1/4).
Slice this in two, and discard one half.
This represents land that is inhospitable to people: deserts, swamps, high mountains, land covered by ice.

Q: What fraction do you now have left? (1/8).
Slice the 1/8 into four final segments, and dispose of three.
These 3 × 1/32 segments are areas that are too rocky, too cold, too steep, still covered by (fast-disappearing) rain forest, or with soil too poor to actually produce food. They also include cities, suburban sprawl, roads, shopping centres, schools, factories, car parks.

Q: What fraction now? (1/32).
Carefully peel the last 1/32 slice.
This tiny bit of apple peel represents the skin of the Earth's crust, which is the topsoil on which all humankind and much of the biosphere depends. It averages only a few feet deep. Due to human activities (erosion, over-farming, pollution) we lose an average 25 billion tons of it per year. With more and more people sharing the land, each person's share gets ever smaller.

Adapted from the Activity Guide supplied with World Population Dots, *a superb DVD available from* www.popconnect.org.

and sea and in the air. Numberless species of animals and plants will be known by our grandchildren only through museums and video-recordings. They are not, as the townies of our civilization may suppose, an 'optional extra'. We co-exist with a vast assemblage of living organisms, the biodiversity that has evolved over almost 4 billion years of our planet's history. This forms a 'web of life' upon whose continuing health the very life-support systems of the earth depend. Systems which we humans require as much as any other species: crucial in the maintenance of clean air, clean water, and fertile soils.

Human population growth is coming to represent, in Professor Aubrey Manning of Edinburgh's biological terminology, a 'voracious monoculture, . . . a deadly combination of human numbers, human aspirations, and technology is . . . leading through habitat destruction to extinction rates up to 10 000 times the base-rate through geological time'.

Humanity's environmental impact, < *I* >, has just three components, expressed in the equation:

$$I = PAT$$

where:

- *P* is *Population*, number of persons
- *A* is per person *Affluence*, with inevitably linked 'effluence' which is pollution/resource consumption per person, and
- *T* is the per person *Technology* factor. This is higher where the net impact of all production technologies is the more consuming and polluting, and can be lowered by 'greener' technologies, such as the use of renewable energy and better building insulation.

I think this is the most important equation in the world! To reduce <*I*> we must obviously reduce the <*T*> factor by applying scientific research better—and by the 5 Rs of the environment (refusing/reducing/reusing/repairing/recycling, and *bicycling!*). But scientists foresee future advances as being inadequate to compensate for humanity's profligate use of resources, including fossil fuels—which are causing climate change and anyway are running out.

What about the <*A*> for affluence factor? This can, indeed must, be lowered by reduced per person energy use, resource consumption, and waste, mainly in the northern industrialized countries. Their (our) collective track record is, to put it mildly, not encouraging. We are all, let's face it, addicted to our affluence. In their lifetime, the impact on the environment of an average child born in the wealthy 'North', through car ownership, etc., will cause up to 200 times as much damage to the planet as one born in the country of my own birth (Burundi). Globally, the mirror image of affluence is poverty, blighting almost 3 billion people out of the 6.4 billion already present *plus* almost all the close to 80 million added each year. Think of it, a city, or rather, slum for 1 million has to be built somewhere every five days! And to relieve this degrading poverty, as we surely must, through development—however sustainable—must lead to an *increase* in global per capita Affluence. Hence, inevitably, more consumption and effluence.

With <*T*> set to fall only minimally, and with the global <*A*> factor per person certain to actually increase—not only wrongly, through ever-rising affluence of the already affluent, but also as a human right, through poverty relief for the world's poorest (as just described)—what remains? There are only three factors in the equation. The single remaining one is the <*P*> factor, human numbers: largely neglected yet of crucial relevance

Box 11.2 Population and birth planning are key component variables in all the following

- Use of fossil fuels—and climate change
- Human rights/violence/genocide
- Mass asylum-seeking and economic migration
- Disease, including HIV
- Maternal mortality
- Infant mortality
- Poverty, per head, even with 'development'
- Shortage of water and of food
- Shortage of other basic resources (and energy)
- Pollution of the environment
- Biodiversity and survival in the natural world

Source: Dr Timothy Black (Marie Stopes International)

to meeting all human needs without all but extinguishing the planet's biodiversity. Overpopulation by just one species (humans) is, to quote myself elsewhere, 'not the sole cause of most major world problems, but it is the unrecognized *multiplier* of them'. See Box 11.2, adapted from a presentation by Dr Timothy Black (Marie Stopes International).

Stabilizing/reducing our numbers will not be *sufficient* to solve all these, but it is the one element of any solution which is absolutely *necessary*. Indeed without it we won't survive.

None of this is new: our leaders just disregard it all! Politicians, who are much more concerned about the next election than their grandchildren's future, if they recognize a problem at all they commission demographers to study populations trends in each country. Without even discussing how many might be optimum, they then think they can *predict and provide* (always, for however many, and for ever!). Haven't they heard of the pill? They are very like a man jumping out of an aeroplane and reaching for an altimeter rather than a parachute.

> It takes a long time to realize that as far as looking after the future of humankind and the earth is concerned, there is no one at the controls; but once achieved, the realization is remarkably disquieting.
>
> (John Davoll, *Lecture to the Conservation Society*, 1970)

So, if the '*P*' of the *I* = *PAT* equation urgently needs stabilizing/reducing: as well as helping far more than now to provide (voluntary) reproductive health care for the majority 'South', most countries in the densely-populated and over-consuming minority 'North' would themselves benefit—in a world of increasing resource scarcity—by adopting a (lower) population policy. What a 'green and pleasant land' England might still be, if we had not overshot our own optimum by so much! Let us set a good example to other countries—see www.optimumpopulation.org.

What about poverty? Surely poor people need lots of children as 'social security' and to compensate for so many child deaths?

Very true, but it's an over-simplification. I know a bit about this at first hand, being Africa-born and spending all my early life in Burundi, Rwanda, Uganda, and Kenya. The answer is to 'take care of the people and the population will take care of itself', which is what Fig. 11.1 here depicts. But that definitely must include making *certain* that women have education, and choices in contraception (two of the most neglected items in the Figure).

When I first heard about this 'population bomb' in 1959 there were 3000 million on the planet, of whom around 50 per cent or 1500 million were in dire poverty. Now there are over 6 billion, of whom still about

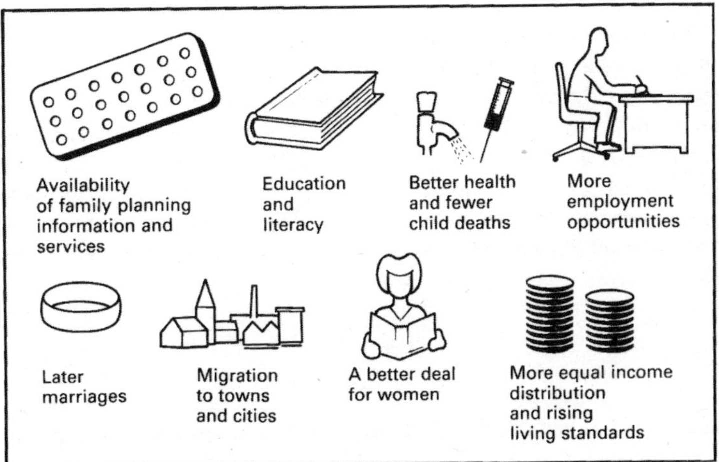

Fig. 11.1 What changes birth rates?

Source: Population Concern, The Shape of Things to Come.

50 per cent are in poverty (some even in 'rich' countries). So what have we done, really, in these 40+ years?

Crudely put, *we have proved that it is possible to give everyone in the 1959 world a 'good life' (in the short term, probably unsustainably in the long term)—that's 3000 million—not a bad effort. But we have simultaneously allowed another entire 1959 world of 3000 million souls to arrive into total misery and violence! And, tragically, it was to a great degree avoidable, with no coercion, if we had simply helped millions of people, especially women, in many vital ways (Fig. 11.1), including contraceptive choices and good education.*

The 'top' 2–3000 million of us continue with the *growth* philosophy, what Sir Crispin Tickell (former UK Ambassador to the United Nations [UN]) so truly calls 'the philosophy of the cancer cell'. We continue to treat this fragile and finite planet (deliberately mixing my metaphors here!) like a bottomless cess-pit and an inexhaustable milch cow—which it is so obviously not.

The net effect of OXFAM and all the other poverty-relief agencies and of FOE and all the dedicated environmental activists in these years (worthy organizations, and I am a committed 'standing order' supporter of both) has thus been, sadly, nullified and then actually reversed by population growth. All largely avoidable, if there had not been such culpable neglect of world reproductive health and women's choices and rights.

As UNICEF said, in 1992: 'Family planning could bring more benefits to more people at less cost than any other single technology now available to the human race.' Moreover, they went on to say: 'This would still be true even if there were no such thing as a population problem.'

Or (my own summary): *the condom, the pill, and the intrauterine device ought to be as much symbols for the Green and sustainable development movements as the photo-voltaic cell and the bicycle!* Just look at Ethiopia if you want one of the clearest examples of unsustainable population growth. (see Box 11.3).

Now, many continue to assume that someone like me must be for some kind of compulsion, that 'any quantitative concern for population is necessarily and intrinsically coercive' of poor people. Not so, compulsion in reproductive health is wrong-headed and except in one highly unusual country (China) has proved counter-productive anyway. Forget coercion, so long as we go on not adequately doing the voluntary things, primarily *ensuring that any woman on the planet who wants a modern contraceptive method to be used by self or partner has easy access to it, as her human right.* Indeed, to continue—as now—doing that so inadequately is arguably the best way to ensure that more future governments will legislate for compulsory birth control.

Others distrust this concern of mine as inevitably being *exclusive* of many other key interventions: social justice, relieving poverty, education,

Box 11.3 Ethiopia: some facts

Year	Population* (millions)
• 1950	18
• 2004	70
• Increase in the last 12 months	1.7
• Expected, therefore, by 2050	173
• Calculated sustainable carrying capacity, given available resources, especially water (based on a 'modest European lifestyle')	8.1 million!

**Ethiopia's numbers never went down, not even in the 'Geldof' years when millions died during the wars and the famine of the 1980s.*

or improving child survival. Not so, again we are talking not 'either–or' here but 'both–and'. Just look again at Fig. 11.1!

Worldwide 150 million couples do not realistically have any modern contraception available to them and 350 million, more than one-third, of all couples that there are, do not have access to the full range we enjoy in the UK. It is true that for cultural and 'social security' reasons many still want large families, yet large-scale social surveys have proved that at least 50 per cent of women wish at the time of questioning to prevent another pregnancy.

'Every minute in the world 380 women become pregnant, and of those 190 did not plan to do so' (UNFPA 2002). We are failing to push at this open door marked 'Contraception'! Indeed, since in the same every minute one woman dies through unsafe induced abortion or childbirth, around 550 000 per annum, the figures suggest that half are being killed by pregnancies they would have avoided *if* they had only had the contraceptive choices we take for granted.

I keep seeing headlines about declining birth rates and a 'birth dearth'?

So do I, and it's certainly good news that the UN has found lower than expected birth rates in many countries. Small thanks, of course, to the vociferous opponents of voluntary birth planning who are often loudest in suggesting the impossible, that there's no limit to the numbers the planet could hold! But the headlines about an impending fall below replacement fertility refer mainly to Europe, and in all to only about 60 out of over 180 countries. In the others (including, mainly through inward migration, the greatest per-person polluter of all, the USA) the numbers are definitely still going up. Every four weeks India has to provide for around a million extra! And there's a population momentum (due to loads of young people already born) that means there is a c.60-year time-lag between average family sizes reaching replacement and any population stabilizing.

What about HIV/AIDS, especially in Africa?

The devastation this causes, which I have seen at first hand in Rwanda and South Africa, is certainly no argument for continuing to leave Africa to 'solve its own population problem'—perish the very thought! Quite the reverse, it is another central argument for *prevention*, as in Fig. 11.1, through holistic and comprehensive reproductive and sexual health care (i.e. meaning among things *dual protection*, using condoms as well, p. 218). Regardless of the above issues of numbers and sustainability, HIV/AIDS prevention and treatment should be fully funded, as a human right and a key intervention for improving the health of women, their partners, and their children.

So what's the 'bottom line'?

Yes, it is very much a *financial* bottom line; there are COSTS which the present-day 'haves' in all countries have been unwilling to pay on behalf of billions of present and future 'have-nots'.

The founder of my faith said 'we should love our neighbour'. Few people of any faith, or claiming none, would dispute that as an ideal for all humankind. But, I say, how can we (as 'haves' rather than 'have-nots') be really loving our neighbours if we don't show practical love to:

- our neighbours *abroad*
- our *future* neighbours, and thirdly
- our *biological* 'neighbours'—the other species—deserving of protection since they were made by our Creator, if you are a theist; and if you are not, simply because this bountiful, beautiful, biodiverse world is all you have and you wish to leave it in good shape for generations to come.

It's an obvious fact of physics that there's a finite maximum number of people this planet/country/region/telephone box can hold! Moreover, the optimum is likely to be less than (and more pleasant to live in than) the out-and-out maximum. So we simply cannot allow ever more and more of our one species 'Homo sapiens (rapiens?)' to arrive, without in the long term imperilling all the other species with which we share the planet—and of course our own selves.

I end with a long quote that explains itself, my Introduction to a little commemorative booklet called 'The Promise':

The eco-time-capsule project, 1994–2044

Usually, time capsules record a particular time and place for posterity, and are buried without any future date for 'unburying' in mind. These that we buried in 1994 were different. The concept came to me through that well-known saying 'we did not inherit the earth from our grandparents, we have borrowed it from our grandchildren'. I reflected on how angry they are likely to be if we continue (and there has been no obvious let-up 10 years later) to wreck their loan to us. With 25 years as the usually accepted average duration of a generation, 'our grandchildren' meant people living 50 years ahead. So this project was addressed to the people of 2044. It was linked to the United Nations World Environment Day, in the Year of the Family, and comprised an apology, a pledge, a competition for school children, a media event, and a family party.

The time capsules contained environmentally relevant items and were buried with explanations and letters of apology at significant sites around the world. In the UK these were Kew Gardens in London and the University of Liverpool's Ness Gardens in South Wirral. Over the same weekend in June 1994 similar time capsules were sealed and buried in Mexico (Fundidora Park, Monterrey and at two other sites) and in the botanical gardens of Pietermaritzburg, South Africa, the Seychelles, and Mount Annan near Sydney, Australia.

Children were—and still are—central to this project, since they are the prime stakeholders for a decent, sustainable future. In 1994 they were invited to enter two competitions: one for the best brief letter or poem addressed to the finder in 2044; the other for the most striking and original ideas for appropriate artifacts to go in the capsules. At Kew the selected objects included: sealed capsules of the cleanest available 1994 air, water and garden loam (each as a reference for comparison in 2044!), and a petrol cap, labelled as representing one of our most environmentally damaging items. My own choices for sustainability symbols were a bicycle pump and a packet of contraceptive pills, since contraceptives are really the ultimate in eco-friendly devices.

We felt it was essential to apologize. But more important and empowering for all concerned at that time and since was the *pledge*: to do all we could to save the planet by individual and united action 'according to our talents and opportunities', influencing those in power and changing as necessary our own lifestyles—with the goal that the finders of each time capsule in the year 2044 will wonder why we apologized!

Since 1994 there have been regular gatherings at the time capsules on or about World Environment Day, annually at Ness gardens. Over the years we have had the enthusiastic support of many distinguished people, including Sir Crispin Tickell (former UK Ambassador to the UN), Susan Hampshire, David Bellamy, and the Conservation Foundation.

The project is ongoing (www.ecotimecapsule.com). Other countries and other groups and concerned individuals are cordially invited to join in any year, to organize a similar time-capsule ceremony, still to be addressed to the people of 2044 and containing the same letters of apology, translated as necessary.

Reader, join us! Come one sunny day if you can to Kew or to Ness and read the above-ground inscriptions. Together, today, we still need to face up to our own over-consumption of limited natural resources; greenhouse gas production and mismanagement of other waste and pollution; global poverty and injustice; and gross under-funding of sexual and reproductive health as a human right for all. As we campaign together on these interconnected issues, why should not apologies to all our grandchildren become truly superfluous?

It is better to light a candle than to curse the darkness!

(Adlai Stevenson)

The pill and responsibility in sex

Anyone coming to a family-planning doctor for advice should be met on their own ground. In all but the most unusual case, if an unmarried couple are having intercourse regularly it would be alienating as well as useless to recommend abstinence. Circumstances vary, but the main thing is to help people avoid the nightmare of an unwanted pregnancy. My own views are often different from those to whom I prescribe the pill, but saying so, except if they ask, will risk losing the opportunity to help them (often not just with their contraception). 'A gram of empathy beats a kilogram of knowledge' (and a tonne of being judgemental) every time.

So I do regularly prescribe the pill to unmarried people; and also, with counselling—not moralizing—to young teenagers. We live in the real world and my medical practice must be relevant to that world as it really is.

That said, a 'real world' whose philosophy can be encapsulated as 'if you can't eat it, wear it, sleep with it, or drive it, it's no damn use' has some real problems: every year ever more divorces or breakdowns of other relationships where there are vulnerable children; single-parent families; induced abortions; not to mention prescriptions for tranquillizers for more and more insecure people, who have lost the ability to trust each other. The 'copulation explosion' lies behind the epidemic of STIs, including AIDS; and also, we now know, of abnormal cervical smears and the risk of cancer of the cervix.

So it is no more than sound factual medicine, telling it how it is, to inform young people that one of their *options* is still not to have sex with this person, or at all maybe, until they are sure they have met 'Mr or Miss Right', and after that to be loyal; or to reinforce perhaps a teenager's wish, if she has it, *not* to be given the pill just yet despite being pressurized by her boyfriend. In the UK, let's face it, we live in a post-Christian society which has thrown out old values but can offer only emptiness instead: in the words of Gladys Mwiti, a Tear Fund worker in Nairobi, 'You cannot fill a values vacuum with condoms.' It is a society where most young people receive little guidance, and plenty of bad examples from unhelpful role models. The pressures on them from the media and their friends are enormous, so it really seems to be abnormal not to be having sex at 16. Or, as a family doctor has said, 'Sex at 16 may be legal but it is not yet compulsory!'

Concerned as they rightly are with harm reduction, to prevent unplanned pregnancy, schoolteachers, doctors, and nurses can sometimes be caught up in these same social pressures. They can find that their promotion of family planning is being seen as almost implying an official seal of approval for teenage sex.

The young will laugh at an arbitrary 'not at all', but will at least listen to a case for a range of choices, one of which being 'not yet', provided it is factual and not linked to taboos or a negative attitude to sex. They need to know that responsible sex means more than just avoiding pregnancy and STIs. At risk are self-respect, respect for others, and a lot of potential grief: getting *hurt*, or else becoming emotionally *hard* and less able to bond in a committed way thereafter. This applies to boys as well as to girls. The sexual 'double standard' is offensive and must be abolished! But there are also relevant medical facts: all contraceptives *can* fail, and the possible long-term risks may include infertility, AIDS, and even cancer of the cervix (see p. 116).

The stakes are high for everyone. In the book *I Married You* (Inter-Varsity Press, 1972), Walter Trobisch describes sexual love as being like the glue between two pieces of paper (old-fashioned Gloy, not the glue of Post-it notes!):

> If you try to separate two pieces of paper which are glued together, you tear them both. If you try to separate husband and wife who cleave together, both are hurt—and in those cases where they have children, the children, the

> children as well. Divorce means to take a saw and to saw apart each child, from head to toe, right through the middle.

The powerful bonding function of love-making between two humans should come as no surprise, it is what the Designer intended. Like Trobisch, I believe the sexual behaviour that we were designed for can be summed up in the one word *loyalty*; 'a one-man woman making love only with her one-woman man—and for life'.

Some people think that the only things that show whether somebody has been sexually responsible are the two negatives: if he or she has (*a*) not caused an unwanted pregnancy and (*b*) not acquired a sexually transmitted infection. But making love is something a bit more positive and special and exciting than that. It is, surely, nature's physical 'seal of approval' on a committed, caring relationship between two people. The sex itself is better then. I remember well an article in, surprisingly, *Cosmopolitan* about 10 years ago headed:

LOVE + COMMITMENT = EXPLOSIVE ORGASMIC SEX

It was written by a woman who described how their love-making was totally like her headline (only) when she and her partner decided they were going to commit together, for life. Most who have tried it both ways will agree that sex is best when your lover is equally your 'best mate' as well—and, by the way, how can you ever know that on the first night?!

The inventor of sex must, first, have a great sense of humour; and, secondly, must intend it to be, in the right circumstances, supremely enjoyable! (I like to tell the kill-joys in some faith communities that the God who made the clitoris—an organ that Science has never found any function for, except for pleasuring during foreplay and intercourse itself—must *want* his creatures to enjoy themselves.)

A sexual experience which pre-dates a loving experience is a pale shadow of the real thing. Consider this quote from Dr Esther Sapire (from her book *Contraception and Sexuality in Health and Disease* [McGraw-Hill, 1990]):

> Sex is part of oneself to accept and live with comfortably and enjoy. It is not something that comes in from outside and takes over the body and flies off. It is something we *are* not something we *do* as a physical act and it cannot be isolated from the total relationship. Sex is an expression of love, and is only one aspect of it which enhances the relationship. . . . There is a time when one is ready for sexual experiences, but if the process is hastened unduly without allowing the natural process to 'unfold' at its own pace, it may never function well. This can be likened to a closed, exquisite rosebud being pulled

open by someone impatient to see it in its fully glory—only to find the petals bruised and torn in the process, and that it does not fulfil its potential of giving pleasure.

Love says, 'What can I give?' much more than, 'What can I get?' As a *minimum*, I think that responsible sex means asking these three questions before any couple make love: 'Do we want, and can we care for, a baby?'; 'If not, are we using a reliable method of family planning, such as the pill, maybe with a condom also for safer sex?'; and, most important, 'Will making love with this person lead to anyone, my partner, myself, or any third party, being hurt?' Having realized that someone might very well get hurt, some young people even in the 21st century do actually decide not to have sex *even with precautions*. They are using what has been described as the 'safest of all oral contraceptives'—namely, the word 'No'. They feel empowered to assert their rights over their own body and with whom to share it. To quote Esther Sapire again: 'They can choose when and by whom to be touched without shame or guilt, and they have the right to say "No" if they so desire without feeling old fashioned or freakish.' Worth a thought.

I fully accept that many will consider much of the above incredibly old-fashioned. They reject all or most of it and believe they can avoid unwanted pregnancies and STIs, and succeed in practising 'serial monogamy' without hurting each other or third parties, and, most importantly, can in due course bring their children up in secure homes based on mutual trust. All I would say is, are not these good outcomes more *likely* down the other road?

Yet, I join them in agreeing wholeheartedly that anyone who thinks that 'abstinence education' will suffice for *all* our modern young people must be living on another planet! I go on to say the following:

The 'best' must not be allowed to be the enemy of the 'good'

What is 'the good'? I say it is not just 'sex education'. I am opposed to that! What we all should favour is really good sex *and relationships* education (SRE). This should start (ideally) from age one through to 10, and be delivered to begin with by the child's parents, answering their questions in an unembarrassed and age-appropriate way. It should then continue at school and include contraceptive services delivered to young people in a 100 per cent *confidential* and straightforward way and in a user-friendly environment: leading, after all questions are answered, to the provision of their choice from methods like the pill, implant, and condom—and emergency contraception. Moreover, as one youngster said in a focus group, when asked who would be the best provider of such services: 'Someone with a smile would be your best bet!'

Part of 'the good' is still, surely, to encourage longer-term rather than shorter-term relationships, and monogamy within each. Sociological research has regularly shown that so-called *integrated* relationships with sharing and communication have a much better track record, even just for avoiding an unwanted pregnancy, than do the non-sharing, often short-term *segregated* type. Couples in integrated relationships consider and discuss contraception as part of their sexual relationship, and so it is arranged first. Contraception in segregated relationships is seen as entirely the woman's business, and she gets around to it *after* sex starts happening, if then. Connected with this is another well-established fact, that *most unplanned conceptions happen at the start and at the end of relationships.* At the start, couples without good lines of communication are often inhibited from actually discussing contraception. And at a 'bust-up' there seems no point in continuing to take the pill; but often there is at least one attempt at reconciliation along with sex—and the condom is either not available or seems truly a 'barrier'. Whatever the explanation, those are the times when most unwanted conceptions happen. If so, there's a pretty obvious conclusion, but few experts in this area are prepared to come out with it. If unwanted conception is such a big feature of the start and finish of relationships, surely it is much better *purely on contraceptive grounds* to have loyal, long-term relationships and thus fewer contraceptively dangerous partner changes!

What about the pill in all this? It cannot be expected to be a cure-all of society's ills. Nor should it be blamed for too many of them—they are caused by people, not by the pill. Certainly it can enable some people to behave irresponsibly, people who forget that bodies also have feelings and emotions attached. Even then, at least a disastrous pregnancy will be avoided.

A child has the best chance in life if born to parents who trust each other and because of their commitment are prepared to keep *working* on their relationship, so as to ensure an emotionally secure and happy home for all the years he or she needs to reach maturity. And then the pill and other methods can help that home not to be overwhelmed by more new arrivals than the family, or the family's country and world, can properly care for!

There are many types and many different outlooks in this troubled world. This postscript was written so that you, reading this book, might know where I stand.

100 frequently asked questions about the Pill

Introduction

The answers to the FAQs here are deliberately very brief and hence sometimes over-simplified. Please refer to the pages mentioned for more details. The two main types of pill are: POP = progestogen-only pill, COC = combined oral contraceptive pill. As in the rest of this book, the COC is often just called the Pill, and because it is much more widely used than the POP, most of the questions and answers below refer to it. Moreover, nearly always what I say here applies also to the others in the group of *combined hormonal methods*: EVRA, the skin patch (p. 172) and the vaginal NuvaRing (p. 173) – since as we saw earlier they are also combined hormone products, *very* similar to two COCs (Cilest and Mercilon respectively).

In fact I think that the only questions that do not apply at all to users of EVRA or the NuvaRing are nos. 7, 23, 25–9, 33–4 . . . (aside from all questions about the POP and other obviously-different progestogen-only or male methods . . .).

(a) Types of pill and how they work

1. What is the combined oral contraceptive pill (COC)?

This contains an estrogen and a progestogen and is usually taken daily, for 21, 22, or 23 or 24 days out of every 28. One or other type of tricycling is also a possible option (pp. 29–31), including 'Seasonale' in the USA.

2. How does it work?

Chiefly by stopping maturing and release of eggs (Chapter 1).

3. What is the 'mini-pill'/progestogen-only pill (POP)?

As its (better) second name suggests, this contains only a progestogen in very low dose, and is taken every single day of the year without breaks

(Chapter 8). Being estrogen-free means it has none of the risks of the COC that are connected with that hormone.

4. How does the POP work?

The old-type POP chiefly works by altering the cervical mucus to stop sperm entering the uterus, but also by blocking egg-release. Cerazette blocks egg-release more efficiently, so needs to use the mucus effect less often, as back-up. See Chapter 8 for more details about both types of POP.

5. How effective are pills against pregnancy?

Very, if regularly taken. The failure rate of the COC is <1 but in less good pill-takers can go up to 3 or more pregnancies per 100 woman-years (p. 13). The figures for the POP range from <1 to 1 per 100 women per year for Cerazette and from 1 to 4 per 100 woman-years for the old-type POPs, (p. 177). Cerazette is believed to have more "margin" for error (p. 182).

6. Are all the combined pills the same?

No, there are differences between the brands, but we do not know for certain which is the 'best buy' (p. 155). It seems best to take the lowest acceptable dose of both hormones and *normally* to start with one containing levonorgestrel (LNG) or norethisterone (NET) as the progestogen (p. 156). But every woman is different: some need slightly higher doses, or different progestogens.

7. What about phasic pills?

These are COCs giving a daily dose of both progestogen and estrogen, but the ratio of one hormone to the other varies stepwise (see pp. 160–3 for details). They may be either biphasic (two phases) or triphasic (three phases).

(b) Availability of the Pill

8. How can I get a supply of the Pill?

In Britain over 95 per cent of family doctors will prescribe it. If your doctor will not, you should be able to obtain it from another local doctor, even if he or she is in a different practice; or from a Family Planning Clinic (addresses in the telephone directory, or through the FPA on 0845 3101334).

9. But I am under age . . . Will they insist on telling my parents?

NO. They will recommend to you that *you* involve a parent, but no pressure. Their duty of care and complete confidentiality is just the same as for adults, pp. 22–3. The slogan is "Here to listen not to tell!"

10. Can my partner come to the clinic or surgery with me?

Certainly and, if you ask, he can usually also come in with you when you see the doctor or nurse.

11. Do I have to be examined internally at the first visit?

Almost never. The internal examination should only be done if you have a particular medical reason on the day (pp. 21–2). Even after that, once you are a pill-taker, regular checks of blood pressure and of headache pattern are the two main things (p. 152). Cervical smear tests are 'well-woman' checks, not specially connected with the Pill, and the policy now is that they should normally only start being done at the age of 25. Breast examinations ought only to be done if you have found a lump or *some other change that concerns you.*

12. How often should I have a smear test done?

The national guidelines now say once every three years, from the ages of 25 to 49. Above the age of 50, 5-yearly is the routine, stopping altogether at 65 (above that, doing it only if none has been done since age 50). That frequency is safe even if you both smoke and take the Pill (p. 116), but smears will probably be recommended more often if you ever have an abnormal one.

13. They have asked me to come back for a smear test in only three months: what does this mean? Can I continue on the Pill?

No reason to panic. This may be because the first test picked up too few of the right kind of cells for the lab to check they were completely normal, so they want to look again. Or, some abnormal cells were found in your previous smear. Quite often these are got rid of by the body without any further treatment anyway, and so are not seen when you have the repeat done. Otherwise the doctor will discuss the whole matter with you. He or she will explain that even persistent changes in the smear can be readily dealt with, and actual cancer of the cervix—which in any case would not occur for many years—can be prevented altogether by minor treatment, usually as an out-patient (pp. 116, 151). And yes, you should continue on the Pill until you see your doctor, while you are having any treatment, and usually for as long thereafter as you wish (see p. 151).

14. How often should I attend the clinic or surgery for my tablets?

This will usually depend on the number of packets you are given at each visit. Commonly you will be seen three months after first starting on the Pill, then regularly every six months for about two years; and then if your blood pressure is normal and you have no risk factors you may be given 13 packs at a time (p. 152). However, you must feel free to come back sooner than your next routine visit if you ever have any anxiety about using the Pill or about any side-effect it seems to be having on you. See also below, about special medical supervision.

(c) Practical pill-taking

15. Which diseases that I have ever suffered from should I be sure to mention to the doctor?

The main thing to mention is any past thrombosis, also any disease or disorder affecting the circulation (pp. 67–78). These include diabetes, high blood pressure and especially migraine. If you get those headaches, be sure you describe to the doctor or nurse any "aura" you have: mainly this is a "bright" loss of vision on one side beginning before the headache itself starts (pp. 84–6). How many you smoke and any past liver troubles should be mentioned; the other important short- and long-term disorders are to be found on pp. 137–51. Don't forget any regular medicines you take, including ones you buy over the counter: St John's Wort is very relevant (see p. 45/55). Allergies, especially to drugs, should always be entered in your case notes.

16. What diseases in my family are important?

Any history in your immediate family of thrombosis (blood clots) in veins or arteries, heart attacks, and any kind of stroke; or of any other family problem (such as raised blood pressure or diabetes, or 'Factor V Leiden' – p. 143) that you have been told makes some kind of thrombosis more likely. A true family history is mainly if it affected a parent, brother or sister at a young age (under the age of 45). Mention also if there is a family tendency to breast cancer, especially in mother or sister under 40 years-old. When in doubt, also mention any unusual family complaint, like porphyria (p. 140).

17. Who should never take the Pill (WHO 4)?

In the light of any diseases in your own past or still affecting you, or those which run in your family, the final decision about this will be taken by your doctor or specialist nurse, always in consultation with you. See pp. 137–143, and the Box about the WHO scale we now use to sort out who may use a method like the Pill, ranging from "always" (WHO 1) to "never" (WHO 4).

18. Who should be very cautious about taking the Pill and then only with special medical supervision?

Again, this will depend mainly on your own medical history and that of your family (pp. 143–151). If one of these 'relative contra-indications' applies, either WHO 3 (cautiously usable) or WHO 2 (broadly usable), it is more important than usual to use a COC giving the minimum possible dose—or even one of the POPs instead (p. 178). WHO 3 also then means special medical supervision thereafter.

19. What is 'special medical supervision', then?

It means being seen by the doctor more often than usual, being told what to look out for so as to return earlier if necessary, and sometimes having special tests done. It also means being ready to discontinue the Pill should some condition worsen, or a new risk factor or relevant disease appear, or you reach age 35 (pp. 145–6).

20. There seems to be no medical objection, so how do I start taking the Pill?

There are two main ways, but you should usually start on day 1 of the period (pp. 33–4 and Fig. 3.2, also 161). The POP should almost always be started on day 1 (p. 180). See also pp. 35–6 and 180 for how to start COCs and POPs after any kind of recent pregnancy.

A useful tip: if you happened to start taking your *first pill ever* on a day in the second half of the week, such as Thursday, your 'periods' (really withdrawal bleeds, pp. 14–16) will then always affect your week-ends. This could go on for years. But see p. 31 for how to shorten one pill-free interval and they will then always happen on week-days . . .

21. Which pill is best if I plan to breastfeed my baby?

The old-type POP—but read carefully the discussion on pp. 191–2. And you could also choose a non-hormonal method if you prefer, instead.

22. How soon after starting hormonal methods am I protected against pregnancy?

At once, if either the COC, or NuvaRing, or EVRA or the POP is started early enough after a full-term baby (pp. 35, 180); or if any are started by the day after a miscarriage or termination of pregnancy, or on day 1—or even up to day 3—of the menstrual cycle. Otherwise, for maximum reliability alternative precautions such as the condom should be used, just until seven tablets have been taken (p. 39).

23. How do I take the pills after that?

You take twenty-one consecutive daily pills followed by a seven-day break for all the COCs except the 22- or 24-day types available in some countries or if you have been advised to use one of the 'tricycle' schemes (pp. 29–31). Every Day (ED) pills contain dummies to be taken during the Pill-free week. Like them, POPs are taken every single day including during periods. With *all* pills tablet-taking should best continue following the daily routine, even if there is a side-effect like nausea or some unexpected bleeding (pp. 164–6) – since they so often settle if you keep going. (But of course, take advice early on if the side-effect really bothers you).

24. Is it safe to make love on the regular days when COCs or other combined hormones are not taken?

Yes: *but only* if no pills have been missed (or not absorbed) towards the end of the previous pill packet, and you do in fact start another packet on time after the Pill-free week (p. 31). The safety of this time depends on the NEXT PACKET (or patch or ring) as much as on the one that came before. This vital need to restart on time after those 7 days without the contraception is something just as true of EVRA and NuvaRing as well!

25. Do I have to take pills at the same time of day, and if so what time is best?

For COCs, any regular time will do, morning or evening, within a couple of hours, but more than one day late means loss of protection. POPs (all kinds) should ideally be taken within around an hour of the same time each day, and being late by as little as three hours means loss of protection.

26. How can I ever remember to take my pills?

I am a great believer in the Every Day packs of COCs (pp. 29, 161), like Microgynon ED, which contain twenty-one active tablets and seven dummies, so there is no need to remember when to stop and start successive courses. Ask your doctor – they cost exactly the same to the NHS! A useful tip is to get your pill-taking routine linked with something else that you do regularly every day. For instance, you could use a rubber band to tie your packet of COCs to your toothbrush. For the POP I strongly recommend setting an alarm on your mobile phone, so it reminds you at the same time of day even when your routine may be different at week-ends. I am quite sure I would need an alarm reminder if there were a male pill!

27. I have forgotten to take a pill: am I in big trouble and sure to get pregnant?

No, especially if you are on the COC, and with both types of pill if you do not rely on pills alone, taking extra precautions for the recommended time.

28. What shall I do?

According to the new advice (2004), if it was a missed <u>COC</u>, and you are *more than* 24 hours late in pill-taking, take the missing pill(s) and then continue in all respects as usual with your pill-taking routine. On top of that, if you are more than one day late in re-starting, so as to lengthen the Pill-free time to *more than* 8 days, or you missed any two or more of tablets 1–7 in a pack, you need emergency pills *as well*—see p. 52 – and should either not have sex or use condoms until you have taken 7 daily pills. *If and only if* you find you have missed one or more of the last seven pills in the packet, go straight on to the next packet when you finish the current one. That's all, unless you have missed more than 4 tablets: see Fig. 3.4 and pp. 39–42 for further details. See pp. 172–4 for EVRA and NuvaRing.

If it was a missed **POP**, if you are only three hours late (12 hours for Cerazette) in taking one or more tablets, abstaining or extra precautions are advised (now) until you have taken two daily pills (pp. 181–2). And if you (have) carried on love-making in the whole time between when you first missed the first tablet through until those two new tablets are on board, the emergency pill treatment would be advisable *as well* (p. 183).

29. What shall I do if I have a stomach upset?

As far as your body is concerned, vomiting is just like missing a tablet. But if you take another within 2 hours and it stays down, that's sufficient to replace it. See pp. 43–4, 181 for what to do if you keep on vomiting, with either COCs or POPs. But with EVRA and NuvaRing since they do not enter via the stomach at all, there's no problem here!

30. Can other medicines affect the reliability of COCs, EVRA, NuvaRing, all the POPs and hormonal EC?

Yes, this is an important way every one of these could be made to fail. The main medicines involved are rifampicin and rifabutin, and a number that are used in the treatment of epilepsy and HIV/AIDS (p. 44). St John's Wort ("Nature's Prozac"), a treatment that you may have decided to buy for yourself, is particularly important, since the CSM's advice is always to use another reliable method and not the COC or POP at all. With the others the Pill or EC maybe could still be used (WHO3) in a special way (pp. 46–155). Bleeding on COC-taking days may be an early warning sign (pp. 164–6).

31. Can hormonal methods affect the actions of other medicines?

Ciclosporin (used after transplant surgery) is a rare example where the new treatment might need to be modified for this reason. Women who have to take warfarin to thin their blood, such as after a thrombosis, should have their special INR blood test checked more often at first, if they are given the POP, the emergency pill or (most unusually) any combined hormonal method.

32. Should I always make a special point of telling any doctor who sees me that I am on the a combined hormonal method or the POP?

Yes. This is vital, not only as just mentioned because of the potential problem of interaction between drugs, but also because laboratory tests may be affected (pp. 60–3). Moreover the knowledge that you are on COC, EVRA, NuvaRing or a POP may also help when making a diagnosis or planning any surgery.

33. If a change to a different brand of COC is recommended, are there any special rules?

Yes. If moving to a pill definitely on the same 'rung' of Fig. 7.1 (p. 155), or higher, just take the usual seven-day break between old and new packets. But if moving *down* to a lower-dose pill, or if in doubt, it will always be contraceptively safe to follow one of the 'rules': *either* to start the first new packet without any break after the old one (pp. 47–8), *OR* to take the usual break and use condoms for the subsequent seven tablet-taking days. See p. 161 for the rules for phasic pills, and p. 180 if moving to the POP, or from the POP to any other method.

34. If I lose my COCs half-way through a packet and my friend has a spare packet of a different brand, is it safe to take them?

This could be a very muddled situation if either yours or hers are phasic pills (pp. 160–3). Even if they are of the fixed-dose type, it is *not* recommended. However, if there seems no alternative, perhaps when you are away for a weekend, then you should certainly check that the Pill is on an equivalent rung of the ladders of Fig. 7.1. If it is higher, protection will be maintained, but if it is lower, then protection may be reduced and you should preferably follow the seven-day loss-of-protection rule, using condoms as well as taking the new pills. (The same rule, or running on the packets as described above and on pp. 47–8, is best followed when you return to your normal pill from a borrowed higher-dose one.)

35. What shall I do if I need some more pills (or any hormonal method) when in a foreign country?

Look up your variety of pill or the other method on the website www.ippf.org.uk (p. 267) or pp. 269–77 here. You should then be able to use the name of the nearest equivalent locally available brand when you visit the doctor or a chemist.

36. If my partner goes abroad, or if I get a bad side-effect, can I stop the Pill or patch or ring in the middle of a packet/cycle ?

First of all, it must be beyond day 7, because of that rule on p. 39, that "7 days of Pill-taking puts the ovaries to sleep" reliably. Even then, with the COC/patch/ring it is best to complete the sequence, otherwise you will get a bleed prematurely. But if the reason for stopping is one of the possibly serious symptoms mentioned on p. 50–1, you should still be able to avoid a pregnancy if you transfer *immediately* to using another method, such as the condom.

POPs almost never need to be stopped in a hurry: they are best stopped during a period (p. 180) so this could be before the end of a packet.

37. When I am stopping the Pill, patch, or ring to take a break for a while, can I assume protection for the next 7 days like in the usual hormone-free break?

Emphatically NOT! See Q 24 above. In fact, if your decision to stop the Pill is made any time during the seven-day gap between packets (or even before 7 new tablets have been taken after it) *and* you carry on making love during those seven days: then you really shouldn't stop, you should take one more packet. This is to put back to sleep your ovary, which you remember might always be close to releasing an egg after 7 no-pill days. Or you could take the emergency pill. The same approach applies to EVRA and NuvaRing. This is all explained on pp. 37–41.

38. Does it matter if I take the Pill or other combined hormonal method for short spells of a few months at a time, according to need?

No, so long as the rules for starting and stopping are followed each time (see Questions 22, 23, and 36). But this still risks getting "carried away" when you are no longer protected and is probably why so many unwanted conceptions happen at the start and finish of relationships (p. 242). So, many modern women, especially in the Netherlands, are so confident in the safety of the Pill that they stay on it even when their partner is away or between relationships.

39. If I want a baby, can I just stop the Pill or other hormones? Or should I use another method like condoms for a while?

See pp. 102–3 for the answer to this one and to Question 75 (about pill-taking *during* pregnancy). It seems that previous use of the Pill does not increase the chance of having an abnormal baby (above the background risk, which there always is of course). A really important thing is to take a 0.4 mg folic acid tablet daily while you are 'trying', and not just after you conceive.

40. I am going into hospital for an operation—should I stop the Pill or combined ring or patch? and if so, when? And when can I take it again?

Much depends on whether this is for a major or a minor operation (pp. 139, 147). If it is ANY treatment for varicose veins (p. 73), or ANY operation on the legs (including arthroscopy), or you are told the operation somewhere else in the body will:

- last for more than thirty minutes and
- you will be in bed for at least the first twenty-four hours in hospital after it, then you should whenever possible transfer from the COC, EVRA or the NuvaRing to another effective estrogen-free method (like Cerazette or Depo-Provera, for example) four weeks beforehand. However major the surgery, there is normally no need to discontinue any of the POPs in this way (because it is EE-free (p. 187).

If there are no complications, if you have not had sex you can restart the Pill by "Quick start" (p. 35) with precautions for 7 more days, any time which is at least two weeks following full mobility after the operation. Otherwise start on Day 1 of the first period which comes, again, not less than two weeks afterwards.

41. Does being sterilized count as a major operation?

Not if done by modern laparoscopy techniques (p. 147). Therefore there is no need to stop any of the combined hormonal methods, and usually it is best to continue after the operation until the end of the current packet/cycle of treatment. The POP is continued for at least 7 days and usually until the next period.

42. I am going ski-ing and I take the COC. What should I do if I break a leg?

Most people realise that the COC should be stopped if you become suddenly bed-bound due to illness, accident, or major surgery as an emergency. But not enough know that even if only a leg has to be pinned or completely fixed in plaster after a fracture, once again the Pill – or EVRA, or NuvaRing – should be avoided or stopped. There is a real risk of thrombosis in that leg: so as well as stopping the combined hormonal method immediately, inform the surgeon who will probably decide to give you blood-thinning (anti-coagulant) medication – if s/he wasn't going to anyway.

43. How long can I stay on the Pill or other combined hormone method? Should I make a break every two years? Or after five years?

The effect of the length of pill-use on the risks of diseases of the circulation and cancer is fully discussed on pp. 121–2. The short answer is that breaks usually do more harm than good, and normal pill-taking gives you sufficient breaks anyway (one week in every four). However, if you want a break (switching to some other good method) for your own reasons, that is certainly your right. The uncommon infertility problem of amenorrhoea—absent periods for many months—after stopping the Pill is no more likely after long-term than short-term use (p. 102).

However, it could be acceptable for you to use a 20 mcg COC or NuvaRing right up to 51, which is the average age of the menopause, if you wish to and are a slim, healthy non-smoker with no migraines (pp. 79, 121, 159). EVRA – and some other COCs – would be a bit high-dose for this use.

The risks, if any, of long-term use of the POP are thought to be so low that it can be used well into the 50s, beyond the very slightest risk of any egg-release (p. 189).

(d) Pills and periods, or no periods

Combined oral contraceptive pill (COC) and all other combined hormonal methods

44. What causes 'periods' on the COC/ring/patch? Are they really periods at all?

The natural menstrual cycle is abolished whether or not you have any bleeding. It is replaced by the combined hormone cycle in which bleeding is caused in a quite different way, by withdrawal of the hormones from the blood supply to the uterus for (usually) seven days out of every twenty-eight. So they are not true periods (pp. 14–16).

45. I have very irregular periods naturally (only three or four a year) or have missed them altogether for months at a time—can I take the Pill?

This depends: special tests may be required. If your ovaries are not producing enough estrogen and you need contraception, or if you have PCOS (p. 98) one of the combined hormonal methods might actually be good for you, the best choice (149–50).

46. I have missed a 'period'—what shall I do?

If you have no reason to suspect loss of protection by the Pill (pp. 42–3), you should start a new packet after the Pill-free week in the usual way. However, if the next pill withdrawal bleed also fails to come—i.e. you miss two 'periods' in a row—you should do a pregnancy test and see your doctor before starting another packet. Same applies to EVRA or NuvaRing.

47. If I don't see much of a 'period' on any of the combine hormonal methods, or if I see no bleeding at all in the hormone-free week, is blood collecting inside me?

No: as explained on pp. 16, 167–8, if you have no bleeding it simply means that there is no blood to come away. After a check to make sure you are not pregnant, you can continue with the Pill or other combined method if you wish (Fig. 7.3*b* and p. 168).

48. Can I avoid having monthly bleeding altogether—e.g. when going on holiday?

Yes: the best way is to take two packets in a row (p. 31). But there are special rules for phasic pills (pp. 162–3). Even if there is no special reason, it is also a choice you have after discussion with the doctor to *tricycle* (see below). This will mean having at most only 4 or 5 'periods' in a year. . . .

49. What is the tricycle pill?

This is actually the ordinary pill, but 'tricycling' means a way of taking it: usually four, sometimes three, packets in a row followed by a break of seven or sometimes fewer days (pp. 29–31). This produces only four or five hormone withdrawal bleeds a year and has some important uses. NB Do not confuse this with the triphasic pill—see pp. 160–3.

50. I am bleeding like a period on days of pill-taking: should I stop in the middle of a packet?

The golden rule of pill-taking is to carry on taking your pills according to the routine, usually twenty-one days on, seven days off, irrespective of the pattern of bleeding or no-bleeding which may occur. See p. 166 (Fig. 7.3*a*) and the Box on p. 164 and make an early appointment to discuss this with your doctor, particularly if it is a new problem. It could be wise to have a Chlamydia test, particularly if you have recently had a change of partner.

To control a bad breakthrough-bleeding problem, provided you have taken at least seven tablets to make your ovaries inactive, your doctor may sometimes suggest stopping altogether for a maximum seven days and then restarting. This often works.

51. I not only get spotting on pill-taking days, I have also had no expected bleeding during the last seven days of no pills. What shall I do?

Actually, this is quite a common combination of problems. If you have no reason to suspect loss of protection from the Pill, and this is the first missed 'period', then follow the advice at Question 46 above and start taking your next packet on the correct day. If you persevere, taking your pills regularly, there is a good chance that the correct bleeding pattern will be established. If not, you should make an early appointment to discuss things with your doctor (Fig. 7.3 and pp. 165–8).

Irregular bleeding like this is more likely to happen after erratic pill-taking, or some other reason for loss of protection like a new medicine you've been given (pp. 44–8). If that is a concern, see Fig. 3.4 (p. 38) and perhaps take your doctor's advice before starting another packet.

As before, the advice in this answer *(and in Qs 44–50, above)* applies with minor adjustment also to EVRA and NuvaRing.

Progestogen-only pill (POP)

52. What causes periods on the POP?

Quite unlike the bleeds that occur while taking the COC, if periods happen while using old type POPs these are like natural ones—due to the loss of the natural progesterone and estrogen, as egg-release and formation of a corpus luteum usually occur (p. 176). But Cerazette nearly always blocks egg-release, *and* an old type POP-user may be among the 40 per cent or more who similarly have their cycle stopped. In either case any bleeds that occur during long periods of no bleeding at all are of the "breakthrough"- type (BTB).

53. Does it matter if I see no periods on the POP?

Yes and no. First check you are not pregnant. If not, this means you are as protected against pregnancy as if you were on the COC (pp. 183–4). It may mean your natural menstrual cycle is particularly easy to stop; but neither kind of POP will harm your fertility and so can be continued. See pp. 184–5 and discuss the matter with your doctor.

54. What should I do if I get erratic bleeding and spotting on the old-type POP or Cerazette?

Continue daily pill-taking: if the bleeding pattern is unacceptable, see your doctor.

Periods after stopping the Pill—either COC or POP

55. Although I had very regular 'periods' on the Pill (or ring or patch), I stopped taking it some months ago and have seen no periods yet. What does this mean?

It means that your natural menstrual cycle, with egg-release and periods, has not yet been restored. It usually will be, without treatment, but if more than six months go by some tests should be arranged (pp. 101, 185 and Question 56).

56. We have been trying to have a baby since stopping the Pill (or ring or patch) with no success yet. Was it to blame and should we have tests done?

Between 10 and 15 per cent of all couples are not pregnant after 'trying' for a whole year. So it *could* be a coincidence, especially if you're a bit older now (since not starting to try till above age 35 tends to mean taking longer). Discuss referral for tests with your doctor if you have been without periods for six months or more, but if:

- the periods have returned *and*
- *you have no bad pain symptoms* (which could be due to endometriosis) and
- you are under 30

it is usually fine to keep trying for up to a year before being investigated for a possible fertility problem.

57. Could using the Pill for a long time make my menopause happen earlier? or later?

Neither a combined hormonal method nor the POP (nor not ovulating for months on end because of having lots of babies and breastfeeding them all) seems to have any effect at all, whether to make the final period come later or earlier. This happens when your ovaries' supply of eggs runs out—something predetermined for each woman.

58. If I am on the POP, how do I find out that I have reached the menopause?

As well as your periods stopping, which can happen on the POP anyway, you may start getting symptoms like hot flushes. It may sometimes be possible to confirm the menopause by a blood test—discuss this with your doctor and see p. 189 and Question 74. But there is no rush to change to another method, since it is so safe just to continue with the POP.

(e) Problems with the Pill

59. How dangerous, really, is the COC?

Like any drug it has risks, but these have often been exaggerated. See Chapter 6! One very good point is that no harm is likely to be caused by a large overdose (p. 59). And it's difficult even to try to do that with EVRA or a NuvaRing!

60. How dangerous is the POP?

Probably even safer than the remarkably safe COC!

61. What side-effects will I notice?

Often none at all. If you do, it is nearly always worth persevering with the COC, EVRA or NuvaRing, or the POP (but see Question 62), at least for three months. Even then, do not give up the method too easily; there are other brands which might be tried.

62. What symptoms should make me see a doctor at once?

These are listed on pp. 50–1, but, apart from abdominal pain (pp. 186–7), they do not apply to the POP. Even with the COC, EVRA or NuvaRing they are very rare, so do not let the list worry you!

63. Won't I put on a lot of weight?

Usually none with the POP, and very little if any with the modern ultra-low-dose combined hormonal methods. But you may need to control it by diet and exercise. Some of the weight gain noticed by young teenage pill-takers is now known to be due just to growing up, since the same is observed in non-users of the COC. If you are already overweight, see pp. 139, 146, 178–9, and 189.

64. Could the Pill be causing my headaches?

This is possible, especially on the Pill-free days. This could be a good reason for tricycling (pp. 29–31), which can be done even for migraines at that time if they are the kind *without* aura. Bad headaches, especially migraines which change their symptoms, should always be discussed with your doctor (pp. 83–8).

65. I get so depressed these days: how likely is it that the Pill is to blame?

There may sometimes be a clear-cut link with the Pill (pp. 81–2), or with being on a more progestogen-dominant kind (p. 171), so a change of pill may help – but it may not. Vitamin B6 (p. 82) is sometimes worth a try: it takes 2–3 months to produce any benefit.

66. I seem to have lost interest in sex too; would stopping or changing the Pill help?

Not very often. Could there be something wrong within your sexual relationship, for which some counselling might even help? If you are on the pills with an anti-androgenic progestogen (Yasmin and Dianette) and have this loss of libido without being depressed at all, it may help to switch to a less estrogen-dominant one (p. 170). If depression is perhaps a more important feature, I would recommend a *more* estrogen-dominant pill (p. 171). The POP especially Cerazette is also worth trying.

If the problem is partly a feeling of vaginal dryness or soreness, arrange a check-up (preferably at a GUM clinic, as they are the specialists. Often the cause is thrush (Candida), which is a great turn-off for sex, is not a sexually transmitted infection and is easily treated. After that you could try a lubricating jelly (see p. 83).

67. Could the brown blotches I have started to get on my face be due to the Pill?

Yes they could; they are given the name chloasma (p. 106). This is unfortunately very hard to get rid of, whether it starts during a pregnancy or use of a hormonal contraceptive. It has to be "treated" mainly cosmetically.

68. Since starting on the Pill, I feel sick and dizzy and have too much vaginal discharge—what shall I do?

All these may well improve after two or three courses of pills. Nausea is often worse in the first few days after each pill-free interval, but then happens on fewer and fewer days with each new packet. It can also often be reduced by taking the pills last thing at night.

Otherwise these and other symptoms, which seem to be due to too much estrogen effect in comparison with the progestogen effect, can be helped by using a progestogen-dominant pill, or by the progestogen-only pill (Cerazette, if you are under 45-years-old and greatest available efficacy is important to you, p. 190).

69. Thrombosis sounds very worrying: I am told it means clots, so does it mean that I can't use the Pill if I have clots with my periods?

Far from it: clots with the periods just mean that they are heavy, and could well improve dramatically if you went on the Pill (pp. 15, 27) or the ring or patch. Tricycling (p. 29–31) would also be a thought.

70. What are the facts about thrombosis and other troubles of the circulation?

Chapters 4 and 7 are mainly about this. In brief, the risk is primarily in people who have other risk factors, listed on pp. 143–8. Smoking is the most common and main one, and becomes even more important as age increases (pp. 79–80).

71. Which reduces this risk more, to stop the Pill or to stop smoking?

For anyone smoking fifteen or more cigarettes a day, the risks of all the currently available pills are much MUCH less than those of smoking. However long you have been a smoker, your chances of survival are always greater if you stop (p. 80).

72. I smoke at least twenty cigarettes a day: how can I be helped to stop?

In Britain, ASH (Action on Smoking and Health— www.ash.co.uk – can give you loads of practical advice and there may be an anti-smoking clinic you could attend locally. Quitline is particularly useful (p. 268). Smoking substitutes give your body the powerful (strong as heroin) drug of addiction it so craves, in a much cleaner way than along with all that carbon monoxide and carcinogenic tar. Some find the nicotine inhaler good, as it gives you something to do with your hands.

But there is no magic method and you will never succeed unless:

- you really want to give up,
- you are prepared to work hard to do so, and you need to
- get your partner to join you if he is a smoker.

73. At what age should I stop the Pill?

You must stop the COC, or EVRA or NuvaRing at 35, according to UK policy, if you cannot *completely* stop smoking, or have a similar risk factor (pp. 145–6). Otherwise healthy non-smokers may if they so choose take one of the lowest-dose pills until their menopause (pp. 146, 159–60). The POP (including Cerazette), the implant and IUDs may be used by both smokers and non-smokers until then and even longer. See pp. 188–9, Table 10.1 (pp. 215–21), and discuss with your doctor or nurse.

74. I am near that 'change of life', and I have been given treatment for hot flushes, the Pills are in a packet which looks like 'the Pill' and I take them the same way. Are they contraceptives?

No! If you were still having periods, even irregularly, up to the time of starting this treatment, which is known as 'hormone replacement therapy', you should not rely on it. The dose system is different, and it may not be effective in preventing pregnancy.

See also Q 43 and pp. 159–60, 190: for how, if you are a *completely* healthy slim non-smoker without migraines, it might sometimes be OK for you to use a 20 mcg pill or NuvaRing until age 51 anyway, so getting contraception as well as the extra estrogen you may need. Even better for many women is to combine the LNG-IUS with natural estrogen by any chosen route (p. 226).

75. If I got pregnant and did not realize, would continuing to take the Pill harm the baby?

The risk of this is very low indeed, if it exists at all (p. 102). But when possible it is always best to avoid exposing any pregnancy to hormones or any drug.

76. Does the evidence we have so far suggest that the overall risk of cancer is greater in pill-users than those who never take the Pill?

No: see pp. 116–19. Overall, the risks may even be reduced, depending on the outcome of ongoing research into breast cancer (pp. 110–15).

77. Have the risks of the Pill sometimes been exaggerated?

Yes. Even more commonly, the problems of the Pill are not put in perspective against its benefits, or in comparison with the risks and problems of alternatives, of using no method at all, and of life generally (pp. 127–34).

78. What about the risks for people in developing countries?

These are probably less than in 'over-developed' countries, the risks of alternatives and of pregnancy also tend to be greater. But much more research is needed.

79. Are there still things we don't know about the Pill, particularly about long-term risks?

Yes: see pp. 119–123, 135–6. This book can do no more than give a consensus or majority view on the known facts about the Pill. Very preliminary findings are not mentioned, because it would be as wrong to cause false fears as it would be to raise false hopes.

80. After all that, what good effects does the Pill have?

See p. 27 and the Table 6.1 (pp. 126–7). Main advantages are that it is so highly effective, acceptable, unrelated to intercourse, and almost 100 per cent reversible; but in most women the Pill also has good effects on the menstrual cycle and provides protection against two or may be three cancers (pp. 116–8).

(f) People in special categories (if your situation is not mentioned here, please use the index)

81. Does it affect my choice of pill that I am very underweight?

Underweight women (with a BMI below 19 (see Glossary p. 279)) are more likely to have side effects like menstrual cramps, nausea, and breast discomfort, and to have a long delay in return of their periods after stopping the Pill. Hence they should try either a combined pill with the lowest possible dose, or perhaps the POP.

82. What about being overweight?

See BMI in the Glossary (p. 279) again. If the BMI is really high, 40 or above, this is WHO 4 "do not use", for the Pill and also EVRA and NuvaRing. Above 30 is WHO 3 for all on the combined hormones, but with EVRA there is the extra point that weighing above 90 kg (regardless of height) seems to make it less effective (p. 172). Even a BMI of 25 up to 30 is WHO 2, broadly usable, yes: but wouldn't it be even better to get down if at all possible to achieving WHO 1, below 25?!

83. Can I take a combined pill, patch or ring if I have varicose veins?

Yes, if you have not suffered from clotting within them, on their own these rarely mean that you must avoid the method. See p. 73. They are WHO 3 if you have them badly and have suffered a condition called phlebitis in them in the past since this connects somewhat with thrombosis. And they are WHO 4 while you are actually having either medical or surgical treatment for them.

84. Can I take the Pill if I am a diabetic?

Sometimes, but only if you do *not* smoke, at all, have no other risk factors and no diabetic complications, and then with special medical supervision for the shortest possible time (pp. 144, 138). The POP could be a better choice of pill for you, but the IUS('Mirena') is perhaps the best method altogether (pp. 224–6).

85. I am troubled by acne, does this affect which pill I should take?

Yes it does: you should use a relatively estrogen-dominant pill (pp. 108), and if it's moderately severe it may be best to start with or switch to Yasmin or Dianette (pp. 157–8) since they contain anti-androgenic progestogens. (Really bad acne may need referral to a hospital dermatologist).

86. Can I use contact lenses if I take the Pill?

Probably: with modern lenses and modern ultra-low-dose COCs (and POPs). But if your eyes ever become sore do not use the lenses until you have seen your optician again for them to be examined, and for advice (p. 90).

87. I tend to be anaemic, can I take the Pill?

It depends. If you have one of the commonest kinds of anaemia, due to heavy periods, the Pill will be a great help (p. 99). But if you have sickle-cell anaemia (an inherited blood disease that occurs primarily in black people) discuss the matter with your doctor (p. 149). Depo-Provera would usually be a better choice.

88. Does the fact that I have recently had infectious hepatitis (jaundice) mean that I cannot ever again take the Pill?

No, but it does mean that you must have blood tests done to check when your liver is functioning normally, and you will usually be advised to stay off both the COC and the POP for as long as you must avoid alcohol, normally at least three months (p. 140).

89. What about the very itchy mild jaundice that I had in pregnancy?

This, like other conditions which are probably affected by any type of sex hormones (p. 141), means the pill is WHO 3 (cautiously usable, but stop at once of course if jaundice recurred). You should always avoid the

Pill (WHO 4) if you had so-called "cholestatic" jaundice (p. 140) in the past while taking the COC, and it was thought to be the cause.

90. Does it matter that I had high blood pressure (toxaemia) in pregnancy?

This must be mentioned to your doctor, and your blood pressure will need to be checked more often than usual. But most women with this history do not have any trouble on the Pill, provided that they avoid *smoking* (p. 145). If they do smoke real caution is necessary (WHO 3).

91. I had a funny kind of miscarriage, and am now having regular blood tests. Why?

This sounds like trophoblastic disease—ask your doctor, and see p. 117–8 for a full explanation. If so, in the UK, you will generally be advised to avoid *all* hormonal methods: but only until you are given the 'all-clear' by your doctor, based on the hCG tests.

(g) Miscellaneous

92. Should I avoid any foods or alcohol, or take extra vitamins while on the Pill?

As a rule, no (p. 64). It's just not that bad, to need anything like that! But see also p. 102.

93. I am going on a long scheduled flight to Australia. I am on the Pill, are there any precautions I should take?

Yes there are. High altitude increases the risk of thrombosis. Even though the plane will be pressurized to the equivalent of 2,000 metres, thrombosis in the veins of your leg is indeed more likely. Take a maximum amount of fluid and a minimum of caffeine and alcohol which cause the kidney to produce more urine: as the risk is greater if you are dehydrated. If you are at all overweight, special below knee support stockings are advised.

There is no usually no need to actually come off the Pill—many flight attendants use it all the time. But follow their example and take some exercise during the flight by walking around the plane every hour or so.

94A. Are there any problems for long-haul air travellers in pill-taking itself through crossing time-zones?

Yes, it is certainly easy to become confused about regular pill-taking because of passing through different time zones. The effectiveness problem is when flying due West, since the new bed-time pill might be late, hours more than the official 24 hours after the preceding one. One solution is a watch which gives the time in the departure city as well as local time, and any way to base pill-taking on the time where your journey began.

On arrival at a new destination pill-users should always err on the side of taking a pill too early rather than late.

Suppose you fly to London from Auckland and normally take your pill at bed time, if you then switch to taking it at the London bed-time you could have a 36-hour interval between tablets. This increases the risk of pill-failure though not much for the COC: it would be completely unacceptable for ordinary old-type POPs. With both types of pill it increases the risk of irregular or breakthrough bleeding (BTB). So what should you do?

- While on the flight or during any stopover you should continue taking your tablets at the correct hour *based on your departure time zone.* Nothing else needs to be done.
- Upon arrival, as the journey was westbound, after your regular COC or POP has been taken at 24 hours – on the departure time basis – *take an extra tablet (use the last one in that pack) at the next London bedtime.* This will be after only 12 more hours in the Auckland to London situation, but only 8 hours later if the trip was London to Los Angeles, for example. Not a problem.
- And if the journey was actually eastbound, taking that day's pill at the correct local time will shorten the actual pill-taking interval and this is always contraceptively safe.
- If this is done no extra precautions are needed and, with both types of pill, the risk of either BTB or breakthrough conception should be negligible.

95. What shall I do, my 3-year-old daughter has just swallowed all the Pills in my next packet?

Nothing—provided you are sure that this is all she took. She may vomit, and within the next day or two she may have some painless bleeding from her uterus, like a light period. This sounds alarming but is actually no cause for concern (p. 60).

96. If the Pill stops release of eggs, what happens to the eggs?

They stay in the ovary, just as they would in a woman who was perpetually pregnant. However, there is always a steady loss of egg cells within the ovary, from before birth right through to the menopause (p. 2 and see Question 57).

97. What is the injection/jab/jag/shot?

These words and others are used to describe the valuable injectable contraceptive called Depo-Provera, (pp. 222–3). Don't forget Implanon, another progestogen-only method which many people also find highly acceptable (p. 223) – it's a bit like an injectable with the injection only every 3 years instead of 3 months!

98. What is the 'morning-after' pill?

This is a rather bad name for the oral hormonal method that can be used after intercourse to prevent pregnancy (pp. 54–8). A better name, because it does not make people think wrongly that it would be too late if they got the treatment later than the next morning, is 'the emergency pill'. Though it is even more effective when taken within 24 hours rather than 72 hours.

99. What about the male pill?

This is still very much in the future. There is no safe, acceptable pill for men now, nor is there likely to be one for years to come. See Chapter 9.

100. What if I have any other questions about *ANYTHING*?

Ask them and keep on asking them: pertinent or impertinent questions! It is your body, and you have a right to know. Never hesitate to go back to whoever prescribed your pills to discuss all aspects of pill-taking. But remember that some facts simply are not yet available.

Further reading

If you would like more information about ALL methods of contraception, the following book will be useful:

Szarewski, A, Guillebaud, J, *Contraception: A User's Guide* (Oxford University Press, 2000). This provides up-to-date information about *all* the marketed types of contraception, including the newer barrier, implanted, applied or inserted and natural methods, and male and female sterilization.

I would also recommend three medical books which, though written primarily for health-care professionals, are readily understandable and often used by general readers:

Belfield, T, *The FPA Contraceptive Handbook: The Essential Reference Guide for Family Planning and Other Health Professionals* (Family Planning Association, 1997).

Guillebaud, J, *Contraception—Your Questions Answered* (Churchill Livingstone [Elsevier] 2004).

Guillebaud, J, *Contraception Today—A Pocketbook for General Practitioners* (Martin Dunitz [Taylor & Francis], 2004).

Miscellaneous, also relevant:

Cooper, E, Guillebaud, J, *Sexuality and Disability* (Radcliffe Medical Press,1999).

Djerassi, C, *The Politics of Contraception: Birth Control in the Year 2001.* (Freeman, 1981).

Ehrlich, P, Ehrlich, A, *The Population Explosion.* (Arrow Books, 1991).

Skrine, R, Montford, H, *Psychosexual medicine – an introduction.* (Arnold, 2001).

FPA's own publications and their excellent leaflets can be ordered through 0845 122 8600. Their Helpline is **0845 310 1334**

'Believable' web addresses in reproductive health

www.fpa.org.uk: Comes first, because so often all you need can be accessed here, or you can find out by phoning their superb Helpline – **0845 310 1334**. The FPA specialises in client/user information generally, including essential leaflets on all the methods – and on many related subjects like STIs and abortion. Can also tell you how to access locally, near where you live, appropriate (for your problem) sexual and reproductive health.

www.brook.org.uk: Similar to FPA in some ways, but mainly for the under-25s. Has a secure On-line enquiry service, and a free Helpline 0800 0185023.

www.margaretpyke.org: Has a useful search engine for the most common frequently asked questions (FAQs) about contraception. Also the Margaret Pyke Centre itself is a busy open-access clinic in central London.

www.ippf.org.uk: Online version of the Directory of Hormonal Contraception, with names of equivalent Pill brands and other hormonal contraceptives as used throughout the world.

www.fertilityuk.org: The fertility awareness and NFP service, including teachers available locally.

www.ruthinking.co.uk: Home page starts with "Sex – are you thinking about it enough?" A website that fully informs, plus makes it really easy for young people to access services: with a good search engine giving details of their local clinics, both for contraception and sexual health with testing and treatment for STIs. Supported by the Teenage Pregnancy Unit.

www.likeitis.org.uk: Sexual and reproductive health for lay persons by Marie Stopes and fronted by Geri Halliwell.

www.sexplained.com: Slogan is "From the clinic to the street." Very frank and accessible website for young people.

www.teenagehealthfreak.com: FAQs as asked by teenagers, on all health subjects, not just reproductive health – from anorexia to zits!

www.relate.org.uk: Enter postcode to get nearest Relate centre for relationship counselling and help for psychosexual problems. Many publications also available.

www.ffprhc.org.uk: Includes Faculty of Family Planning's Guidance on Emergency Contraception (April 2003) and other authoritative reports.

www.who.int/reproductive-health: WHO's Eligibility Criteria and new Practice Recommendations for health care professionals, and informed lay persons, worldwide.

www.ash.org.uk: Website for Action on Smoking and Health, providing excellent help for pill-takers who want to make it (even) safer to take the pill! There is extra support available by phoning the Quitline: 0800 002200; and also email support from stopsmoking@quit.org.uk

www.the-bms.org: Research-based advice to help an older age group through the hormonal minefield of the menopause. . . .

www.ecotimecapsule.com
www.optimumpopulation.org
www.peopleandplanet.net
} John Guillebaud's websites re: Apology to the *Future* (Eco-time-capsule) project and related issues.

www.popconnect.org: for DVD "*World Population Dots*", mentioned on p. 230

World directory of hormonal contraceptives

What do you do if you are travelling to another country for a long holiday or "Gap year" and need to know whether you can continue to get supplies of your same contraceptive? The answer for many years was to look it up in the Directory of Hormonal Contraceptives, complied by Ronald Kleinman and published by the International Planned Parenthood Federation (IPPF). More recently the IPPF has put this directory in its entirety on its website, www.ippf.org.uk. This is accessible to all, free for the first 2 months and thereafter for a small annual subscription. It is comprehensive, regularly updated and very easy to access.

I have listed below the ***pill brands*** that are currently (in 2004) available in the UK, USA, and Canada, and their international equivalents: which means in fact that most countries' pills are featured. Sometimes a formulation is unique to one country, particularly the USA, but something similar should still be identifiable. The groups by letter A to F are those used in Fig. 7.1 (p. 155), Table 7.1 (pp. 153) and Table 8.2 (p. 178), so that a pill brand identified here can be fitted into the scheme described in Chapters 7 and 8.

Caution: The same or a very similar name is used in different parts of the world for quite different formulations. So recheck the stated formulation of a pill in the list here against that of any previously used packets which you are attempting to match, and if in doubt cross-check with a doctor or pharmacist. He or she can also tell you if one of the ideal 28-day (Every Day) versions is available.

Abbreviations

Estrogens	ethinylestradiol	EE
	mestranol	MEE
Progestogens		
Group A	drospirenone	DSP
Group B	norgestimate	NGM
Group C	gestodene	GSD

Group D	desogestrel	DSG
Group E	levonorgestrel	LNG
Group F	norethisterone	NET
	(In N. America this is always called norethindrone)	

There are also some close relatives in Group F which actually become NET in the body (pp. 154, 178):

norethisterone acetate	NEA
etynodiol diacetate	EDA

Cyproterone acetate (CPA) is yet another progestogen, used in Dianette and Diane 35: these are primarily treatments for acne and hirsutes but they do also act as useful contraceptive pills and are appropriate for some women (pp. 157–8). Their alternative names are also listed below.

NB Other brands exist worldwide, but only those which are identical or similar to UK, USA, or Canadian brands are listed here. Those available in the UK are in *italics*, those in the USA are **bold**, and those in Canada underlined.

Combined pills, containing estrogen

Unless otherwise stated, the active pills are taken for 21 days. Many versions (not always mentioned here) also contain 7 days of placebos, especially in the US and Canada. Where Fe appears at end of a pill's name, this means the placebos contain iron (as for example in Estrostep Fe).

Group A (drospirenone, DSP)

Micrograms	*Micrograms*	
EE 30	DSP 3000	***Yasmin***, Petibelle

Group B (norgestimate, NGM)

Micrograms	*Micrograms*	
EE 35	NGM 250	Anele, *Cilest*, Cyclen, Effiprev, Effiprev 35, Mactex, Neofam, **Ortho-Cyclen**

Triphasic formulae

EE 35	NGM 180 . . . 7 days	**Ortho Tri-Cyclen**, Pramino, Tri-Anele, Tri-Cilest, Tricilest, Tridette, Tri-Mactex, Vivelle
EE 35	NGM 215 . . . 7 days	
EE 35	NGM 250 . . . 7 days	

EE 25	NGM 180 . . . 7 days	**Ortho Tri-Cyclen Lo**
EE 25	NGM 215 . . . 7 days	
EE 25	NGM 250 . . . 7 days	

Group C (gestodene, GSD)

Micrograms	*Micrograms*	
EE 30	GSD 75	Ciclomex, Evacin, Feminol, Femodeen, Femoden, *Femodene*, Femodene ED, Femovan, Gestodeno, Ginera, Ginoden, Gynera, Gynovin, Gynovin CD, Lerogin, *Minulet*, Minulette, Moneva, Myvlar
EE 20	GSD 75	Ciclomex 20, Diminut, Fedra, Femiane, Feminol-20, *Femodette*, Gynera 75/20, Gynovin 20, Harmonet, Lerogin 20, Logest, Meliane, Meloden, Melodene, Microgen, Minifem, Minigeste
EE 15	GSD 60	Meliane Light, Melodene 15, Melodia, Minesse, Mirelle

Triphasic formula

EE 30	GSD 50 . . . 6 days	Milvane, Phaeva, *Triadene*, Triciclomex, Trievacin, Tri-Femoden, Tri-Gynera, Trigynera, Trigynovin, *Tri-Minulet*, Triodeen, Trioden, Triodena, Triodene
EE 40	GSD 70 . . . 5 days	
EE 40	GSD 100 . . . 10 days	

Group D (desogestrel, DSG)

Micrograms	*Micrograms*	
EE 30	DSG 150	Ciclidon, Cycleane 30, Desmin 30, **Desogen**, Desolett, Desoran, Desorelle, Frilavon, Gynostat, Lovina 30, *Marvelon*, Marvelon 28, Marviol, Microdiol, Novelon, **Ortho-Cept**, Planum, Practil 21, Prevenon, Prevenon 28, Regulon, Varnoline

EE 20	DSG 150	Ciclidon 20, Cycleane 20, Desmin 20, Desoren 20, Femilon, Femina, Gynostat-20, Lovelle, Lovina 20, Marvelon 20, *Mercilon*, Microdosis, Myralon, Novynette, Primera, Securgin, Segurin, Suavuret

Phasic formulae

EE 20	DSG 150 . . . 21 days	**Mircette**
Placebo	. . . 2 days	
EE 10	. . . 5 days	
EE 25	DSG 100 . . . 7 days	**Cyclessa**
	DSG 125 . . . 7 days	
	DSG 150 . . . 7 days	

Group E (levonorgestrel, LNG)

Micrograms	*Micrograms*	
EE 50	LNG 250	Anfertil, Anulette, Anulit, Contraceptive HD, Daphyron, Denoval, Denoval-Wyeth, D-Norginor, Duoluton, Duoluton L, Duotone, Dystrol, Euginon, Eugynon, Eugynon 0.25, Eugynon 50, Eugynon CD, Eugynona, Evanor, Evanor-d, FMP, Femenal, Fertilan, Follinette, Follinyl, Gentrol, Gravistat, Gravistat 250 Mithuri, Mithuri Red, Monovar, Neogentrol, Neo-Gentrol 250/50, Neogynon, Neogynon 50, Neogynon 21, Neogynon CD, Neogynona, Neo-Primovlar, Neovlar, Noral, Nordiol, Nordiol Norginor, Normanor, Novogyn 21, Novogynon, Ologyn, Ovadon, Ovidon, Ovlar, Ovoplex, **Ovral**, Ovral 0.25, Ovran, Pil KB, Planovar, Preven, Primovlar, Primovlar 50, Stediril, Stediril-d Tetragynon
EE 30	LNG 250	Combination 5, *Eugynon 30*, Neogynon 30, Nordiol 30, Ovran 30, Primovlar-30
EE 30	LNG 150	Anna, Anovulatorios, Microdosis, Anulette C.D., Anulette, Anulit, Ciclo 21, Ciclon,

		Combination 3, Confiance, Contraceptive LD, Duofem, Egogyn 30, Femenal, Femigoa, Femranette mikro, Follimin, Gestrelan, Gynatrol, Innova CD, **Levlen**, Levonorgestrel Pill, **Levora 0.15/30**, Lo-Femenal, Lo-Gentrol, **Lo-Ovral**, Lo-Rondal, Lorsax, Mala D, Marvelon 28, Microfemin, Microfemin Cd, Microgest, Microginon, Microgyn, Microgynon, Microgynon 21, Microgynon 28, *Microgynon 30*, *Microgynon 30 ED*, Microgynon CD, Microgynon ED, Microgynon ED 28, Microvlar, Minibora, Minidril, Minigynon, Minigynon 30, Minivlar, Min-Ovral, Mithuri Green, Monofeme, Neo-Gentrol 150/30, Neomonovar, Neovletta, Nociclin, Nordet, **Nordette**, Nordette 150/30, Nordette 28, Norgestrel Pill, Norgylene, Norvetal, Nouvelle Duo, Ologyn-micro, Ovoplex 3, Ovoplex 30/150, Ovoplexin, Ovral L, Ovranet, *Ovranette*, Ovranette 30, Perle Ld, R-den, Riget, Rigevidon, Sexcon, Stediril-d 150/30, Stediril 30, Stediril 30/28, Stediril-M, Suginor
EE 30	LNG 125	Minisiston
EE 20	LNG 100	**Alesse**, Anulette 20, Aprll, Leios, **Levlite**, Loette, Loette 21, Lovette, Microgynon 20, Microgynon Suave, Microlite, Miranova

Triphasic formula

EE 30 EE 40 EE 40	LNG 50 . . . 6 days LNG 75 . . . 5 days LNG 125 . . . 10 days	Fironetta, Levordiol, *Logynon*, *Logynon ED*, Logynon 21, Modutrol, NovaStep, Triagynon, Triciclor, Triette 21, Trifas, Trifeme, Trifeminal, Trigoa 21, Trigynon, Trikvilar, **Tri-Levlen**, *Trinordiol*, Trinordiol 28, Trionetta, Tri-Stediril, Triovalet, Triovlar, **Triphasil**, Triquilar, Triquilar ED, Tri-Regol, Trisiston, Triviclor, Trivora, Trolit

Group F (Norethisterone = Norethindrone, NET)

Micrograms	*Micrograms*	
MEE 50	NET 1000	Anogenil, Combiginor, Conceplan, Conlumin, Floril, **Genora 1/50**, Gulaf, Maya, Mithuri Blue, **Necon 1/50**, Nor-50, **NEE 1/50, Nelova 1/50**, NorFor, Noriday, Noriday 1+50, Norimin, Norinyl, *Norinyl-1*,Norinyl 1/50, **Norinyl 1+50**, Norit, Novulon 1/50, Orthonett, Orthonett 1/50, Ortho-Novin, Ortho-Novin 1/50, Ortho-Novum, **Ortho-Novum 1/50**, Ortho-Novum 1+50, Perle, Plan mite, Regovar, Regovar 50, Ultra-Novulane
EE 50	NET 1000	**Intercon 1/50**, Non-Ovlon, **Norethin 1/50M**, Norinyl 28, **Ovcon 50**
EE 35	NET 1000	Brevicon 1+35, Brevinor-1, Genora 1+35, **Genora 1/35**, Gynex 1/35, **Intercon 1/35**, Kanchan, Membrettes, **NEE 1/35, Necon 1/35, Nelova 1/35E, Nelova 1/35**, Neocon, *Neocon 1/35*, Neo-Norinyl, Norcept-E1/35, **Norethin 1/35E**, *Norimin*, **Norinyl 1+35,** Norinyl 1/35, Norquest, Norquest-Fe, Ortho 1+35, Ortho 1/35, Ortho-Novum 1+35, **Ortho-Novum 1/35**, Orthonovum, Ovysmen, Ovysmen 1/35, Secure, Select 1/35
EE 35	NET 600	No 1 oral pill [China only]
EE 35	NET 500	**Brevicon**, Brevicon 0.5+35, Brevicon 20. *Brevinor*, Conceplan mite, **Genora 0.5+35**, Gynex 0.5/35E, **Intercon 0.5/35**, Mikro Plan, Moda Con, Modacon, **Modicon**, NEE 0.5/35, **Nelova 0.5/35E, Necon 0.5/35**, Neo-Ovopausine, Nilocan, Norminest, Norminest-Fe, Ortho 0.5+35, Orthonett Novum, Ovacon, *Ovysmen*, Ovysmen 0.5/35, Perle LD
EE 35	NET 500	Micropil, **Ovcon-35**, Oviprem

Biphasic formula

EE 35	NET 500 . . . 7 days	*Binovum*, **Jenest-28**, NEE 10/11, **Necon 10/11, Nelova 10/11**, Ortho 10/11, **Ortho-Novum 10/11** (The last six are equivalent to UK's Binovum but give 10 days rather than 7 days at the first [lower] dose of NET)
EE 35	NET 1000 . . . 14 days	

Triphasic formulae

EE 35	NET 500 . . . 7 days	Ortho 7/7/7, Ortho 777-28, **Ortho-Novum 7/7/7**, Triella, *TriNovum*
EE 35	NET 750 . . . 7 days	
EE 35	NET 1000 . . . 7 days	
EE 35	NET 500 . . . 7 days	Improvil, Synfase, Synfasic, *Synphase*, Synphasec, Synphasic, **Tri-Norinyl**
EE35	NET 1000 . . . 9 days	
EE 35	NET 500 . . . 5 days	

Group F continued (norethisterone acetate, NEA)

Micrograms	*Micrograms*	
EE 30	NEA 1500	*Loestrin 30*, Loestrin 1.5/30, **Loestrin 21 1.5/30, Loestrin Fe+ 1.5/30**, Logest 1.5/30, Minestril-30, Zorane 1.5/30
EE 30	NEA 1000	Econ 30, Econ mite, Mala N, Milli-Anovlar, Trentovlane
EE 20	NEA 1000	Loestrin, *Loestrin 20*, Loestrin 1/20, **Loestrin 21 1/20 Loestrin Fe 1/20**, Minestril-20, Minestrin 1/20, Norgest, Zorane 1/20

Triphasic formula

EE 20	NEA 1000 . . . 9 days	**Estrostep, Estrostep Fe+**
EE 30	NEA 1000 . . . 7 days	
EE 35	NEA 1000 . . . 5 days	

Group F (etynodiol diacetate, EDA, see p. 270)

Micrograms	*Micrograms*	
EE 30	EDA 2000	Conova, Demulen 30
EE 35	EDA 1000	**Demulen 1/35, Zovia 1/35E**

Cyproterone acetate (CPA) containing pills

micrograms	*micrograms*	
EE 35	CPA 35	Anuar, Brenda 35, Diane, Diane 35 DIARIO, Diane Mite, Diane Nova, Diane-35, Dianette, Dianette Generic, Dixi 35, Evilin, Gynofen 35, Juliet-35 ED, Lady-Ten 35, Minerva, Preme, Selene, Tina.

Continuous progestogen-only pills (POPs)

Group A	DSP	not yet available
Group B	NGM	not yet available
Group C	GSD	not yet available

Group D (desogestrel, DSG)

Micrograms	
DSG 75	*Cerazette*

Group E (levonorgestrel, LNG)

Micrograms	
LNG 37.5	Monofem, *Neogest*, Norgeal, **Ovrette**
LNG 30	28 mini, Follistrel, Levonorgestrel, Microlut, Microlut 35, Microluton, *Microval*, Mikro-30, *Norgeston*, Nortrel

Group F (norethisterone = norethindrone, NET)

Micrograms	
NET 350	Conceplan-Micro, Dianor, Locilan, Micronett, ***Micronor***, Micro-Novum, Micronovum, *Noriday*, Noriday-1, Noridei, **Nor-QD**

NET 30	Conludag, Gesta Plan, Mini-Pe, Mini-Pill, Monogest

Group F (etynodiol diacetate, see p. 270)

Micrograms

EDA 500	Continuin, *Femulen*

Emergency Contraceptive (EC) Pills

Levonorgestrel (LNG) as single dose, as early as possible after conception risk

Micrograms

LNG 1500	Duofem (ECP), Estinor, *Levonelle*, *Levonelle 2*, Madonna, Norlevo, **Plan B**, Postinor, Postinor-2, Rigesoft, Vikela

Glossary

abortion loss of a pregnancy at any time before independent existence apart from the mother is deemed to be possible. Abortion may be spontaneous (= miscarriage) or induced, meaning caused to happen either legally or illegally. The general public often uses the word 'abortion' on its own to mean a legal induced abortion, but doctors prefer to use either that phrase or termination of pregnancy

allergy abnormal reactivity of an individual to a specific substance, following previous exposure to the same or a closely related substance

A similar process to *immunity*, but the *antibodies* produced are unwanted and can be harmful

amine an organic compound which contains nitrogen. The ones referred to in this book are present in the brain and believed to be important in its functions, both in health and disease

anaemia a decrease in the blood of a substance haemoglobin, carried by the red blood cells, which transports oxygen round the body

androgenic masculinizing, the effect of an androgen like testosterone

antibodies substances produced by the body as a reaction to a foreign protein, or a substance which the body treats as foreign. Antibodies can be beneficial (as in *immunity*) or harmful (as in *allergy*)

BMI, Body Mass Index. This is the *weight* of a person in kilograms divided by *height* in metres squared. It gives the best measure of being overweight (or underweight) as related to one's height. The normal range of BMI is 19–25; 25–30 is in my opinion WHO 2 (see p. 26), over 30 up to 39 is WHO 3 but above that is WHO 4

BTB, breakthrough bleeding any unexpected bleeding on the combined pill happening on tablet-taking days, between the hormone-withdrawal bleeds ('periods')

cervix the narrow lower end of the *uterus*, containing the entrance to it. Sometimes called 'the neck of the womb'

Chlamydia the commonest cause of sexually transmitted infection of the fallopian tubes, also known as salpingitis or pelvic infection, with pelvic pain as a possible symptom. Sometimes it causes bleeding between periods, or what gets called "breakthrough bleeding" in pill-takers. It can also be very 'silent', not causing symptoms. Yet with or without symptoms it can lead to ectopic pregnancies (below) or sterility, through damaged or blocked fallopian tubes. Well worth avoiding!

chloasma (also known as **melasma**) abnormal facial skin pigmentation occurring in some women during pregnancy or when taking the combined Pill

chromosome one of the microscopic thread-like structures visible in the nucleus of any body cell when it divides, carrying the genes. Each gene controls, alone or more usually with others, the inheritance of a special characteristic of the individual—e.g. blood group or colour of the eyes

COC (combined oral contraceptive) contraceptive which is taken by mouth and contains two hormones: one a *progestogen* and the other an *estrogen*. Usually called the Pill

cone biopsy a minor operation under general anaesthesia to remove some skin at the entrance to the uterus in order to treat some abnormal cells found by cervical smear. A similar excising of the tissue with the abnormal cells is now more often done using a so-called 'large loop', as an out-patient under local anaesthetic

contraception prevention of pregnancy by a reversible method. This definition excludes the other two types of birth control, which are sterilization and abortion (though a few people label some contraceptives as 'causing abortion', see pp. 207–10)

contraceptive any substance or device which reversibly prevents conception (while allowing intercourse)

contraindications medical reasons to avoid a contraceptive. In this edition these are now classified on the WHO's 1–4 Scale, see p. 26 for a full explanation)

corpus luteum the yellow body formed in the ovary during the menstrual cycle, formed from the largest follicle after it has released its egg

cystitis inflammation of the urinary bladder, usually caused by infection, provoking a desire to pass urine more frequently and often a burning sensation on doing so

D&C (Dilatation and Curettage) with hysteroscopy, a common minor operation in which the cervix is dilated, or enlarged sufficiently to allow a scope and/or a curette to be passed. The inside of the uterus can then be inspected, tissue obtained for laboratory examination (see also *endometrial biopsy*), or it can be completely emptied—e.g. after a miscarriage or induced abortion which has been incomplete

diabetes strictly, should be diabetes *mellitus*—a disturbance of body chemistry causing an increase in the level of glucose in the blood after food, due to lack of the hormone insulin, or reduction in its effectiveness. These changes can lead to long-term complications affecting the arteries, nerves, kidneys, and eyes

EE (ethinylestradiol) the main artificial estrogen used in the Pill, not to be confused with the natural estrogen used in HRT

ectopic pregnancy a pregnancy in the wrong place—i.e. anywhere other than in the cavity of the uterus. The commonest site is in the uterine (fallopian) tube. It leads to the need for urgent operation, because the growing pregnancy can cause internal bleeding. The damage to the tubes that leads to the risk of an ectopic is nearly always caused by a previous pelvic infection, usually with Chlamydia (see above). This may not have been noticed at the time (often no symptoms).

ejaculation the spurting-out of semen (sometimes called the ejaculate) from the end of the penis when a man has a climax

embolism transfer in the bloodstream of a mass, such as a blood clot from a vein, to lodge elsewhere, generally in the lungs (pulmonary embolism)

embryo name given to the early pregnancy from the day of fertilization for about two months (then called the *fetus*)

endometrium the special lining of the uterus, which is prepared by the hormones of the menstrual cycle in readiness for implantation of an embryo—or otherwise is shed at the menstrual period

endometrial biopsy sampling of the endometrium as an outpatient through a special plastic tube used via the cervix

enzyme a biological catalyst, which is a chemical which promotes the process of transformation of one substance to another within the body

epididymis a long tube coiled on itself to form a small linear structure attached to the testicle, and connecting it with the vas deferens

estrogen the female sex hormone produced by the ovary throughout the menstrual cycle. It is the hormone required to bring animals 'on heat', which occurs at the time called oestrus—hence the name estrogen

estrogen-dominant Pill a combined pill whose biological effects on the body are due to the relatively stronger effect of the estrogen it contains than to the progestogen

fertilization the union of sperm and egg cell. The fertilized egg divides to produce an embryo and eventually a new individual

fetus correct name (rather than foetus) for any growing baby after eight weeks of intrauterine life

fimbriae the seaweed-like fronds which surround the outer end of each uterine tube, like a fringe

follicle a small fluid-filled balloon-like structure in the ovary, containing an egg cell. Only one, out of about twenty which enlarge in each menstrual cycle, normally releases a mature egg

FSH (follicle stimulating hormone) the hormone, produced by the pituitary gland which stimulates the growth of follicles in the ovary; and hence causes the production of estrogen and the maturing of an egg cell in the largest follicle

GTT (Glucose Tolerance Test) a test for *diabetes* and similar body states, in which glucose is taken, usually by mouth, and subsequent blood tests measure how its level rises and then falls in the blood

GUM (genitourinary medicine) the branch of medicine which specializes in treating STIs

hCG (human chorionic gonadotrophin) the hormone, produced by an early pregnancy, which travels to the ovary in the bloodstream and causes its corpus luteum to continue producing estrogen and progesterone beyond its usual fourteen-day life span. When LH levels drop, this saves the embryo from being lost in the next menstrual flow.

GnRH (gonadotrophin releasing hormone) the hormone which travels in so-called pulses from the *hypothalamus* to the pituitary gland down its stalk, and so causes it to release important hormones of its own (FSH and LH) into the bloodstream

HELLP syndrome a not-fully-understood problem in late pregnancy, in which there is Haemolysis (red cells being destroyed in the blood), Elevated Liver enzymes (*enzymes* being released from damaged liver cells) and Low *Platelets* (i.e., low blood levels). After full recovery following delivery, HELLP does NOT mean the Pill must be avoided thereafter

HIV/AIDS Human Immuno-deficiency Virus/the sexually transmissible cause of Acquired Immune Deficiency Syndrome, which leads without treatment to lack of immune resistance to infections and, eventually, death

hormone a chemical substance produced in one organ and carried in the bloodstream like a 'chemical messenger' to another organ or tissue, whose function it influences or alters

HRT (hormone replacement therapy) treatment with *natural* estrogen, often along with a progestogen, given when women lack sufficient from their own ovaries—e.g. after the menopause.

hypertension high blood pressure, above the level which is accepted as normal (pp. 77–8)

hysterectomy an operation to remove the uterus

hypothalamus the structure at the base of the brain which releases GnRH in pulses to stimulate the pituitary gland so it releases FSH and LH

immunity resistance of the body to the effects of a foreign substance or microbe, resulting from the production of *antibodies* which are not harmful and often beneficial—unlike those produced as a result of *allergy*

implantation the process of the embedding of the developing embryo in the *endometrium*

IUD (intra-uterine device) a small plastic contraceptive device, which usually carries copper in the form of wire or bands and is inserted into the uterus to prevent pregnancy

IUS (intra-uterine system) a plastic contraceptive device slowly releasing a *hormone*, currently always a *progestogen*, into the interior of the uterus over several years

LH (luteinizing hormone) the hormone produced by the pituitary gland which causes egg-release, and the production and maintenance of the corpus luteum

libido the internal drive and urge of the sexual instinct, making either sex want foreplay and intercourse

lipids fats and associated chemical substances, carried in the blood

mcg (microgram) this abbreviation is used of the metric unit which is one millionth of a gram in weight

menopause cessation of the menstrual periods due to failure of ovulation and hormone production by the ovaries. Often used inaccurately for the climacteric or the peri-menopause time, which is several years before and after periods actually cease

menstrual cycle the cycle of hormone and other changes in a woman's body which leads to a regular discharge of blood from the non-pregnant uterus

mestranol the now rarely used one of two artificial estrogens which are used in combined oral contraceptive pills

mucus slippery fluid produced by mucous glands on the surface of a body structure. Cervical mucus is mucus produced by the glands of the cervix. Progestogens change it so it impedes sperm when they try to enter the uterus

ovary the female sex gland in which ova (egg cells) are developed and which is the main source of natural sex hormones

ovulation release of the ovum or ova from the ovary—more often called egg-release in this book

PCOS (polycystic ovarian syndrome) a condition (described on p. 98) in which *multiple* small cysts develop around the outside of the ovary and the woman has *androgenic* effects like acne or unwanted hair growth. This is *different from just having polycystic ovaries* showing up on an ultrasound scan, with no symptoms; and also different from having a *solitary* cyst on the ovary (p. 97)

phlebitis thrombosis and inflammation involving a vein—usually a superficial vein of the leg—which causes it to become hard and very tender

pituitary gland the gland, about the size of a pea, on a stalk at the base of the brain, which produces many important hormones including FSH and LH

placenta (afterbirth) the structure on the wall of a pregnant uterus in which the mother's bloodstream is brought into close proximity with that in the fetus, so allowing nutrition for the growing baby and elimination of its waste products

platelets tiny particles circulating in the blood which are important in the early stages of thrombosis

progesterone the other main sex hormone produced by the ovaries (see *estrogen*). This hormone is produced only in the second half of the menstrual cycle, by the corpus luteum. It prepares the body, especially the uterus, for pregnancy. It is *one of* the general class of progestogens

progestogen: a number of artificial progestogens that are chemically related to natural *progesterone* are used along with an artificial estrogen to produce the combined pill

progestogen-dominant Pill a combined pill whose biological effects on the body are due more to the relatively higher dose of progestogen it contains than to the estrogen

POP (progestogen-only Pill) as the name suggests, a pill with only the one hormone present, an artificial progestogen. Is even safer than the COC, since it is EE-free

prolactin a hormone produced by the pituitary gland which stimulates the breasts to produce milk and is also involved in the menstrual cycle

prostaglandins natural substances manufactured and released within many tissues of the body. Some natural prostaglandins cause the uterus to contract, and these and other artificial variants can therefore be used to cause an induced abortion

puberty the time when a boy or girl begins to develop secondary sex characteristics and then becomes fertile. In a girl, the most significant event is the onset of periods, correctly called the menarche

pyridoxine this is another name for Vitamin B_6

SLE (systemic lupus erythematosus) a strangely-named disease caused by developing a kind of *allergy* to the person's own connective tissues, in many organs and systems of the body. If the patient goes on to develop an acquired pre-disposition to *thrombosis*, they must not use the Pill (WHO 4)

spermicide a substance which is capable of killing sperm. Recommended, generally, for contraception along with another method such as the diaphragm/cap, rather than used alone

STIs (sexually transmitted infections) There are many of these, including *Chlamydia* – usually best treated at a GUM clinic

sterilization an operation in a person of either sex which permanently prevents pregnancy, and which is either impossible or difficult to reverse. The definition therefore includes removal of the uterus, or of both ovaries or testicles, though these are only done when necessary because of some disease. More usually, sterilization is achieved by blocking a woman's uterine tubes or a man's vas deferens on each side (*vasectomy*)

subarachnoid haemorrhage this is serious bleeding from a localized weakness of the wall of an artery in the brain, damaging the brain and leading to blood appearing in the surrounding cerebro-spinal fluid. It can be fatal or cause prolonged loss of consciousness, but recovery is possible, sometimes with the aid of surgery

testicle (testis) the sex gland of the male in which spermatozoa (sperm) develop, and which also manufactures male sex hormones (androgens), especially testosterone

thrombosis the formation of a blood clot within a blood vessel (can be an artery or vein). Arterial thrombosis can produce *heart attacks* or *strokes*, venous thrombosis in the legs can spread to the lungs to cause *pulmonary embolism* - see p. 68.

uterine (fallopian) tubes the tubes which in the female convey the egg to the uterus, and within which fertilization by a sperm usually occurs

uterus (womb) the hollow organ in women, like other mammals, in which the young develop during pregnancy

vagina the distensible passage way which extends from the cervix to the vulva, into which the penis is inserted during intercourse, and which also forms the main part of the birth canal during delivery of a baby

vas deferens the tube in the male which conveys the sperm from the epididymis to the base of the penis. It is the tube that is divided at *vasectomy* (*male sterilization*)

vulva the name given to the female external genital structures

WTB (withdrawal bleeding) bleeding from the uterus caused by the woman herself when she stops the supply of hormones to it, by taking a break at the end of each packet as (usually) instructed. It occurs during the *Pill-free interval.*

[100] woman-years a measure of the frequency of an occurrence such as pregnancy. For example, a pregnancy rate of one per 100 woman-years for a given method means that one pregnancy can be expected among 100 women using it for one year

index

When several page numbers are listed under a topic, any which appear in ***bold italic*** *represent a more extensive section of text devoted to that topic*